second edition

PHARMACY PRACTICE

for technicians

Don A. Ballington, M.S.
Midlands Technical College
Columbia, South Carolina

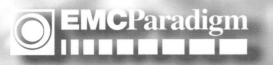

EMCParadigm

Developmental Editor	Christine Hurney
Editorial Assistant	Susan Capecchi
Copy Editor	Katherine Savoie
Mathematics Copy Editor	Susan Gerstein
Cover and Text Designer	Michelle Lewis and Jennifer Wreisner
Desktop Production	Parkwood Composition
Photography	Tova Wiegand Green
	(Specific photo credits follow index.)
Indexer	Nancy Fulton

Publishing Management Team

George Provol, Publisher; Janice Johnson, Director of Product Development; Tony Galvin, Acquisitions Editor; Lori Landwer, Marketing Manager; Shelley Clubb, Electronic Design and Production Manager

---

Library of Congress Cataloging-in-Publication Data

Ballington, Don A.
    Pharmacy practice for technicians / Don A. Ballington—2nd ed.
      p. cm.
    Includes index.
    ISBN 0-7638-1535-7 (text)
    1. Pharmacy technicians. 2. Medicine—Formulae, receipts, prescriptions. I. Title.
    [DNLM: 1. Pharmacy. 2. Pharmacists' Aides. 3. Pharmaceutical Services—United States.]

    RS122.95 .B35 2003
    615'.1—dc21   2001054472

Text ISBN 0-7638-1535-7
Product Number 01565

© 2003, 1999 by Paradigm Publishing Inc.
        Published by **EMC**Paradigm
        875 Montreal Way
        St. Paul, MN 55102
        (800) 535-6865
        E-mail: educate@emcp.com
        Web site: www.emcp.com

Contents

CHAPTER 7
Dispensing, Billing, and Inventory Management 143

CHAPTER 8
Extemporaneous Compounding.......169

CHAPTER 9
Human Relations and Communications.................................185

CHAPTER 10
Hospital and Institutional
Pharmacy Practice 197

CHAPTER 11
Your Future in Pharmacy Practice....237

Preface

Pharmacy Practice for Technicians, Second Edition is designed to introduce the pharmacy technician student to the techniques and procedures necessary to prepare and dispense medications in both the institutional and community pharmacy setting. Preparing medications involves using sterile and nonsterile techniques to count, measure, and compound drugs. The text covers reading the order/prescription; procedures for preparing, packaging, and labeling the medication; and information regarding maintaining the patient profile. Other medication and nonmedication pharmacy-related activities are introduced, including billing and inventory management.

This text offers the pharmacy technician educator and students the tools to achieve the competencies needed to obtain certification. This text supports the following goals.

General Operations
- ◇ Perform pharmacy technician duties within the scope of the position and ethics of the industry.
- ◇ Perform the roles and responsibilities of the pharmacy technician and comply with performance standards established for the community and hospital pharmacy settings.
- ◇ Perform record-keeping functions associated with dispensing pharmaceuticals, processing insurance claims, and maintaining drug inventory.

Drug Dosage and Knowledge
- ◇ Demonstrate a working knowledge of drug dosages, routes of administration, and interactions within the scope of the pharmacy technician responsibilities.
- ◇ Read and understand drug labeling, packaging, and dosage information and dispense as prescribed.
- ◇ Use drug references to accurately identify generic and brand equivalents.
- ◇ Use the medical terms, abbreviations, and symbols essential to prescribing, dispensing, administering, and charting of medications correctly and precisely.

Accurate Drug Calculations and Measurement
- ◇ Follow the correct procedures related to compounding and admixture operations.
- ◇ Perform calculations required for the usual dosages and solution preparations.
- ◇ Perform basic calculations to determine inventory and purchasing needs, profit margins, and inventory control.
- ◇ Perform accurate conversions between measurement systems.

Administrative and Customer Relations
- ◇ Translate prescribed dosage and administration instructions to ensure patient understanding.
- ◇ Assist the pharmacist in all matters of customer relations and support.

Improvements to the second edition include:

◇ Full-color design features and expanded art and photo program.
◇ Web links and Internet research assignments on important sources of information about drugs and diseases.
◇ Web links provided as avenues to continually expand and update chapter material.
◇ Communications skills and role playing exercises provided for "authentic" communication practice.
◇ Expanded coverage of pharmacy calculations, including business math.
◇ Expanded coverage on law and ethics including federal, state, court, and voluntary standards.
◇ A new workbook with exercises for each chapter; expanded medical terminology, calculations, and prescription practice; and in-the-lab activities.

Each chapter begins with learning objectives and concludes with a chapter summary. These pedagogical tools help students focus their study and enhance their learning review. End-of-chapter questions reinforce the information presented in the chapter, and provide opportunity for discussion and communications skills practice. The Pharmacy in Practice exercises require students to apply the theory to hands-on pharmacy scenarios. In addition, Internet Research exercises provide an opportunity to do further topic investigation on the Internet.

The appendixes provide valuable reference material including common abbreviations for student reference (Appendix A), a conceptual list of common drug categories and their actions (Appendix B), and reference lab values (Appendix C). Appendix D lists valuable resources, including pharmacy organizations and journals, as well as references for additional information on health and anatomy, drug information, pharmacy practice, law and ethics, and certification. When available, Web sites are listed for these resources. Appendix E provides a list of guidelines to help the pharmacy technician avoid errors in the pharmacy.

Resources for the Student

Students are encouraged to use the workbook to reinforce the information taught in the text. The new workbook that accompanies *Pharmacy Practice for Technicians, Second Edition* includes extensive exercises, vocabulary review, and in-the-lab practice.

Online self-guided quizzes and additional valuable resources are available on the Internet Resource Center for this title at www.emcp.com.

Resources for the Instructor

In addition to suggested course syllabus information, the Instructor's Guide that accompanies *Pharmacy Practice, Second Edition* includes answers for all end-of-chapter and workbook exercises. It also provides teaching hints for each chapter and ready-to-use chapter quizzes as well as midterm and final examinations.

Course tests and assessments are available at the password-protected section of the Internet Resource Center for this title at www.emcp.com.

WebCT and Blackboard Web course management systems are available to support this product. Each comes preloaded with course information, chapter outlines, and quizzes.

Paradigm Publishing Inc. also publishes *Pharmacology for Technicians, Second Edition*, and *Pharmacy Calculations for Technicians, Second Edition*. Both of these titles are supported with instructor's guides, testbanks, and Web course management systems. A workbook is also available for the *Pharmacology for Technicians, Second Edition* title.

About the Author

Don A. Ballington, M.S., serves as program coordinator for the pharmacy technician training program at Midlands Technical College in Columbia, South Carolina. He has served as president of the Pharmacy Technician Educators' Council and consulting editor for the *Journal of Pharmacy Technology*. Over the course of his career at Midlands Technical College, he has developed and refined a set of training materials. These materials became the foundation of the manuscripts that were developed into *Pharmacy Calculations for Technicians, Pharmacology for Technicians*, and *Pharmacy Practice for Technicians*. All of these books are now available in second editions.

Acknowledgments

The author would like to thank the editorial team at Paradigm Publishing as well as the following list of reviewers for their expert advice and opinions on how to make this textbook an effective learning tool.

Tova Wiegand Green
Ivy Tech State College
Fort Wayne, Indiana

Mary M. Laughlin, Pharm.D., M.Ed.
Regional Medical Center
Memphis, Tennessee

Neal F. Walker, R.Ph
University Medical Center—Mesabi
Hibbing, Minnesota
University of Minnesota College of Pharmacy
Minneapolis, Minnesota

The author and editorial staff would like to offer a special thank you to Tova Wiegand Green for her substantive contributions to this edition of *Pharmacy Practice for Technicians*. Her dedication to producing a quality text was impressive.

The author and editorial staff invite your feedback on the text and its supplements. Please reach us by clicking the "Contact us" button at www.emcp.com.

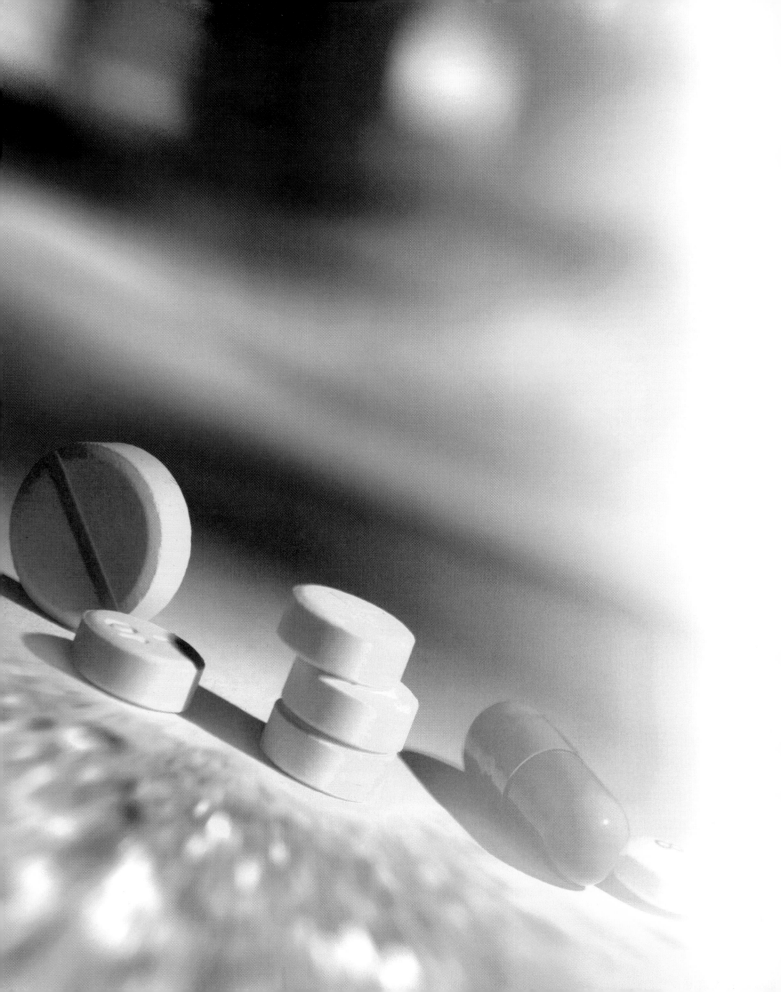

The Pharmacy Technician

Learning Objectives

◇ Describe the origins of pharmacy.

◇ Describe three stages of development of the pharmacy profession in the twentieth century.

◇ Enumerate the functions of the pharmacist.

◇ Differentiate among the various sub-fields within the profession of pharmacy, including pharmaceutics, pharmacognosy, pharmacology, and clinical pharmacy.

◇ Explain the licensing requirements for pharmacists.

◇ Identify the duties and work environments of the pharmacy technician.

◇ Differentiate among the various kinds of pharmacies.

From its ancient origins in spiritualism and magic, pharmacy has evolved into a scientific pursuit involving not only the compounding and dispensing of medications but also the provision of accurate information and counseling about a wide range of medication-related issues. The contemporary pharmacy technician provides a wide variety of essential services to pharmacy customers and patients, to supervising pharmacists, and to such healthcare professionals as physicians and nurses. In recent years, pharmacy technicians have made tremendous strides toward recognition of their status within the ranks of highly skilled paraprofessionals.

ANCIENT ORIGINS

The word *pharmacy* comes from the ancient Greek word *pharmakon,* meaning "drug." The use of drugs in the healing arts is older than civilization. Modern archaeologists, exploring the five-thousand-year-old remains of the ancient city states of Mesopotamia, have unearthed clay tablets listing hundreds of medicinal preparations from various sources, including plants and minerals. Already, at the dawn of civilization, a traditional pharmacological lore existed, probably reflecting practical experience dating back for centuries or even millennia. The ancient Egyptians compiled lists of drugs, known as formularies, dispensatories, or pharmacopeias, along with directions for creating them from natural sources using such simple equipment as the scale, the sieve, and the mortar and pestle. The peoples of ancient India attributed the miraculous and curative powers of the gods and of their priestly shamans to an intoxicating drug, still unidentified but possibly derived from a mushroom, that they referred to as *soma.* The word *soma* was picked up by the ancient Greeks and came to mean "body." It is with this meaning that it was later used as a root in such English words as *psychosomatic.* Predictably, early recipes for drug preparation are freely mixed with incantations, rituals, and imitative magic.

To the ancient Greeks, and particularly to the fathers of medicine, Hippocrates and Galen, we owe the beginnings of a nonmagical, scientific approach to the arts of healing and to drug use. Hippocrates, who was born on the Greek island of Kos

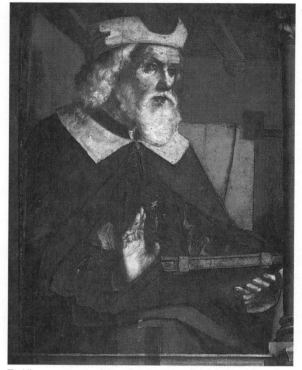

To Hippocrates, traditionally viewed as "the father of medicine," the ancients ascribed the creation of approximately 70 works dealing with the identification and treatment of disease. Today, Hippocrates is remembered for the Hippocratic Oath, by which physicians pledge, among other requirements, "to give no drug . . . for a criminal purpose."

around 430 B.C., established the theory of humors, which was to dominate medicine for almost two thousand years. According to this now long-discredited theory, health involved harmony among four fundamental bodily fluids, known as humors. Each humor was associated with particular personality characteristics. The humors were blood, phlegm, yellow bile, and black bile, and were associated, respectively, with cheerfulness, sluggishness, irritability, and melancholy.

Galen, born around A.D. 129 in Asia Minor, expanded on the theory of humors and produced a systematic classification of drugs for the treatment of pathologies involving want, excess, or corruption of the bodily humors. The greatest of the ancient pharmaceutical texts, however, was *De Materia Medica (On Medical Matters),* written by Pedanius Dioscorides in the first century A.D. Born in what is now Turkey, Dioscorides served in the Roman army during the rule of Nero and traveled widely, gathering knowledge of medicinal herbs and minerals from Persia, Africa, Egypt, Greece, and Rome. His book served as the standard text on drugs, primarily herbal remedies, for fifteen hundred years.

Although drugs from herbal and mineral sources have been used for millennia, *pharmacy* as a distinct professional discipline devoted to creating, storing, dispensing, and providing information about drugs is a relatively young field. In 1231, Emperor Frederick II of Germany was the first to officially recognize pharmacy as a distinct professional category. Since that time, the profession of the dispenser of drugs, the pharmacist, or, in older terminology, the apothecary, chemist, or druggist, has grown concurrently with that of the modern, scientifically trained physician. Until the nineteenth century, the dispensary that distributed drugs to patients was usually owned by a physician, but gradually it became an independent entity owned and operated by the pharmacist.

THE ROLES OF THE PHARMACIST

The modern pharmacist has two primary roles. The first of these is to dispense drugs prescribed by physicians and other healthcare practitioners. The second is to provide information to patients, physicians, and other practitioners on the selection, dosages, interactions, and side effects of medications.

Evolution of the Pharmacist's Roles

During the twentieth century, the pharmacy profession evolved through three stages: from the traditional era, dominated by the formulation and dispensing of drugs from natural sources; through a scientific era in mid-century, dominated by scientific training in the effects of drugs on the body; to a clinical era at the end of the cen-

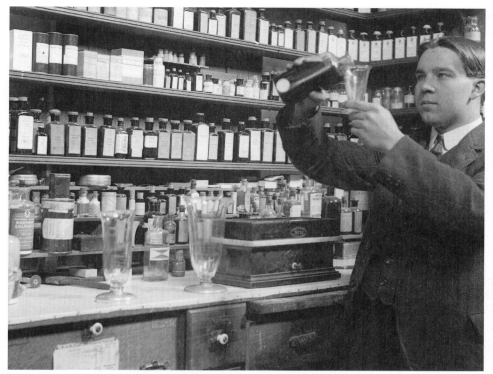

Dr. Emil King prepares medicine in his pharmacy in Fulda, MN, 1905.

tury, which combined these traditional roles with a new role as dispenser of drug information.

Prior to the 1940s, the job of the pharmacist/apothecary consisted almost entirely of pharmaceutics, the science of preparing and dispensing drugs. Important aspects of the traditional profession included pharmacognosy, knowledge of the medicinal functions of natural products of animal, plant, or mineral origin, and galenical pharmacy, knowledge of the techniques for preparing medications from such sources. A nineteenth-century apothecary not only sold drugs but also manufactured them.

The emergence of the pharmaceutical industry in the twentieth century created a crisis for the profession of the pharmacist. As the manufacturing of drugs moved from the apothecary shop to the labs and factories of the pharmaceutical manufacturers, the pharmacist increasingly became a drugstore operator, a dispenser of drugs who was more a businessperson than a healing arts professional. This situation soon changed, however, as the educational institutions that trained pharmacists turned to scientific studies on drug effects and interactions, researches that were largely funded by pharmaceutical companies. Pharmacology, the scientific study of the site and mode of action, the side effects (including the adverse side effects, or toxicology), and the metabolism of drugs by the body, became part of the pharmacy curriculum, along with physics, chemistry, and physiology.

By the late 1950s and 1960s, many pharmacists began to feel that their training had shifted too far in the direction of scientific knowledge isolated from actual pharmacy practice. At the same time, many felt that pharmacists were being underutilized. Pharmacists constituted a highly knowledgeable, scientifically trained professional class with vast pharmacological knowledge, and yet they devoted the bulk of their energies to running businesses rather than interacting with patients and other professionals. Then, in 1973, the American Association of Colleges of Pharmacy established a study commission under Dr. John S. Millis to reevaluate the mission of the pharmacy profession. The 1975 Millis Report, titled *Pharmacists for the Future*, defined *pharmacy* as a primarily knowledge-based profession and emphasized the role of the pharmacist in sharing knowledge about drug use. This report led to a new emphasis in the profession on what is known as clinical pharmacy—the sharing of information about drugs with patients and healthcare practitioners as well as monitoring drug therapy to ensure optimal patient outcomes. The modern pharmacist thus carries out the important role of advisor and counselor to physicians and patients, as well as the role of dispenser of drugs.

Duties of the Pharmacist

Today, compounding, the mixing of ingredients to create tablets, capsules, ointments, solutions, and the like, is but a small part of the pharmacist's actual practice. The pharmacist who works in a community, or retail, pharmacy (the "drugstore") counsels customers, asking about their medical histories and what other medications they are currently taking, providing information about over-the-counter medications and making recommendations for these, describing possible adverse reactions and drug interactions related to prescriptions, and giving advice about home healthcare supplies and medical equipment. Of course, the pharmacist still compounds and dispenses drugs, and the community pharmacist still commonly functions as a businessperson, hiring and supervising employees, selling merchandise not directly related to health, and otherwise serving as the manager of a retail operation.

The pharmacist who works in a hospital or clinic dispenses medications and advises medical staff on drug selection and effects. Other typical tasks for the hospital pharmacist include monitoring drug regimens, preparing sterile solutions, purchasing medical supplies, and providing prerelease counseling on drugs to patients about to be discharged. The pharmacist who works in home healthcare may prepare medications and intravenous infusions, or IVs, for home use and may also monitor patients' drug therapies. (For more information on intravenous infusions, see Chapters 4, 5, and 10.)

Whether working in community, clinical, long-term care, or home healthcare settings, pharmacists typically keep records of patients' drug therapies, in part to prevent adverse interactions among prescribed medications. Some pharmacists teach and some function as consultants with expertise in particular fields of drug use, such as the diagnostic application of radioactive drugs, intravenous nutrition, or drug therapy for psychiatric, pediatric, or geriatric patients.

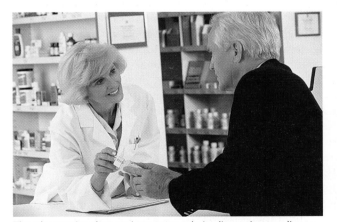

The pharmacist plays an important role in dispensing medications as well as instructing patients about side effects of medications, food and drug interactions, and dosing schedules.

Education and Licensing Requirements for Pharmacists

One indication of the professional status of pharmacy is the stringent licensing and educational requirements placed on practitioners. In the United States, all states require pharmacists to be licensed. Obtaining a license involves graduating from an accredited college of pharmacy, passing a state certification examination, and serving an internship under a licensed pharmacist. In addition, in most states, pharmacists must meet continuing education requirements in order to renew their licenses. Most states have reciprocal agreements recognizing licenses granted to pharmacists in other states. Licensing and general professional oversight are carried out by state pharmacy boards, self-monitoring professional organizations in each state. Most colleges of pharmacy offer six-year programs, culminating in the Doctor of Pharmacy (Pharm.D.) degree. Most colleges of pharmacy require one or two years of prepharmacy education, including chemistry, physics, and biology. Some colleges require that applicants take the Pharmacy College Admission Test, or PCAT. Some have master's and PhD programs in pharmacy that prepare pharmacists for specialization and for teaching.

Web Link

Learn more about the PCAT at www.tpcweb.com/pse/g-conts0.htm

THE ROLES OF THE PHARMACY TECHNICIAN

A pharmacy technician, sometimes referred to as a pharmacy technologist, assistant, or aide, is someone who, under the supervision of a licensed pharmacist, assists in a wide variety of skilled activities necessary for the dispensing of drugs and drug information. A central defining feature of the technician's job is accountability to the pharmacist for the quality and accuracy of his or her work. While the technician carries out many of the duties traditionally performed by pharmacists, his or her work must always be checked by the pharmacist. As a paraprofessional, or skilled assistant to a professional person, the pharmacy technician bears a relationship to the pharmacist similar to that of an x-ray technician to a radiologist or a medical technologist to a pathologist. A pharmacy technician assists the pharmacist with routine technical and nontechnical functions but leaves most judgment calls and decision making to the pharmacist. The technician functions in strict accordance with standard written procedures and guidelines. The pharmacist, in turn, takes final responsibility for the technician's actions. It is important to note that the essential differences in the duties of a pharmacist and a technician are regarding accountability and making decisions about the patient's healthcare. The pharmacist is responsible for providing a certain standard of care to the patient, and the technician is there to assist in that duty.

Work Environments and Conditions

Pharmacy technicians are employed in most of the same settings as pharmacists, including community pharmacies (drugstores), hospital pharmacies, home healthcare, and long-term care facilities. These will be discussed in more detail later in this chapter. Pharmacy technicians, like pharmacists, usually work in clean, well-lighted, well-ventilated environments. For the most part, their work requires standing, often for long hours. Because people's health needs know no clock, both pharmacists and pharmacy technicians work days, nights, weekends, and holidays. At any time, 24 hours a day, some number of the estimated 81,000 pharmacy technicians currently employed are on the job.

Characteristics of the Pharmacy Technician

A successful pharmacy technician must possess a wide range of skills, knowledge, and aptitudes. He or she must have a broad knowledge of pharmacy practice and a dedication to providing a critical healthcare service to customers and patients. In addition, the pharmacy technician must have high ethical standards, eagerness to learn, a sense of responsibility toward patients and toward the healthcare professionals with whom he or she interacts, willingness to follow instructions, an eye for detail, manual dexterity, facility in basic mathematics, excellent communication skills, good research skills, and the ability to perform accurately and calmly in hectic or stressful situations. The ability to "multi-task," or work on several projects at the same time, is a skill that will be useful in every pharmacy environment.

Training, Certification, Pay, and Job Outlook

At present, no federal requirements and few state requirements exist for the training and credentialing of pharmacy technicians, although some states have begun to require registration of pharmacy technicians. In the past, most pharmacy technicians learned their trade on the job, and it is still possible to gain employment as a pharmacy technician with only a high school diploma. However, many pharmacy technicians have associate degrees or one-year certificates, and many are also nationally Certified Pharmacy Technicians, or CPhTs.

In 1995, several professional organizations, including the American Pharmaceutical Association (APhA), American Society of Health-System Pharmacists (ASHP), Michigan Pharmacists Association, and Illinois Council of Health-System Pharmacists, came together to create the Pharmacy Technician Certification Board (PTCB). This board in turn created the Pharmacy Technician Certification Examination. It also established guidelines for recertification every two years, which involves ten hours of continuing education each year. Increasingly, hospitals and drugstore chains are requiring technicians to be certified. However, it remains uncertain the extent to which certification will become mandatory across the United States. Most states do not require certification. A few do either by the PTCB or their own state certification examinations. Some require only that pharmacy technicians be registered with the state and undergo supervised on-the-job training.

The job outlook for pharmacy technicians is superb. One school that trains pharmacy technicians estimates that the number of technicians nationwide will grow to about 109,000 by the year 2005. In 2001, wages for first-level pharmacy technicians ranged from around $19,000 to about $26,000 per year, with hospitals, on the whole, paying higher wages than community pharmacies and higher salaries being paid to certified technicians. In a 2001 PTCB survey, 65% of certified pharmacy technicians were paid between $9 and $20 per hour. Pharmacy technicians can expect to receive additional pay for working off-hours and for overtime. Hospitals and chain store pharmacies tend to have excellent benefits packages, including medical and dental plans, retirement plans, paid sick leave, and tuition reimbursement for those considering pursuing a Pharm.D. degree.

Web Link

Go to the Pharmacy Technician Certification Board (PTCB) site at www.ptcb.org or salary.com for information on pharmacy technician salaries.

THE PHARMACY WORKPLACE

Pharmacists work primarily in community and hospital pharmacies after graduating from pharmacy school. A few will go on to pursue further education and higher degrees, and others enter fields such as home care, long-term care, and pharmacy sales.

Community, or Retail, Pharmacies

Three-fifths of all pharmacists in the United States work in community, or retail, pharmacies. Some of these pharmacies are independently owned small businesses, while some are part of large retail chains, and still others are franchises. A franchise combines characteristics of an independent business and a large retail chain. Franchise agreements vary, but typically they involve a large retail company, the franchiser, that grants exclusive use of the company name and rights to sell company products to an owner/operator of a drugstore, the franchisee. An example of such a franchise operation is The Medicine Shoppe. Most community pharmacies are divided into a back prescription area offering prescription merchandise and related items and a front area offering over-the-counter drugs, toiletries, cosmetics, cards, and so on.

Web Link

Visit The Medicine Shoppe at www.medicineshoppe.com

Typical duties of the pharmacy technician in a community pharmacy are to aid the pharmacist in the filling, labeling, and recording of prescriptions; to operate and be responsible for the pharmacy cash register; to stock and inventory prescription and over-the-counter (OTC) medications (those not needing a prescription); to maintain computerized or written patient records; to prepare insurance claim forms; and to order and maintain parts of the front-end stock. The last of these duties might involve interaction with a front-end manager responsible for the nonpharmacy area of the drugstore.

Hospital Pharmacies

A quarter of all pharmacists work in hospital settings. According to the American Hospital Association definition, a hospital is an institution that offers 24-hour healthcare service; that has six or more beds, a governing authority, and an organized medical staff; and that offers nursing and pharmacy services. Hospitals are classified by type of service into general and specialized hospitals; by length of stay into short-term care (under 30 days) and long-term care (30 days or more) hospitals; and by ownership into governmental and nongovernmental hospitals, and into for-profit and nonprofit hospitals. In addition, hospitals are often described according to bed capacity. The functions of a hospital include

- diagnosis and testing
- treatment and therapy
- patient processing (including admissions, record keeping, billing, and planning for post-release patient care)
- public health education and promotion, done through a variety of programs, including smoking cessation programs, weight loss programs, support group programs, and screenings of community members (including mammographies and testing of blood pressure and cholesterol)
- teaching (training health professionals)
- research (carrying out programs that add to the sum of medical knowledge)

Traditionally, hospitals are run by a president who reports to a board of directors. Reporting to the president or to an executive vice president, in a typical hospital, are vice presidents of

- ambulatory services
- community services
- fiscal services
- human and educational services
- management services
- medical services

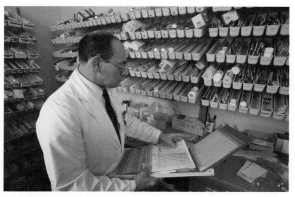

The pharmacy provides an important service to the hospital. Here, a pharmacist reviews a patient's chart.

- nursing services
- planning and program development
- professional services

The vice president for professional services usually oversees the departments responsible for anesthesiology, clinical services, laboratory testing, medical records, psychiatry, radiology, rehabilitation, respiratory care, social services, and pharmacy.

Similar to a community pharmacy, the hospital pharmacy carries out the functions of maintaining drug treatment records and ordering, stocking, compounding, repackaging, and dispensing medications and other supplies. It also prepares sterile intravenous medications (IVs), prepares 24-hour supplies of patients' medications, stocks nursing stations, and delivers medications to patients' rooms. The pharmacy technician in a hospital setting may take part in all of these functions. In addition, he or she may operate manual or computerized, robotic dispensing machinery.

In addition to the functions described in the preceding paragraph, a hospital pharmacy typically carries out numerous clinical functions, the purpose of which is dispensing not drugs but information. These clinical functions include providing drug information to healthcare professionals, monitoring drug therapy profiles, educating and counseling patients about their drug therapies, conducting drug usage evaluations, collecting and evaluating information about adverse drug reactions, participating in clinical drug investigations and research, providing in-service drug-related education, auditing for quality assurance, and providing expert consultation in such areas as pediatric pharmacology (the effects of drugs on babies and children) and pharmacokinetics (the absorption, distribution, and elimination of drugs by the body).

As part of their clinical functions, hospital pharmacies typically operate Drug Information Centers, the purpose of which is to collect and provide information and literature about drugs and their effects. The technician working in a Drug Information Center may be responsible for maintaining and filing correspondence and pharmacy-related literature, including abstracts, catalogs, correspondence, journals, microfilm, and newsletters; for logging information requests and compiling statistics about those requests; and for collating data on drug utilization and adverse reactions.

The staff of the hospital pharmacy may include administrators, staff pharmacists with BA degrees, clinical pharmacists with Pharm.D. degrees, and pharmacy technicians. Hospital pharmacies and drugstore chains are more likely than community pharmacies to require that pharmacy technicians be certified. Some pharmacy employers encourage technicians to become certified by paying for the certification exam and giving raises to those who pass it.

Other Pharmacy Workplaces

In addition to working in community and hospital pharmacies, both pharmacists and pharmacy technicians find employment with home healthcare services; nursing homes and other long-term care facilities; clinics; health maintenance organizations (HMOs); the federal government, including the military services; nuclear medicine pharmacies; mail-order prescription pharmacies; insurance companies; medical software developers; pharmaceutical manufacturers; drug wholesale companies; manufacturing companies in the food and beverage industries; and educational institutions offering training to pharmacists and pharmacy technicians.

HOME HEALTHCARE SYSTEMS   In recent years, spiraling hospitalization costs, regulatory changes, and advances in parenteral therapies (those involving the administration of nutrients and medications through subcutaneous and intravenous injection)

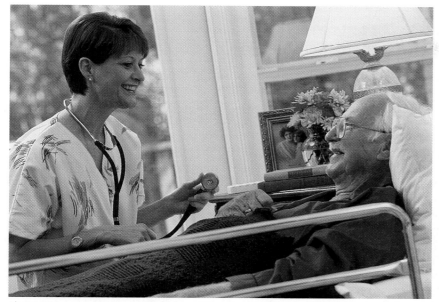

Pharmacists and pharmacy technicians will work with home healthcare workers who provide services to patients who remain at home.

have created an explosion in home healthcare, the delivery of medical, nursing, and pharmaceutical services to patients who remain at home. The home healthcare market grew from less than a billion dollars per year in the 1970s to over 30 billion per year in the late 1990s. Pharmacists and pharmacy technicians working in home healthcare—through a hospital, community pharmacy chain, HMO, or private home healthcare provider—provide educational materials, carry out traditional compounding and delivery functions, prepare and provide infusions and infusion equipment, and often must be available for emergencies on a 24-hour basis.

LONG-TERM CARE FACILITIES Long-term care facilities provide institutional services to elderly patients and to others who cannot provide for themselves, including infants, children, and adults who suffer from severe birth defects, traumatic brain injuries, or chronic (long-lasting), debilitating illnesses. They also provide adult day-care services for persons with chronic psychiatric or medical disorders. Licensed pharmacists, who can be either employees of the facility or outside consultants, provide to long-term care facilities such services as establishing record-keeping systems related to controlled substances, reviewing the drug regimens of residents, reporting irregularities related to drug treatments or controlled substances, monitoring the on-site repackaging and storage of pharmaceuticals, ensuring that medications are uncontaminated and have not expired, calling attention to medication errors and possible adverse reactions or interactions, educating residents and sometimes their family members regarding drug therapies and self-medication, and providing medications to outpatients or residents on leave. In many of these areas, the pharmacist may play a crucial role in ensuring regulatory compliance by the long-term care facility, as long-term care is a highly regulated industry. For example, each patient profile in a long-term care facility must be checked monthly by a licensed pharmacist.

Under supervision by the pharmacist, the pharmacy technician in a long-term care facility may log prescriptions and refill orders via computer, prepare billings, maintain drug boxes or trays for emergencies, package and label medications, deliver medications to nursing stations, maintain records, retrieve patient charts and organize them for the pharmacist's review, conduct regularly scheduled inspections of drugs in inventory and in nursing stations to remove expired or recalled medications, and repackage drugs in unit doses labeled for each patient. Unit dose systems typically make use of a storage bin in a medication cart containing medication for a given resident for a 24-hour period. Some long-term care providers fill medication carts for longer periods—two, three, or five days.

Chapter Summary

The profession of pharmacy has ancient roots, dating to the use of drugs for magical and curative purposes before the beginning of civilization. Starting in the Middle Ages, pharmacy began to disengage itself from medicine and to become established as a distinct profession. Today, pharmacists are highly educated professionals who operate in a variety of settings, including community pharmacies, hospitals, home healthcare systems, and long-term care facilities.

Pharmacy is primarily a knowledge-based profession. As such, it provides not only a dispensatory function, involving the ordering, preparation, and dispensing of medicines, but also a clinical function, involving the provision of information about drugs to patients and healthcare practitioners.

The pharmacy technician is a paraprofessional who, under the supervision of a pharmacist, carries out a wide range of duties related to prescription preparation, communication, and inventory control. The technician also typically has various clerical duties. At present, the job of the pharmacy technician is being redefined, moving away from lay clerical status to paraprofessional status involving education to the Associate degree level and, in many cases, professional registration and certification. Pharmacy technicians work in all the settings in which pharmacists are found, and the demand for competent technicians is expected to grow considerably in the near future.

Chapter Review

Knowledge Inventory

Choose the best answer from those provided.

1. A list of drugs is known as a
   - a. formulary.
   - b. dispensatory.
   - c. pharmacopeia.
   - d. All of the above

2. The humor associated with melancholy was
   - a. blood.
   - b. phlegm.
   - c. yellow bile.
   - d. black bile.

3. In days gone by, the pharmacist was commonly referred to as
   - a. an apothecary.
   - b. a chemist.
   - c. a druggist.
   - d. All of the above

4. Knowledge of the medicinal functions of natural products of animal, plant, or mineral origin is known as
   - a. pharmacognosy.
   - b. pharmacology.
   - c. galenical pharmacy.
   - d. clinical pharmacy.

5. The emergence of the pharmaceutical industry threatened to reduce the traditional role of the pharmacist to that of a
   - a. compounder of medications.
   - b. pharmaceutical scientist.
   - c. drugstore operator.
   - d. toxicologist.

6. The work that heralded the emergence of modern clinical pharmacy was the
   - a. Code of Ethics of the American Pharmaceutical Association.
   - b. Millis Report.
   - c. Report of the President's Commission on Controlled Substances.
   - d. Kefauver-Harris Amendment to the Food, Drug, and Cosmetic Act of 1938.

7. A technician who has completed the national certification examination is known as a
   - a. Pharm.D.
   - b. CPhT.
   - c. RPhT.
   - d. PCT.

8. Another name for a community pharmacy is a
   a. retail pharmacy.
   b. long-term care facility.
   c. home healthcare pharmacy.
   d. health maintenance organization.

9. The purpose of clinical pharmacy is to
   a. dispense medications.
   b. compound medications.
   c. report adverse reactions or interactions to medications.
   d. provide information about medications and monitor drug therapy to ensure optimal patient outcomes.

10. Licensing and general professional oversight of pharmacists and pharmacies is carried out by
    a. colleges of pharmacy.
    b. the American Pharmaceutical Society.
    c. the United States Pharmacopeial Convention.
    d. state pharmacy boards.

Pharmacy in Practice

1. Go to the library and find a copy of the latest edition of the federal government's *Occupational Outlook Handbook.* Using information from this handbook, prepare a short report on the work conditions, duties, training, salaries, and job outlook for one pharmacy-related profession.
2. Call some local drugstores and hospital pharmacies and arrange to interview two practicing pharmacy technicians about their job duties. Compare your findings with the description you researched in Exercise 1. Prepare an oral report for your class.
3. Contact the admissions department of one college of pharmacy and ask them to send you information on admissions policies, degrees, and programs offered at the school. Based upon the information that you receive, do a report on the various degrees and programs open to people in the pharmacy field.

Improving Communication Skills

1. Pharmacy as a profession and the pharmacist have been at the top of many surveys which rank the public's trust. For many years, pharmacy has been the number one profession that inspires trust in the public. Pharmacists and those who work in a pharmacy strive to behave in a professional manner, and communicate effectively with the patients they serve. Make a list of ten things that you have noticed about pharmacy and/or a particular pharmacist that make you feel the trust is warranted.
2. The culture of the United States is changing constantly and becoming more diversified. Patients are often influenced by a wide variety of factors in their culture, religion, and community. Explain in writing why it is important for a pharmacist and the pharmacy employees to get to know individual patients, their families, and their cultural beliefs. Include three examples or case illustrations in your explanation.

Internet Research

Exercises in this section focus on Web research and information retrieval. The information you access on the Web needs to be thoughtfully reviewed and evaluated. As you complete the Internet questions in this and later chapters, use the questions below to help you determine the reliability and validity of information.

- Who created this site and who are the sponsors of the site? From whose perspective is the material written?
- Who are the intended audiences of the site?
- What special knowledge do the site authors and contributors have?
- Is the material factual or does it seem biased? Can the information be validated by secondary source?
- When and how often is the Web site updated?
- Is this site easy to navigate? Can you find new information quickly and efficiently?
- Will you bookmark this site and use it regularly?

1. Visit the Pharmacy Technician Certification Board Web site at www.ptcb.org. Locate the test site most convenient to you, and dates for the application deadline and exam over the coming year. Place these important dates in your calendar. Then, make a list of the subjects covered in the exam and examine the sample questions. Be prepared to participate in a class discussion concerning the content of the certification exam.

2. Visit one of the many online news services such as MSN, CNN, ABC, Reuters, mayohealth, or prnewswire. Search these sites and find at least three news items about a medical treatment or new drugs. Print out and summarize the articles and present them to the class.

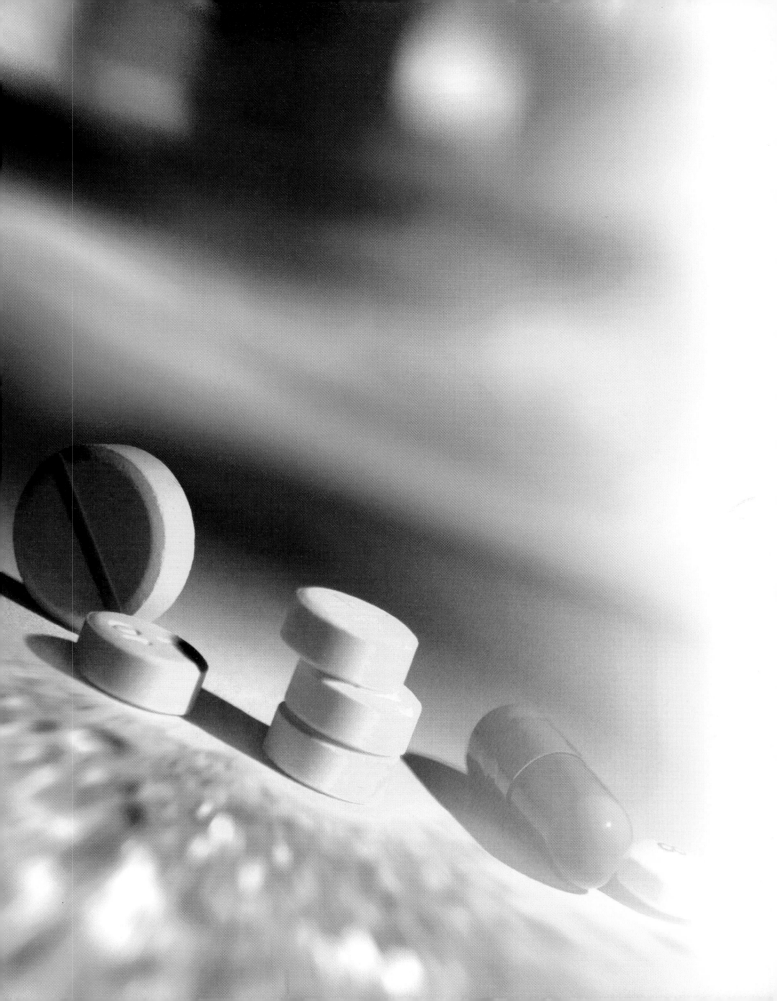

Pharmacy Law, Standards, and Ethics for Technicians

Learning Objectives

◇ Distinguish among common law, statutory law, regulatory or administrative law, ethics, and professional standards.

◇ Explain the potential for tort actions under the common law related to negligence and other forms of malpractice.

◇ List and describe the major effects on pharmacy of the major pieces of statutory federal drug law in the twentieth century.

◇ Enumerate the major principles of the Code of Ethics for Pharmacists of the American Pharmaceutical Association and the Code of Ethics of the American Association of Pharmacy Technicians.

◇ Enumerate the duties that may legally be performed by pharmacy technicians in most states.

The practice of pharmacy is controlled by a variety of mechanisms. These include common law—the system of precedents established by decisions in cases throughout legal history; statutory law—laws passed by legislative bodies at the federal, state, and local levels; regulatory law—the system of rules and regulations established by governmental bodies such as the FDA and state boards of pharmacy; professional standards—guidelines established by professional associations; and codes of ethics—rules for proper conduct, again established by professional associations. The complex system of interrelated laws, regulations, standards, and ethical guidelines helps to ensure that drug therapies and merchandising are carried out safely and in the public interest.

THE NEED FOR DRUG CONTROL

Not until 1951, with the passage of the Durham-Humphrey Amendment to the Food, Drug, and Cosmetic Act of 1938, was the distinction made under U.S. federal law between drugs that can and drugs that cannot be purchased without a prescription from a physician. In some countries yet today, any drug can be dispensed or sold by any person without legal restriction. To persons working in pharmacy in the United States today, such laxity of control over drugs seems astonishing, for pharmacy has become, in our time, one of the most highly proscribed professions. The contemporary pharmacy is subject to many kinds of control at the federal, state, and local levels. Controls on contemporary pharmacy are exercised by various groups and organizations, including

◇ state boards of pharmacy
◇ courts
◇ federal, state, and local legislative bodies such as the United States Congress, state legislatures, and municipal governing councils
◇ federal and state regulatory agencies such as
  • the Food and Drug Administration (FDA), with general authority to regulate the manufacture and sale of drugs
  • the Drug Enforcement Adminstration (DEA), with enforcement authority over controlled substances

- the Occupational Health and Safety Administration (OSHA), with authority over workplace safety
- the Federal Trade Commission (FTC), with authority over business practices
- the Health Care Financing Administration (HCFA) of the Department of Health and Human Services (DHHS), with authority over reimbursement under the Medicare and Medicaid programs
- state health and welfare agencies
- state boards of pharmacy, with licensure and regulatory authority over pharmacy practice at the state level
◇ the private corporation known as the United States Pharmacopeial Convention (USPC), which publishes the compendia setting standards for drug formulation and dosage forms
◇ professional organizations such as the
- American Pharmaceutical Association (AphA)
- American Association of Colleges of Pharmacy (AACP)
- National Association of Boards of Pharmacy (NABP)
- Joint Commission on Accreditation of Healthcare Organizations (JCAHO)
- American Society of Health-System Pharmacists (ASHP)
◇ individual institutions such as community pharmacies, hospitals, long-term care facilities, and home healthcare organizations.

Numerous healthcare organizations have established voluntary standards regarding many aspects of healthcare and its provision. The law offers a minimum level of acceptable standards, and ethics offer guidelines for personal conduct within a profession or certain situation. Some organizations offer additional levels of accreditation beyond what the minimum level of the law requires. The Joint Commission on Accreditation of Healthcare Organizations (JCAHO) is one of these organizations. Many inpatient and some outpatient facilities undergo a rigorous inspection process with JCAHO on a regular basis to maintain their current accredited status. Some insurance carriers require this accreditation for reimbursement when providing services to its members. This accreditation is voluntary under the law, but is required for "doing business" in today's healthcare industry.

A BRIEF HISTORY OF STATUTORY PHARMACY LAW

Many people are familiar, from novels and movies, with the lawlessness that reigned during the nineteenth century with regard to medications. Consider the situation in John Irving's superbly researched novel *The Cider House Rules,* in which a character dies from taking a medication called French Lunar Solution, the label of which makes the following promises: "Restores Female Monthly Regularity! Stops Suppression!" and carries the warning: "Caution: Dangerous to Married Women! Almost Certainly Causes Miscarriages!" *Suppression* was a nineteenth-century euphemism for pregnancy, and the medication, a concentrated fluid extract of an extremely poisonous, or toxic, weed known as tansy, was meant as an aborticide. To combat real-life abuses of this kind—abuses in formulation and labeling—the United States Congress passed, in 1906, the first of a series of landmark twentieth-century laws to regulate the development, compounding, distribution, storage, and dispensing of drugs.

Pure Food and Drug Act of 1906

The purpose of the Pure Food and Drug Act of 1906 was to prohibit the interstate transportation or sale of adulterated and misbranded food and drugs. The act did not

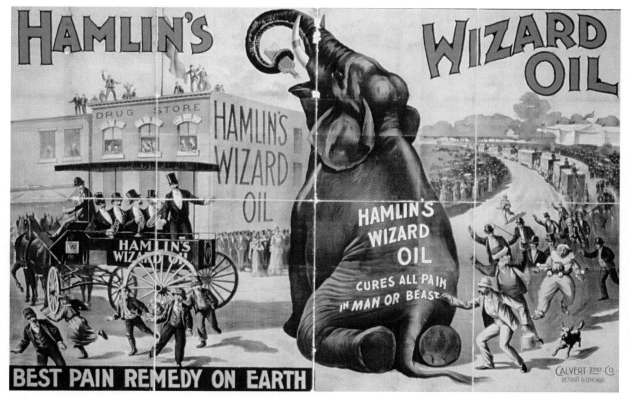

In the late 1800s, there was no control on the sale of pharmaceutical products. Thus, consumers were not protected.

require that drugs be labeled, only that the label not contain false information about the drug's strength and purity. The act, though amended, proved unenforceable, and new legislation was required. In 1937, the need for new legislation was tragically demonstrated by 107 deaths resulting from the sale of a sulfa drug product that contained diethylene glycol, used today as an antifreeze for automobile radiators.

Food, Drug, and Cosmetic Act (FDCA) of 1938

The Food, Drug, and Cosmetic Act (FDCA) of 1938, the most important piece of legislation in pharmaceutical history, created the Food and Drug Administration (FDA) and required pharmaceutical manufacturers to file a New Drug Application (NDA) with the FDA. Under this act, manufacturers must, before marketing a drug product, prove to the FDA's satisfaction that the product is safe for use by humans. To do so, the manufacturer must conduct and submit the results of toxicological studies on animals followed by clinical trials with human beings. Toxicological studies are conducted to determine the degree of toxicity, or danger to living organisms, of a substance. Clinical trials are controlled experiments held to determine the effects of drugs on human subjects. The New Drug Application must detail the chemical composition of the drug and the processes used to manufacture it. The FDCA also extended and clarified the definitions of adulterated and misbranded drugs. It defined adulterated drugs as those

◇ consisting "in whole or in part of any filthy, putrid, or decomposed substance," ones "prepared, packed, or held under insanitary conditions"

- prepared in containers "composed, in whole or in part, of any poisonous or deleterious substance"
- containing unsafe color additives
- purporting to be or represented as drugs recognized "in an official compendium" but differing in strength, quality, or purity from said drugs

The relevant "official compendia" referred to are the *United States Pharmacopeia* and the *National Formulary*. The act defined misbranded drugs, in part, as those

- containing labeling that is "false or misleading in any particular"
- in packaging that does not bear "a label containing (1) the name and place of business of the manufacturer, packer, or distributor, and (2) an accurate statement of the quantity of the contents in terms of weight, measure, or numerical count"
- not conspicuously and clearly labeled with the information required by the act
- that are habit-forming but do not carry the label "Warning—May be habit forming"
- that do not contain a label that "bears (1) the established name of the drug, if any, and (2) in case it contains two or more ingredients, the established name and quantity of each active ingredient, including the quantity, kind, and proportion of any alcohol, and also including, whether active or not, the established name and quantity" [of certain other substances listed in the act]
- that do not contain labeling with "adequate directions for use" and "adequate warnings against use in those pathological conditions or by children where its use may be dangerous to health, or against unsafe dosage or methods or duration of administration or application"
- that are "dangerous to health when used in the dosage or manner, or with the frequency or duration prescribed, recommended, or suggested in the labeling"

Under this act, the FDA has the power not only to approve or deny new drug applications but also to conduct inspections to ensure compliance. The Supreme Court later held that the act applied to interstate transactions as well as to intrastate transactions, including those within pharmacies. Unfortunately, the act required only that drugs be safe for human consumption, not that they be efficacious, or useful for the purpose for which they were sold.

Durham-Humphrey Amendment of 1951

This Durham-Humphrey Amendment of 1951 states that drug containers do not have to include "adequate directions for use" as long as they bear the legend "Caution: Federal law prohibits dispensing without a prescription." The dispensing of the drug by a pharmacist with a label giving directions from the prescriber meets the law's requirements. The amendment thus established the distinction between so-called legend, or prescription, drugs and over-the counter (OTC), or nonprescription, drugs. It also authorized the taking of prescriptions verbally, rather than in writing, and the refilling of prescriptions. However, the refilling of prescriptions subject to abuse was limited. Under the amendment, prescriptions for such substances could not be refilled without the express consent of the prescriber.

Kefauver-Harris Amendment of 1962

The Kefauver-Harris Amendment of 1962 was passed in response to the birth, mostly in other countries, of thousands of infants with severe anatomical abnormalities to mothers who had taken the tranquilizer thalidomide. It extended the FDCA to require that drugs be not only safe for humans but also efficacious. The amendment requires drug manufacturers to file with the FDA, before clinical trials on humans, an Investigational New Drug Application. After extensive trials in which a product is proved both safe and effective, the manufacturer may then submit a New Drug Application that seeks approval to market the product.

Comprehensive Drug Abuse Prevention and Control Act of 1970

The Comprehensive Drug Abuse Prevention and Control Act of 1970, commonly referred to as the Controlled Substances Act, was created to combat and control drug abuse and to supersede previous federal drug abuse laws. The act classified drugs with potential for abuse into five categories, or schedules, ranging from those with great potential for abuse to those with little such potential. The agency made primarily responsible under this act is the Drug Enforcement Administration (DEA), an arm of the Department of Justice. The DEA is charged with enforcement and prevention related to the abuse of controlled substances.

Poison Prevention Act of 1970

The Poison Prevention Act of 1970, enforced by the Consumer Product Safety Commission, requires that most over-the-counter and legend drugs be packaged in child-resistant containers that cannot be opened by 80 percent of children under five but can be opened by 90 percent of adults. The law provides that on request by the prescriber or signed request by the patient/customer, the pharmacist may dispense a drug in a non-child-resistant container. The patient or customer, but not the prescriber, may make a blanket request that all drugs dispensed to him or her be in noncompliant containers. Other exceptions provided for by the law are detailed in Table 2.1.

Table 2.1	Exceptions to the Requirement for Child-Resistant Containers Pursuant to the Poison Prevention Act of 1970

1. Single-time dispensing of product in noncompliant container as ordered by prescriber
2. Single-time or blanket dispensing of product in noncompliant container as requested by the patient or customer in a signed statement
3. One noncompliant size of an over-the-counter product for elderly or handicapped users, provided that the label carry the warning "This Package for Households without Young Children" or, if the label is too small, "Package Not Child Resistant"
4. Drugs dispensed to institutionalized patients, provided that these are to be administered by employees of the institution
5. The following specific drugs:
   ◇ Betamethasone tablets with no more than 12.6 mg per package
   ◇ Erythromycin ethylsuccinate tablets in packages containing no more than 16 g
   ◇ Inhalation aerosols
   ◇ Mebendazole tablets with no more than 600 mg per package
   ◇ Methylprednisolone tablets with no more than 85 mg per package
   ◇ Oral contraceptives to be taken cyclically, in manufacturer's dispensing packages
   ◇ Pancrelipase preparations
   ◇ Potassium supplements in unit dose form, including unit dose vials of liquid potassium, effervescent tablets, and unit dose powdered potassium packets with no more than 830 mEq per unit dose
   ◇ Powdered anhydrous cholestyramine
   ◇ Powdered colestipol up to 5 g per packet
   ◇ Prednisone tablets with no more than 105 mg per package
   ◇ Sodium fluoride products with no more than 264 mg of sodium fluoride per package
   ◇ Sublingual and chewable isosorbide dinitrate in strengths of 10 mg or less
   ◇ Sublingual nitroglycerin (tablets to be taken by dissolving beneath the tongue)

Drug Listing Act of 1972

The Drug Listing Act of 1972 gives the FDA the authority to compile a list of currently marketed drugs. Under the act, each new drug is assigned a unique and permanent product code, known as a National Drug Code (NDC), consisting of ten characters that identify the manufacturer or distributor, the drug formulation, and the size and type of its packaging. The FDA asks, but does not require, that the NDC appear on all drug labels, including labels of prescription containers. Using this code, the FDA is able to maintain a database of drugs by use, manufacturer, and active ingredients and of newly marketed, discontinued, and remarketed drugs.

Orphan Drug Act of 1983

An orphan drug is one that will be used by so few people that developing and marketing it is prohibitively expensive. The Orphan Drug Act of 1983 encourages the development of orphan drugs by providing tax incentives and allowing manufacturers to be granted exclusive licenses to market such drugs.

Drug Price Competition and Patent-Term Restoration Act of 1984

A given drug typically has several names, including its chemical names and its official generic or nonproprietary name (e.g., ibuprofen), both of which are given in official compendia, and one or more brand or proprietary names (e.g., Advil, Motrin) given by manufacturers. A generic drug is one with the same chemical composition as a brand-name drug that can be substituted (under regulations now existing in every state) for the brand-name drug in prescriptions. The Drug Price Competition and Patent-Term Restoration Act encouraged the creation of both generic drugs and innovative new drugs by streamlining the process for generic drug approval and by extending patent licenses as a function of the time required for the drug application approval process.

Prescription Drug Marketing Act of 1987

Passed in response to concern over safety and competition issues raised by secondary markets for drugs, the Prescription Drug Marketing Act of 1987 prohibits the reimportation of a drug into the United States by anyone except the manufacturer. It also prohibits the sale or trading of drug samples, the distribution of samples to persons other than those licensed to prescribe them, and the distribution of samples except by mail or by common carrier. In addition, it requires wholesalers who are not authorized distributors of the manufacturer to notify customers that they are not authorized distributors prior to a sale.

Omnibus Budget Reconciliation Act of 1990 (OBRA-90)

Embedded in this budget bill was legislation with a profound effect on how pharmacy is practiced. The Omnibus Budget Reconciliation Act of 1990 (OBRA-90) requires that, as a condition of participating in the Medicaid program, states must establish standards of practice for pharmacists requiring drug use review (DUR) by the pharmacist. Among other provisions, the act requires "a review of drug therapy before each prescription is filled or delivered to an individual receiving benefits under this subchapter, typically at the point-of-sale or point of distribution. The review shall include screening for potential drug therapy problems due to therapeutic duplication, drug-disease contraindications, drug-drug interactions (including serious interactions with non-prescription over over-the-counter drugs), incorrect drug dosage or duration of treatment, drug-allergy interactions, and clinical abuse/misuse."

Under the law, a pharmacist must make an offer to counsel the patient/customer, but this person may refuse such counseling. The pharmacist must offer to discuss with the patient or the attending healthcare professional all matters of significance, including

◇ name and description of medication
◇ dosage form
◇ dosage
◇ route of administration
◇ duration of drug therapy
◇ action to take following a missed dose
◇ common severe side effects or adverse effects
◇ interactions and therapeutic contraindications, ways to prevent the same, and actions to be taken if they occur
◇ methods for self-monitoring of the drug therapy
◇ prescription refill information
◇ proper storage of the drug
◇ special directions and precautions for preparation, administration, and use by the patient

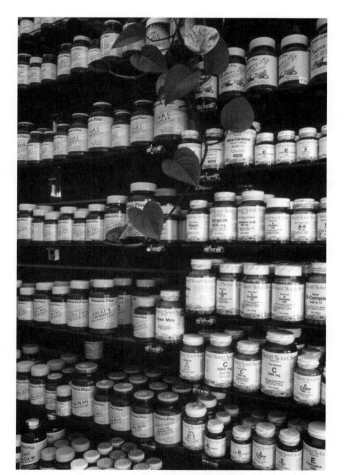

Dietary supplements and vitamins are not strictly regulated like prescription and OTC medications.

OBRA-90 uses the possibility of loss of Medicaid participation to enforce the clinical practices of screening prescriptions and counseling patients and caregivers. It also requires state boards of pharmacy or other state regulatory agencies to provide for the creation of DUR boards for prospective and retrospective review of drug therapies and educational programs for training physicians and pharmacists with regard to the use of medications. The law also requires that manufacturers rebate to state Medicaid programs the difference between the manufacturer's best price for a drug (typically the wholesale price) and average billed price.

FDA Modernization Act

The FDA Modernization Act was passed to update the labeling currently on prescription medications. Currently, the products are labeled "legend" and are to be changed to read "℞ only." Legend is the term that has been used in the past to indicate if a drug was available by prescription or over the counter. The new labeling requirements are to be implemented by 2004.

Dietary Supplement Health and Education Act (DSHEA) of 1994

One area in which the FDA is not permitted oversight is the herbal supplement, nutritional supplement, and vitamin market. A law was passed in the 1994 making the FDA's oversight of this area somewhat tenuous. The FDA is not permitted to require manufacturers of these products to abide by the same laws that apply to prescription and OTC medications. It may only monitor, investigate, and look at false claims advertisements. Manufacturers of these supplements are not permitted to make claims of curing, or treating ailments; they may only state that the products are supplements to support health. If they do make claims, the FDA can then require them to provide the research and proof to back up those claims.

This act defined what a dietary supplement is, and set guidelines for the FDA and industry regarding vitamins, minerals, herbal products, and nutritional supplements. The dietary supplement market does not have FDA oversight, and manufacturers are not required by this law to prove safety, efficacy, or standardization to any governmental agency. If the FDA wants to remove a dietary supplement from the market, it may do so; however it must then hold public hearings, and the burden of proof is shifted to the FDA to prove that the dietary supplement is unsafe.

NATIONAL OVERSIGHT AGENCIES

The federal government has used the acts and amendments passed in the twentieth century to address a broad scope of issues and provide a basic structure for the utilization of drug products, and the practice of pharmacy. The acts and amendments are laws in the true sense of the word, and provide the minimum level of acceptable standards. The details of how the standards of practice are implemented are left up the federal agencies that were created, and the state boards of pharmacy. The two primary agencies that were created by federal legislation are the FDA and DEA. Another national organization with interest in pharmacy law is the NABP, or National Associations of the Boards of Pharmacy. This is an organization that meets regularly to establish general consensus among the member states, and develop model regulations to be taken back to the states and put into place.

Food and Drug Administration (FDA)

Web Link

Visit the FDA at www.fda.gov

The FDA has the primary responsibility of overseeing drug safety in the United States. It has the authority to enforce the law, and the ability to create and enforce regulations that will assist in providing the public with safe drug products. The FDA requires all manufacturers to file applications for investigation and approval, provides guidelines for packaging and advertisement, and oversees the recall of products that are deemed dangerous.

The FDA has regulations for manufacturers to follow while researching new chemical entities and developing those chemicals into drug products. Scientists conduct three phases of drug testing prior to the approval process. Occasionally when a medication appears to be very promising early on in the testing, the FDA may opt to "fast track" the drug, and grant early approval.

Once a drug is approved, the FDA oversight will continue. A manufacturer has very strict guidelines as to how the product may be packaged, advertised, and marketed to physicians, and now the public. A manufacturer may not make speculative claims or false claims about the potential of the product, and it must also disclose the side effects, adverse reactions, contraindications, etc., to those to whom it markets. The FDA has been known to step in and ask a manufacturer to cancel advertising campaigns, and even instruct them to present a new advertisement campaign to clear up any misconceptions. Even the OTC-marketed medications undergo this scrutiny from the FDA, and the label of OTC products must conform to a preferred format for all of the information in order to make it clear to the lay person public.

If a drug is contaminated, of poor quality, or found to have an unsafe record, the drug company may recall the drug. The FDA has the authority to obtain an injunction from the court and force the manufacturer to recall the drug product. Most companies voluntarily recall products when there is a problem as it is in their best interest to do so. There are three classes of recalls, and staff at the FDA determine which class recall is issued from the reports of the manufacturer and healthcare providers. Table 2.2 describes the three types of recalls. The FDA has a medical products reporting program called MedWatch. This program involves voluntary reporting of adverse health events and problems with medical products. The report consists of a one-page form that may be faxed or mailed to the FDA. This form is widely available and published in many drug references. See Figure 2.1.

Drug Enforcement Administration (DEA)

The DEA is one of the agencies responsible for enforcing the laws regarding addictive substances, both legal and illegal. While this agency directs most of its funds and personnel toward the illegal trafficking of C-I drugs, it also has duties relating to legal use of narcotics and other controlled substances. The DEA issues medical practitioners and pharmacies a license (number) that will enable them to write prescriptions for scheduled drugs and, in the case of a pharmacy, order scheduled drugs from wholesalers. Often upon recommendation from the manufacturer and the FDA, the DEA classifies new drugs into a schedule and will even re-evaluate drugs that have been on the market for some time to determine if they warrant being changed to a scheduled drug. A description of the five schedules of drugs is outlined in Table 2.3. Inspections of medical facilities, including pharmacies, is a function of the DEA as well. Inspections are usually limited to facilities where suspicious activity has been detected. The DEA is able to track narcotics from manufacturer, to warehouse, to pharmacy, and can determine which physicians prescribe scheduled drugs. Schedule II narcotics are most highly regulated, and sudden increases in usage in a particular pharmacy may cause the DEA to investigate. A special triplicate form (Figure 2.2 on page 26) must be used when ordering C-II narcotics.

National Association of the Boards of Pharmacy (NABP)

The National Association of the Boards of Pharmacy (NABP) meets several times each year to discuss national trends and issues of importance with the regard to pharmacy law. This organization has no regulatory authority, and indeed there is not a regulatory body that oversees the practice of pharmacy. The FDA deals with medications, and the DEA deals with controlled substances. Individual states have differing laws regarding the practice of pharmacy. Because many of the states

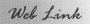

Web Link

Visit MedWatch at www.fda.gov/ medwatch

Web Link

Get MedWatch forms at www. fda.gov/medwatch/ getforms.htm

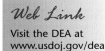

Web Link

Visit the DEA at www.usdoj.gov/dea

Table 2.2	**Recall Classes for Drugs**

Class	Type of Drug
Class I (C-I)	There is reasonable probability that use of the product will cause or lead to serious adverse health events, or death.
Class II (C-II)	The probability exists that use of the product will cause adverse health events that are temporary, or medically reversible.
Class III (C-III)	The use of the product will probably not cause an adverse health event.

Figure 2.1

MedWatch Medical Products Reporting Form

U.S. Department of Health and Human Services

MEDWATCH

The FDA Safety Information and Adverse Event Reporting Program

For **VOLUNTARY** reporting of adverse events and product problems

Form Approved: OMB No. 0910-0291 Expires: 04/80/03
See OMB statement on reverse

FDA Use Only

Triage unit sequence #

Page ____ of ____

A. Patient information

1. Patient identifier	2. Age at time of event: or _____ Date of birth:	3. Sex ☐ female ☐ male	4. Weight _____ lbs or _____ kgs
In confidence			

B. Adverse event or product problem

1. ☐ **Adverse event**   and/or   ☐ **Product problem** (e.g., defects/malfunctions)

2. **Outcomes attributed to adverse event** (check all that apply)

☐ death _____ (mo/day/yr)
☐ life-threatening
☐ hospitalization - initial or prolonged

☐ disability
☐ congenital anomaly
☐ required intervention to prevent permanent impairment/damage
☐ other: _____

3. Date of event (mo/day/yr)	4. Date of this report (mo/day/yr)

5. **Describe event or problem**

6. **Relevant tests/laboratory data,** including dates

7. **Other relevant history, including preexisting medical conditions** (e.g., allergies, race, pregnancy, smoking and alcohol use, hepatic/renal dysfunction, etc.)

PLEASE TYPE OR USE BLACK INK

C. Suspect medication(s)

1. **Name** (give labeled strength & mfr/labeler, if known)

#1

#2

2. **Dose, frequency & route used** #1 #2	3. **Therapy dates** (if unknown, give duration) from/to (or best estimate) #1 #2

4. **Diagnosis for use** (indication) #1 #2	5. **Event abated after use stopped or dose reduced** #1 ☐ yes ☐ no ☐ doesn't apply #2 ☐ yes ☐ no ☐ doesn't apply

6. **Lot #** (if known) #1 #2	7. **Exp. date** (if known) #1 #2	8. **Event reappeared after reintroduction** #1 ☐ yes ☐ no ☐ doesn't apply #2 ☐ yes ☐ no ☐ doesn't apply

9. **NDC #** (for product problems only)
___-___-___

10. **Concomitant medical products** and therapy dates (exclude treatment of event)

D. Suspect medical device

1. **Brand name**

2. **Type of device**

3. **Manufacturer name & address**	4. **Operator of device** ☐ health professional ☐ lay user/patient ☐ other: _____

6. model # _____ catalog # _____ serial # _____ lot # _____ other #	5. **Expiration date** (mo/day/yr) 7. **If implanted, give date** (mo/day/yr) 8. **If explanted, give date** (mo/day/yr)

9. **Device available for evaluation?**   (Do not send to FDA)

☐ yes   ☐ no   ☐ returned to manufacturer on _____ (mo/day/yr)

10. **Concomitant medical products** and therapy dates (exclude treatment of event)

E. Reporter (see confidentiality section on back)

1. **Name & address**	phone #

2. **Health professional?** ☐ yes ☐ no	3. **Occupation**	4. **Also reported to** ☐ manufacturer ☐ user facility ☐ distributor

5. If you do NOT want your identity disclosed to the manufacturer, place an " X " in this box. ☐

FDA

Mail to: **MEDWATCH**
5600 Fishers Lane
Rockville, MD 20852-9787

or FAX to:
1-800-FDA-0178

FDA Form 3500

Submission of a report does not constitute an admission that medical personnel or the product caused or contributed to the event.

Table 2.3	Drug Schedules Under the Comprehensive Drug Abuse and Control Act of 1970	
Schedule	**Types of Drugs**	**Examples**
Schedule I	drugs with no accepted medical use, or other substances with a high potential for abuse	heroin, LSD, marijuana, mescaline, peyote, psilocybin
Schedule II	drugs with accepted medical uses and a high potential for abuse which, if abused, may lead to severe psychological or physical dependence	amobarbital (Amytal), cocaine, codeine (in high doses), Desoxyn, Dexedrine, hydromorphone (Dilaudid), meperidine hydrochloride (Demerol), methadone hydrochloride, morphine, opium, oxycodone hydrochloride (Percodan), oxymorphone (Numorphan), phenobarbital (Nembutal), Preludin, Ritalin, secobarbital (Seconal)
Schedule III	drugs with accepted medical uses and a potential for abuse less than those listed in Schedules I and II, which, if abused, may lead to moderate psychological or physical dependence	certain drugs compounded with small quantities of narcotics and other drugs with high potential for abuse (Tylenol with Codeine tablets), Hydrocodone with acetaminophen (Vicodin, Lortab, Anexsia), certain barbiturates, glutethimide (Doriden), methyprylon (Noludar), nalorphine (Nalline), paregoric
Schedule IV	drugs with accepted medical uses and low potential for abuse relative to those in Schedule III, which, if abused, may lead to limited physical dependence or psychological dependence relative to drugs in Schedule III	barbital, chloral hydrate (Noctec), chlordiazepoxide (Librium), clonazepam (Klonopin), diazepam (Valium), ethchlorvynol (Placidyl), lorazepam (Ativan), meprobamate (Equanil, Miltown), methohexital, oxazepam (Serax), paraldehyde, phenobarbital, propoxyphene hydrochloride (Darvon)
Schedule V	drugs with accepted medical uses and low potential for abuse relative to those in Schedule IV and which, if abused, may lead to limited physical dependence or psychological dependence relative to drugs in Schedule IV	Robitussin A-C syrup

Web Link

Visit the NABP at www.nabp.net

developed laws pertaining to pharmacy over many years as acts and then many amendments, the laws seem to have been put together in an unorganized fashion. A need for a common model developed, and the NABP developed the MSPPA (Model State Pharmacy Practice Act). Individual states can then model their practice acts on the MSPPA and individualize certain aspects of the regulation as needed within the given state. The MSPPA, along with various other recommendations often are taken back to the states and used as the "backbone" for the state regulation that the state board of pharmacy puts into place. The NABP also issues each licensed pharmacy a NABP Number which may be requested by insurance companies on a reimbursement form, or during insurance contract negotiations.

STATE BOARDS OF PHARMACY AND LEGAL DUTIES OF PHARMACY PERSONNEL

State Boards of Pharmacy are usually appointed professionals from the pharmacy community. The board is responsible for a variety of activities, which vary from

Figure 2.2

DEA Form 222
This form is used to order Schedule II drugs to be administered in the pharmacy.

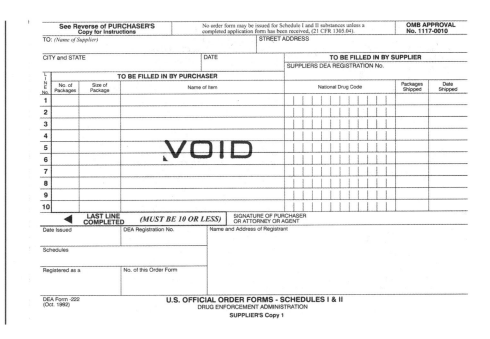

See Reverse of PURCHASER'S Copy for Instructions		No order form may be issued for Schedule I and II substances unless a completed application form has been received, (21 CFR 1305.04).				OMB APPROVAL No. 1117-0010		

TO: *(Name of Supplier)*   STREET ADDRESS

CITY and STATE   DATE   **TO BE FILLED IN BY SUPPLIER**

SUPPLIERS DEA REGISTRATION No.

LINE No.	No. of Packages	Size of Package	Name of Item	National Drug Code	Packages Shipped	Date Shipped
1						
2						
3						
4						
5						
6						
7						
8						
9						
10						

VOID

◄ **LAST LINE COMPLETED** *(MUST BE 10 OR LESS)*   SIGNATURE OF PURCHASER OR ATTORNEY OR AGENT

Date Issued   DEA Registration No.   Name and Address of Registrant

Schedules

Registered as a   No. of this Order Form

DEA Form -222 (Oct. 1992)   **U.S. OFFICIAL ORDER FORMS - SCHEDULES I & II**
DRUG ENFORCEMENT ADMINISTRATION
SUPPLIER'S Copy 1

state to state. Generally, they oversee the regulations already in place, make amendments and new regulations when appropriate, and ensure that pharmacies and pharmacists within the state are practicing according to the state practice guidelines. Occasionally, the board may suspend or revoke the license or registration of a pharmacist.

The State Board of Pharmacy provides regulations regarding refilling of prescriptions, both scheduled drugs and nonscheduled drugs. Although most states have similar laws regarding prescription refills, each state must provide its own regulation as there is not a national "law." Typically, nonscheduled drug prescriptions are refillable for up to one year from the date written. Drugs categorized as schedule III, IV, and V drugs are refillable for up to six months from the date written. Although the law regarding refills on narcotics is covered by The Drug Abuse Control Amendments issued by the federal government, most states have a law that duplicates the federal law. Each state may also regulate certain drugs as to whether or not they are OTC or require a prescription. Insulin, for example is available in most states without a prescription, although it is not advisable for a patient to use insulin without the current care of a physician.

One area of pharmacy practice that differs greatly from state to state is the role and duties of the pharmacy technician. For the most recent information in your state, you should contact your state board of pharmacy. A reference which is useful in comparing duties from state to state is the *Pharmacy Law Digest*.

Definitions of the roles of the pharmacist and the pharmacy technician are in a state of flux. Increasingly, pharmacists are being called upon to perform clinical functions, counsel customers, monitor patient drug regimens, do prerelease and outpatient counseling, and participate in drug studies. As a result, increasing pressure has arisen for legal definition (or, in some cases, redefinition) of the role of the pharmacy technician, who, by assuming additional distribution, compounding, and dispensing responsibilities, could free the pharmacist to undertake his or her clinical duties. However, and this point is extremely important, there is at the present time no statutory federal definition of the role of the pharmacy technician and no uniform definition from state to state. Some states specifically authorize practice by technicians, detailing what duties they may perform. Others do not specifically recognize the technician in state laws and regulations but implicitly define what a technician may or may not do by detailing what the pharmacist must do.

By default, then, duties not required by law or regulation to be done by the pharmacist may be carried out by the technician. As a result of this situation, it is important that a technician become familiar with the applicable statutes and regulations of the state in which he or she practices. In some states, for example, technicians may compound solutions for intravenous infusion under the supervision of a pharmacist. In other states, such compounding may be done only by the pharmacist. In yet others, it may be done, as well, by nurses, but only for use by the nurse doing the compounding. The detailed analysis of state laws and regulations as they impact the practice of pharmacy technicians is beyond the scope of this book, but technicians in training are urged to contact knowledgeable professions in training institutions and/or state boards of pharmacy to learn about state-specific statutes and regulations, particularly those related to registration and/or certification by the state and to the specification of those duties that the technician may lawfully undertake. In most practice situations, a pharmacy has a manual of policies and procedures to dictate the respective duties of the technician and the pharmacist.

Statutes, regulations, and standards of practice vary from state to state, from one locality to another, and even from one community pharmacy or institution to another. A technician in training must learn how these statutes do or do not differ in his or her locality. Generally speaking, as a paraprofessional the technician is expected to work under the supervision of the pharmacist. Table 2.4 lists duties that

Table 2.4	Duties Typically Performed by Pharmacists

A. Dispensing, Record Keeping, and Pricing
receiving a verbal, or oral, prescription in person or by telephone
preparing the written form of the verbal prescription
interpreting and evaluating prescriptions
reviewing patient profile (medication history, duplication of medications, allergies, drug
    interactions, etc.)
verifying and certifying records

B. Preparing Doses of Precompounded Medications
checking/verifying finished prescriptions

C. Preparing Doses of Extemporaneously Compounded, Nonsterile Medications
checking/verifying that drugs were selected properly
calculating weights and measures
verifying that weighing and measuring was done properly
verifying finished product

D. Preparing Doses of Extemporaneously Compounded, Sterile Medications
verifying that drugs were selected properly
calculating weights and measures
verifying use of aseptic equipment and procedures
verifying that weighing and measuring was done properly
checking/verifying finished product

E. Transporting Medications to and from Wards
checking/verifying delivery records
examining returned medications for integrity and reusability
emptying returned medications into stock containers

F. Replenishing Floor Stocks
checking/verifying replenishment of stocks
certifying/checking drug stations
disposing of unused items and discontinued medications

G. Verifying Finished Product Against Original Order or Prescription

typically are performed by pharmacists and may *not* be performed by technicians; Table 2.5 lists duties that typically may be performed by technicians. Because of these variables, these tables may not be completely accurate for a given practice site. In all practice locations, however, all technicians' duties listed, if allowable, *must* be carried out under the direct supervision of a licensed pharmacist.

Table 2.5	**Duties Typically Performed by Technicians**

A. **Dispensing, Record Keeping, and Pricing**
   receiving written prescriptions and conveying them to the pharmacist
   answering telephone calls
   preparing records, including patient profiles and billing records
   some states allow CPhTs to take prescriptions over the phone

B. **Preparing Doses of Precompounded Medications**
   retrieving medications from shelf or supply cabinet
   selecting containers
   preparing labels
   counting or pouring medications
   reconstituting prefabricated medications
   pricing prescriptions

C. **Preparing Doses of Extemporaneously Compounded, Nonsterile Medications**
   retrieving medications from shelf or supply cabinet
   selecting equipment for the compounding operation
   weighing and measuring
   compounding
   preparing labels
   selecting containers
   packaging
   maintaining and filing of records of extemporaneous compounding
   cleaning area and equipment

D. **Preparing Doses of Extemporaneously Compounded, Sterile Medications**
   retrieving medications from shelf or supply cabinet
   selecting equipment for the compounding operation
   using aseptic equipment and procedures
   seighing and measuring
   compounding
   preparing labels
   selecting containers
   packaging
   maintaining and filing records of extemporaneous compounding
   cleaning of area and equipment

E. **Transporting Medications to and from Wards**
   preparing cart, tray, or other means of conveyance
   delivering controlled drugs
   maintaining delivery records
   distributing medications to wards
   organizing medications for administration to patients
   retrieving, reconciling, and recording credit for unadministered medications
   returning unadministered medications to unit-dose bins and injectables to stock
   some states allow a "tech check tech" system where one technician is allowed to check another
      technician's work preparing unit dose carts

F. **Replenishing Floor Stocks**

VIOLATION OF LAW AND REGULATION

When certain violations occur under any level of law—local, state, or federal—a prosecutor or public representative may bring a case against the party who violated the law/regulation. Examples include tax evasion, driving under the influence of alcohol, and more serious cases such as manslaughter, and murder. When a case such as this is filed, it will be filed using terms such as *State vs. John K. Smith.* This type of case is considered a crime or violation against the state or federal government, and it is the prosecutor's duty to see that society is protected from individuals who violate the law.

When cases are filed in court, the party or person filing the case is called the plaintiff, and the party being sued or that the case is against is called the defendant. It is the responsibility of the plaintiff to prove his case, this is referred to as burden of proof. The burden of proof in a case involving crimes against the local, state, or federal government is referred to as "reasonable doubt." This means that the prosecutor or plaintiff must provide convincing evidence that the party committed the act, beyond any "reasonable" doubt of a normal person. If the party is found guilty, the punishment may be monetary fines, probation, or jail time.

If the defendant in a case is a licensed healthcare provider (doctor, nurse, or pharmacist) the appropriate state medical board may look at the case and determine whether or not the party's license should be revoked or suspended. The license may be revoked on ethical grounds, or the board may have a specific regulation that allows them to revoke a license in the event the person is convicted of a felony. It is important to note that the local, state, or federal prosecutor does not have the authority to revoke a license to practice various types of healthcare. Only the appropriate state medical board has this authority.

Civil Law

Civil law is the term given to the types of law that concern the citizens of the United States, and the wrongs they may commit against one another, but not generally against the local, state, or federal government and their respective laws and regulations. Civil law in the US is derived from the precepts of Common Law used in England, and brought here by the settlers. This law covers issues such as wrongs against one another and contracts. A wrong against another is called a tort. Examples of torts include slander, libel, and medical negligence. Another type of law used commonly in civil law is case law and the theory of precedence.

Law of Agency and Contracts

The law of agency is based on the Latin term *Respondeat superior,* which translates to "Let the Master Answer." This law is a general principle that applies to the employee, and employer relationship. The employee is in effect an "agent" for his or her employer, and may enter into contracts on the employer's behalf. This is important in healthcare, because in the medical office, the nurse may act as an agent for the physician, and in the pharmacy, the technician may act as an agent for the pharmacist. This means not only that a contract may be made, but that it is just as valid as if the physician or the pharmacist made the contract. An example of how the contract is made in the pharmacy is as simple as the technician receiving a prescription from the patient at the window and agreeing to get the prescription filled. By doing this, an implied contract now exists, and the pharmacy and pharmacist are obligated to provide the patient with a service. If a mistake is made, the pharmacy and/or pharmacist may be held liable, even though he or she was not the one who entered into the contract to provide service. The pharmacist must therefore "answer" for all of the acts of his or her employees.

Torts

Tort is the term which refers to personal injuries. These are wrongs that one citizen commits against another. In the case of a tort, the injured party sues the party that caused the injury *(Tom Jones vs. Dave's Drugstore, and Dave the Rph)*. The local, state, and federal government do not take part in a lawsuit such as this, as the crime was between two citizens and not against the government and/or its laws and regulations. The simplest is the "broken" contract. Other examples include slander (using spoken words to speak falsely of another), libel (using written words falsely represent another), assault (threatening another with bodily harm), and battery (causing bodily harm to another). Invasion of privacy may be another tort that results in a lawsuit. Medical records, including those in the pharmacy, are considered the physical property of the facility that generates them; however the intellectual property contained in the medical record is the property of the patient. This information may not be divulged to another without consent of the patient, or by subpoena (a legal order). The most common tort in the medical arena is negligence (not providing the minimum standard of care).

Standard of care is the term applied to the level of care expected to be provided by various healthcare providers. Standard of care, when used to judge the type of care provided to a patient, is based on comparisons to other healthcare professionals and what they might have done in the same situation; written guidelines and protocols; and expert testimony. When considering standard of care, two criteria are always taken into account: (1) the level of training the healthcare provider has and (2) the normal practices and protocol for the geographical area in which the healthcare provider works. Only those healthcare providers who work in the same geographical area, and have the same level of training would be compared. For example, a pharmacist in Denver would not be compared with a pharmacist in Boston because practices and protocols may differ by geographical area. Also, a pharmacy technician and a pharmacist would not be held to the same standard because they have a different level of training. A pharmacy technician is not expected to provide the same service or standard of care to a patient as the pharmacist. Similarly, a cardiologist would be expected to provide a different service or standard of care than that of a nurse practitioner at his office.

Malpractice is a form of negligence in which the standard of care was not met. When a case of negligence or malpractice is brought, the burden of proof is on the plaintiff to prove what is known as the "4 D's of Negligence." They are duty, dereliction, damages, and direct cause. The plaintiff must first prove the defendant had a duty to provide care or as there was a contract for care between the two parties. The plaintiff must then prove that the defendant was derelict in his duty, and that this dereliction caused actual damages to the plaintiff, and that the damages were a direct cause of the defendant's derelict. The burden of proof in civil court is lower than in a criminal case. The plaintiff must prove his case by a "preponderance of the evidence," which means that it is more likely than not that the defendant is guilty of the accused act. If the defendant is found guilty, he may be ordered to pay an award of money to the plaintiff. It is not possible for him to be given jail time, as the crime was not against the state but against another citizen.

There are several levels of negligence or malpractice that may be determined during an investigation and subsequent trial. If two or more causes are a factor in the negligence and personal injury to the patient, a case of contributory negligence may be determined. If for example the physician and pharmacist were both responsible for the injury to a patient, each may be found guilty. The award to the plaintiff may then be broken down according to the judge or jury's assessment of the comparative negligence. If the physician was more responsible than the pharmacist, the award may be broken down by a percentage, where the physician must pay 70% of the damages award and the pharmacist must pay 30% of the damages award. There are even cases where the patient himself is found to have contributed to his own injury (for example by not taking medication as directed) and found to be comparatively negligent. In this case, his total award may be reduced by a certain percentage depending on the judge or jury's determination.

There are cases in the news occasionally where a crime is committed in violation of a state or federal law, and the party is prosecuted; and then the victim or his family sue the party in civil court for monetary damages as well. In that case the person may be tried two times, facing two separate plaintiffs. In the criminal case, the defendant may face monetary fines, probation, or prison. The civil case might result in monetary awards to the defendant.

CODES OF ETHICS

Web Link

Visit the AAPT at www.pharmacytechnician.com

Ethics, as a philosophical discipline, is the study of right action or of the nature of good and evil. Both pharmacists and technicians are expected to hold themselves to high ethical standards that both reinforce and go further than specific laws and standards of practice. Tables 2.6 and 2.7 present codes of ethics promulgated by the APhA and the American Association of Pharmacy Technicians (AAPT).

Table 2.6	Code of Ethics for Pharmacists

Preamble

Pharmacists are health professionals who assist individuals in making the best use of medications. This Code, prepared and supported by pharmacists, is intended to state publicly the principles that form the fundamental basis of the roles and responsibilities of pharmacists. These principles, based on moral obligations and virtues, are established to guide pharmacists in relationships with patients, health professionals, and society.

Principles

I. A pharmacist respects the covenantal relationship between the patient and pharmacist.
Considering the patient-pharmacist relationship as a covenant means that a pharmacist has moral obligations in response to the gift of trust received from society. In return for this gift, a pharmacist promises to help individuals achieve optimum benefit from their medications, to be committed to their welfare, and to maintain their trust.

II. A pharmacist promotes the good of every patient in a caring, compassionate, and confidential manner.
A pharmacist places concern for the well-being of the patient at the center of professional practice. In doing so, a pharmacist considers needs stated by the patient as well as those defined by health science. A pharmacist is dedicated to protecting the dignity of the patient. With a caring attitude and a compassionate spirit, a pharmacist focuses on serving the patient in a private and confidential manner.

III. A pharmacist respects the autonomy and dignity of each patient.
A pharmacist promotes the right of self-determination and recognizes individual self-worth by encouraging patients to participate in decisions about their health. A pharmacist communicates with patients in terms that are understandable. In all cases, a pharmacist respects personal and cultural differences among patients.

IV. A pharmacist acts with honesty and integrity in professional relationships.
A pharmacist has a duty to tell the truth and to act with conviction of conscience. A pharmacist avoids discriminatory practices, behavior or work conditions that impair professional judgment, and actions that compromise dedication to the best interests of patients.

V. A pharmacist maintains professional competence.
A pharmacist has a duty to maintain knowledge and abilities as new medications, devices, and technologies become available and as health information advances.

(continues)

Table 2.6	Code of Ethics for Pharmacists—continued

VI. A pharmacist respects the values and abilities of colleagues and other health professionals.
When appropriate, a pharmacist asks for the consultation of colleagues or other health professionals or refers the patient. A pharmacist acknowledges that colleagues and other health professionals may differ in the beliefs and values they apply to the care of the patient.

VII. A pharmacist serves individual, community, and societal needs.
The primary obligation of a pharmacist is to individual patients. However, the obligations of a pharmacist may at times extend beyond the individual to the community and society. In these situations, the pharmacist recognizes the responsibilities that accompany these obligations and acts accordingly.

VIII. A pharmacist seeks justice in the distribution of health resources.
When health resources are allocated, a pharmacist is fair and equitable, balancing the needs of patients and society.

Source: Copyright by the APhA and adopted October 27, 1994. Reprinted with permission.

Table 2.7	Code of Ethics for Pharmacy Technicians

Preamble
Pharmacy technicians are healthcare professionals who assist pharmacists in providing the best possible care for patients. The principles of this code, which apply to pharmacy technicians working in all settings, are based on the application and support of the moral obligations that guide all in the pharmacy profession in relationships with patients, healthcare professionals, and society.

Principles

1. A pharmacy technician's first consideration is to ensure the health and safety of the patient and to use knowledge and skills most capably in serving others.

2. A pharmacy technician supports and promotes honesty and integrity in the profession, which includes a duty to observe the law, maintain the highest moral and ethical conduct at all times, and uphold the ethical principles of the profession.

3. A pharmacy technician assists and supports the pharmacist in the safe, efficacious, and cost-effective distribution of health services and healthcare resources.

4. A pharmacy technician respects and values the abilities of pharmacists, colleagues, and other healthcare professionals.

5. A pharmacy technician maintains competency in practice, and continually enhances professional knowledge and expertise.

6. A pharmacy technician respects and supports the patient's individuality, dignity, and confidentiality.

7. A pharmacy technician respects the confidentiality of a patient's records and discloses pertinent information only with proper authorization.

8. A pharmacy technician never assists in the dispensing, promoting, or distributing of medications or medical devices that are not of good quality or do not meet the standards required by law.

9. A pharmacy technician does not engage in any activity that will discredit the profession, and will expose, without fear or favor, illegal or unethical conduct in the profession.

10. A pharmacy technician associates and engages in the support of organizations that promote the profession of pharmacy through the use and enhancement of pharmacy technicians.

Source: Copyright by the American Association of Pharmacy Technicians. Reprinted with permission.

Chapter Summary

In the modern era, it is generally recognized that governments and professional organizations have a right to exercise control over the manufacture, dispensing, and use of drugs in order to prevent harm to others due to the misuse or abuse of these potent substances. Controls over the use of drugs are embodied in laws, practice standards, drug standards, and ethical standards. All three kinds of law—common law, statutory law, and regulatory or administrative law—have important consequences for the pharmacy profession. In the area of common law, pharmacy is particularly affected by the potential for tort actions due to negligence or other forms of malpractice. In the area of statutory law, major acts passed by the United States Congress with effects on the pharmacy profession include The Food, Drug, and Cosmetic Act (FDCA), the enabling legislation for the major regulatory organization, the Food and Drug Administration; amendments to the FDCA, including the Durham-Humphrey Amendment and the Kefauver-Harris Amendment; the Comprehensive Drug Abuse Prevention Control Act, which established schedules for controlled substances; the Drug Listing Act; the Orphan Drug Act; the Drug Price Competition and Patent-Term Restoration Act; and the Prescription Drug Marketing Act.

In the area of regulatory law, important regulating agencies include the Food and Drug Administration, which approves or denies New Drug Applications and writes and enforces drug-related regulations, and state boards of pharmacy, which license pharmacies, pharmacists, and (sometimes) technicians; promulgate state regulations; and have the power to take administrative actions against people or organizations that violate laws, regulations, and standards. Standards for drugs are set by official compendia, the *United States Pharmacopeia* and the *National Formulary.* Standards for the practice of pharmacy are set by state boards of pharmacy and by various professional organizations. Several professional organizations, including the American Pharmaceutical Association and the American Association of Pharmacy Technicians, also have codes of ethics by which their members are expected to abide. The legal status of pharmacy technicians and their allowable duties vary from state to state, but in all cases, technicians must act under the direct supervision of licensed pharmacists.

Chapter Review

Knowledge Inventory

Select the best answer for the following.

1. The Food, Drug, and Cosmetic Act of 1938 caused the creation of what agency?
    a. DEA
    b. FDA
    c. NABP
    d. State Boards of Pharmacy
    e. Joint Commission on the Accreditation of Healthcare

2. The Kefaver-Harris Amendment required that all new drugs be proved _____ before being marketed.
    a. safe
    b. affordable
    c. effective
    d. both a and b
    e. both a and c

3. A National Drug Code (NDC) indicates
    a. the recall status of a drug.
    b. the effectiveness of a drug.
    c. the drug, packaging, and manufacturer of a drug.
    d. the safety margin the drug had during testing.
    e. the cost of a drug.

4. The OBRA of 1990 legislation requires the pharmacist to
    a. offer patients counseling regarding medications.
    b. fill prescriptions according to FDA guidelines.
    c. report prescription drug errors to the FDA.
    d. provide the DEA with information regarding narcotics.
    e. keep up to date inventory records.

5. What agency is responsible for approving new medications?
    a. Drug Enforcement Agency
    b. Food and Drug Administration
    c. Medicare
    d. Medicaid
    e. State Boards of Pharmacy

6. The Dietary Supplement and Health Education Act took away the FDA's authority to regulate
    a. narcotic prescribing habits of physicians.
    b. manufacturer's advertising claims.
    c. Medicaid payment for prescriptions.
    d. herbal, vitamin, and nutritional products.
    e. the amount of information the pharmacist gives the patient.

7. Which of the following organizations has no legal authority over pharmacy?
   a. Drug Enforcement Agency
   b. Food and Drug Administration
   c. National Association of Boards of Pharmacy
   d. State Boards of Pharmacy
   e. United States Congress

8. Only the _____ has the authority to remove a medical license or registration.
   a. State Boards of Pharmacy
   b. Food and Drug Administration
   c. federal court judge
   d. state court judge
   e. Drug Enforcement Agency

9. If a patient sues a pharmacy, who has the burden of proof in the case?
   a. the pharmacy
   b. the pharmacist and technician who filled the prescription
   c. the patient
   d. the state or local prosecutor
   e. the judge overseeing the case

10. A pharmacist may be sued for _____ if he or she speaks falsely of a physician to a patient.
    a. libel
    b. slander
    c. battery
    d. negligence
    e. malpractice

Pharmacy in Practice

1. A pharmacy technician accidentally chooses the antidepressant drug Prozac instead of the prescribed medication, the antisecretory medication Prilosec, used for treatment of heartburn and gastroesophageal reflux disease. The pharmacist fails to check the medication, and the customer experiences no relief of the heartburn and a rare adverse reaction to the Prozac, rendering him temporarily impotent, a condition that causes the patient great psychological distress. The patient decides to sue the pharmacist and the pharmacy technician for negligence. To establish a *prima facie* case, what four claims must the patient prove and to what degree must he prove these? Given the facts as stated, what arguments and/or evidence can the patient put forward to support each of these four claims?

2. In the case of *Baker vs. Arbor Drugs, Inc.*, which went to trial in 1966, the plaintiff, Baker, was taking the antidepressant drug tranylcypromine, under a prescription that he regularly filled at Arbor Drugs. The patient went to a physician with a cold, and the physician, despite having records indicating that the patient was taking tranylcypromine, prescribed phenylpropanolamine. When Baker came to Arbor Drugs to have his prescription filled, a pharmacy technician was warned by the pharmacy's computer that a potential interaction existed between the new prescription and Baker's prescription for tranylcypromine that had been filled a few days earlier. The technician overrode the computer warning, and the pharmacist filled the prescription, unaware of the potential drug interaction. As a result of taking the phenylpropanolamine, Baker suffered a stroke. Baker brought suit, and on appeal, received a judgment against the pharmacy. Discuss this case with other students. Consider the following questions, given the facts as stated:

   a. Were both the pharmacist and the pharmacy technician guilty of negligence? Consider all four criteria for negligence.

   b. In what ways did the physician, the pharmacy technician, and the pharmacist fail to carry out their duties properly?

   c. What requirement, under OBRA-90, did the pharmacist fail to meet? What relevance does this case have to the expanded clinical role of the pharmacist?

   d. Under what legal principle might Baker sue the pharmacy for the actions of its employees, the pharmacist, and the technician?

   e. Under what legal principle could Baker not sue the manufacturer of the phenylpropanolamine product, given that the physician and the pharmacy had been warned of the dangerous drug interaction?

   f. What role do computers play, in contemporary pharmacy, in helping pharmacists and technicians to meet the counseling requirements of OBRA-90?

   g. Is this a case in which a court could conceivably make a finding of contributory negligence or comparative negligence? Explain.

   h. In what respect was the pharmacist guilty of nonfeasance? In what respect was the pharmacy technician guilty of malfeasance?

3. In the course of his normal duties, a pharmacy technician employed by Hometown Drugs, Inc., discovers from a patient profile that the young man who is dating his daughter is taking a regular prescription for a powerful antipsychotic drug. The technician knows that his daughter and the young man are contemplating getting married. The technician tells his wife about this discovery, who then tells the daughter, who was unaware of her boyfriend's prescription for the drug. Has the pharmacy technician committed a breach of his ethical responsibilities? Explain in writing why you think this is or is not so.

4. In the course of her normal duties, a pharmacy technician employed by Hometown Drugs, Inc., discovers from a patient profile that the young man who is dating her daughter is taking a regular prescription for a powerful antipsychotic drug. The technician keeps this information to herself but, in response to the information, attempts to dissuade her daughter from marrying the young man. Has the technician committed a breach of her ethical responsibilities? Explain in writing why you think this is or is not so.

5. A pharmacist runs a community pharmacy in an area with a 30 percent Spanish-speaking population but does not himself speak Spanish nor employ anyone who speaks Spanish. Might this situation be a breach of the law? Of professional ethics as defined by the Code of Ethics for Pharmacists of the American Pharmaceutical Association?

6. Pharmacists with alcohol or substance abuse problems sometimes fail to seek help for fear that a state board of pharmacy might take some disciplinary action should the problem become known. What might professional associations and state boards do, in your opinion, to combat this problem?

7. Amendments or new legislation are often passed in response to deficiencies in previous legislation. Give three examples from the text.

Improving Communication Skills

1. A pharmacy technician discovers that her employer regularly has been dispensing large amounts of a Schedule II amphetamine to an obviously overweight individual. The prescription is allegedly for control of a rare hyperactivity disorder. However, the technician knows that both the prescribing doctor and her employer's business partner have a financial interest in a local weight loss clinic. The technician asks her employer about this and is told to mind her own business and get back to work.
   a. What legal and ethical obligations do you think that this situation might place on the technician?
   b. What is the technician's responsibility under the Code of Ethics of the American Association of Pharmacy Technicians?
   c. What risk does the technician run if she reports this matter to the state board of pharmacy? How is such a report made?
   d. What would you do in this situation? Write out what you might say to your employer if you were put in this situation.

2. A pharmacy technician is assisting a patient at the pick-up window when she notices that the patient's 17 year old daughter also has a prescription for birth control pills waiting to be picked up. The mother sees her daughter's name on the receipt and wants to know what her daughter is taking.
   a. What are the legal and ethical concerns for the pharmacy?
   b. Write out what you might say to the mother.

Internet Research

1. Visit www.fda.gov/medwatch/index.html. Prepare a summary of what is new in the last two weeks. How is a Med Watch report made? What information is contained in a MedWatch report?

2. Visit www.fda.gov. Find the phone number to report problems in your state. Research recent drug approvals. What are they and for what disease conditions are they generally prescribed?

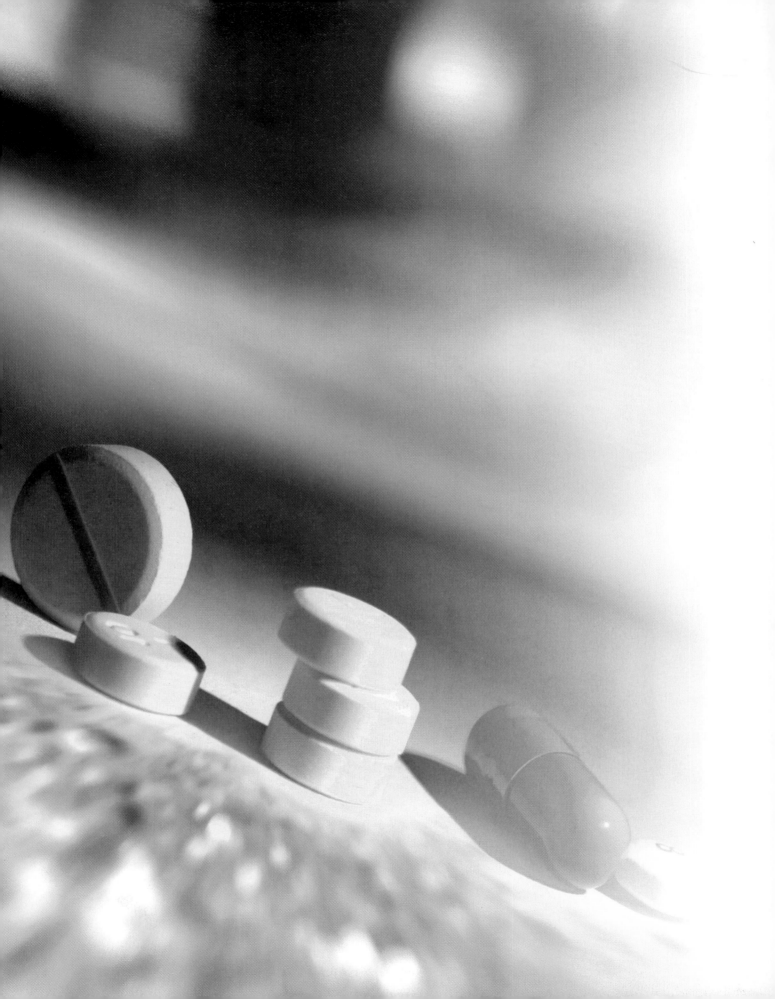

Pharmaceutical Terminology and Abbreviations

Learning Objectives

◇ Identify common Greek and Latin word parts used in medicine and pharmacy.

◇ Define key terms used to describe drugs and their uses, including diagnosis, disease, trauma, disorder, acute, chronic, symptom, syndrome, mitigation, treatment, cure, prevention, generic name, and brand name.

◇ List some common sound-alike and look-alike names of drugs.

◇ List and describe a number of subfields within the field of pharmacy, including clinical pharmacy, pharmacology, clinical pharmacology, pharmacodynamics, pharmacokinetics, nuclear pharmacy, pharmacoeconomics, pharmacogenetics, and pharmacognosy.

◇ Interpret abbreviations and symbols used in prescriptions and medication orders.

◇ Identify common abbreviations and symbols used to describe weights and measures.

Like any profession, pharmacy has its own special language, or jargon. A pharmacy worker needs to be familiar with the wider jargon of health-related occupations in general and with the special abbreviations and symbols used to describe drugs, dosage forms, amounts, administration times, and other essential information on prescriptions and medication orders. Knowledge of these symbols and abbreviations, along with attention to sound-alike and look-alike drug names, can help ensure that medication errors do not occur.

GREEK AND LATIN WORD PARTS

Not so long ago, a dedicated student could go a long way toward mastering the available book-learning (if not the practical knowledge) of his or her culture. Today, all that has changed. Modern education and modern information technologies have created an explosion of knowledge. One consequence of the knowledge explosion is specialization. In the seventeenth century, a single person could comprehend the whole of biological science. In the nineteenth century, that person's descendant could absorb the whole of, say, entomology, the study of insects. Today, as Harvard entomologist E. O. Wilson points out, several lifetimes is not enough time in which to learn all that is known about the behaviors of bees, wasps, termites, and other members of the single order of creatures known as Hymenoptera, which contains over a million known species.

To communicate precisely with other people involved in a particular field of endeavor, people find it necessary to invent new terminology, words, and phrases to describe the particular elements of their field. To communicate quickly as well as precisely, they create abbreviations and special symbols. Sometimes, the specialized words, phrases, abbreviations, and symbols used in a scientific field such as pharmacy or medicine can be intimidating. The name of a lung disease suffered by coal miners, for example, is

pneumonoultramicroscopicsilicovolcanokoniosis

and this is not even the longest of all technical words in chemistry, biology, and medicine! Do not let the foreign-sounding nature of scientific words intimidate you, however. With a little study and practice in the field of pharmacy, you will soon master most of the specialized terms and abbreviations that you need to know. Most are far shorter and far clearer than the word given above.

At the beginning of the scientific revolution, in the Renaissance, most scholars in Western Europe were deeply learned in the Greek and Latin classics, and so it is not surprising that, when inventing new terms to describe their discoveries and observations, they borrowed bits and pieces of these ancient languages. Such coinage, based on Greek and Latin word parts, remains at the heart of scientific naming. Therefore, when you encounter in your practice as a pharmacy technician the names of procedures, parts of the body, drugs, chemicals, and so on, they will often look like this:

Web Link

Visit Medline for a list of online medical dictionaries at www.nlm.nih.gov/medlineplus/dictionaries.html

analgesic from Greek *an,* "without," and *algos,* "pain" (def: pertaining to without pain)

sublingual from Latin *sub,* "under, below," and *lingua,* "language, tongue" (def: under the tongue)

cardiologist from Greek *kardia,* "heart,"-*logia* "the study of," and *ist,* "specialist" (def: person who specializes in the study of the heart)

Some common Greek and Latin word parts encountered in medical and pharmaceutical terminology are listed in the following tables. A root is a word part that forms a major internal constituent of a word. When a word root is combined with a vowel, it is referred to as a combining form. Roots are often combined with other roots and suffixes with the vowel *o.* Common roots and combining forms are listed in Table 3.1. A prefix is a word part added to the beginning of a word, and common examples are listed in Table 3.2. A suffix is a word part added to the end of a word, and common examples are listed in Table 3.3.

You may wish to commit these to memory over a period of many weeks, learning a few at a time. Knowing these word parts will be of considerable value in furthering your education about the effects, toxicity, and interactions of drugs. One effective method of learning medical terminology is to make flash cards using plain index cards and test yourself often over several months. It is most effective to use the flash cards two or three times daily for fifteen to thirty minutes, and sort them regularly into a stack that you know well, and the stack you need more time with. It may help to write several words that contain the word part on the card so that you may associate the word part with its meaning in context. Learn how to use your medical dictionary, and keep it nearby as you are studying medical terms and using drug resources that may utilize unfamiliar terms.

Table 3.1 Common Roots and Combining Forms

Word Part	Meaning	Example
acet/o	vinegar, acid, sharp	acetaldehyde
acr/o	tip, end, sharpness	acromegaly
aden/o	gland	adenoid, adenovirus
adip/o	fat	adipose, adipoma
aer/o	air	aerogel, aerosol
agon/o	contest, struggle	agonist, agony
alb/o	white	albumin, albino
alg/o	pain	analgesia, myalgia
allel/o	one another, mutual	allergen, allergic
amb/i, amph/o	both, two	amphoteric, ampicillin
ambul/o	walk	ambulatory
amni/o	membrane around the fetus	amniotic fluid, amniocentesis
amyl/o	starch	amylase, amylolysis
andr/o	male	androgen
angi/o	vessel	angiogram, angioplasty
anthrac	black	anthrax, anthracosis
aqu, aqua, aque	water	aqueous
arter/o	artery (as opposed to vein)	arterial, arteriosclerosis
arthr/o	joint	arthritis, arthralgia
asthm	shortness of breath	antiasthmatic
atri	entry	atrium
aud, audit/o	hear	auditory, audiometry
aur/o	hear	aural, Auralgan
axill/o	armpit	axillary temperature
bi/o	life	biopsy, biology
blast	sprout, immature cell	erythroblastosis, osteoblast
blephar/o	eyelid	blepharoptosis
bol	throw, create	bolus, metabolism, emboli
brachi	arm	brachial artery
bronch/o	bronchus (pathway from windpipe)	bronchoscope, bronchitis
bucc/o	inside of cheek	buccal membrane
burs/o	pouchlike cavity	bursa, bursitis
calc/o	calcium	hypocalcemia
cap/o, capi,	head, expansion	capillary, capitation
carb/o	carbon	carbohydrate
carcin/o	crab, cancer	carcinogen, carcinoma
cardi/o	heart	cardiology, electrocardiogram
carp/o	wrist	carpal tunnel syndrome
caus	burn	causalgia, caustic
centr/o	center	centrifuge
cephal/o	head, expansion	hydrocephalic
cerebr/o	brain	cerebrovascular accident
cervic/o	neck, cervix	cervicofacial, cervical
chem/o	chemistry	chemotherapy
chir/o	hand	chiropractic
chol/o	bile, cholesterol	cholangiogram, hypercholesterolemia
chondr/o	cartilage; grain	achondroplasia, chondroitin
chron/o	time, long	chronic, chronological
cili	eyelash, hair	cilia, penicillin
coagul/o	clot	anticoagulant

(continues)

Table 3.1   Common Roots and Combining Forms—continued

Word Part	Meaning	Example
collo	glue	colloidal oatmeal
coni/o	dust	pneumoconiosis
core/o	pupil of eye	coreoplasty, coreoplegia
corp/o	body	corpuscle, corpse
crani/o	cranium, skull	craniotomy
cutane/o, cuti	skin	subcutaneous, cuticle
cyan/o	blue	cyanosis, acrocyanosis
cycl/o	circle, wheel	tetracycline, tricyclic antidepressant
cyst/o	bladder, cyst	cystic fibrosis, cystitis
cyt/o	cell	cytologist
dacr/o	tear (crying)	dacryoadenitis
dactyl/o	finger	syndactylism, adactyly
demos	people	pandemic, epidemic
dent/o	tooth	dentifrice, dentalgia
derm, dermat/o	skin	epidermis, dermabrasion, dermatitis
edem, edema	excess fluid in tissues	angioedema, edematous
encephal/o	brain	electroencephalogram, encephalitis
enter/o	intestine (usually small intestines)	parenteral, enteric
erythr/o	red	erythromycin, erythrocyte
esth, esthesi/o	perception	anesthesia, paresthesia
flat	blow	antiflatulent
galact/o, lact/o	milk	galactosemia, lactorrhea
gangl	knot	ganglion
gastr/o	stomach	gastritis
gen	become, beget, produce	antigen, genetic
genesis	origin	pathogenesis, agenesis
ger/o	aged	gerontology, geriatric
gest	produce	gestation
glob	sphere, ball, round body	globule, hemoglobin
gloss/o	tongue	glossectomy, subglossal
gluc/o	sugar	glucose, Glucophage
glyc/o	sugar	hyperglycemia
gnos/o	state of	prognosis, diagnosis
gonad/o	reproductive organ	gonadotropin
gynec/o	female	gynecologist
hem/o	blood	hemostat, hemorrhage
hepat/o	liver	hepatitis, hepatotoxic
hidr/o	sweat	hidradenoma, hidrosis
hydr/o	water	hydrocephalus, hydrophobic
hypn/o	sleep	hypnotic
hyster/o, metr/o	uterus	hysterectomy, endometrium
ichthy/o	fishy, scaly	ichthyosis
immun/o	safe, safe from	immunologist, immune
kera, kerat/o	horned, horny skin cells, cornea	keratolytic, keratin, keratoplasty
kinesi/o	motion	kinesiology, akinetic
labi/o	lip	labia, labial
lachri	tear (from the eye)	lacrimal fluid
leuk/o	white	leukemia, leukorrhea
lingu/o	tongue	sublingual
lith/o	stone	nephrolithiasis
lumb/o	lower back, loin	lumbar, lumbodynia
lymph/o	water, lymph	lymphatic system, lymphoma

Table 3.1 **Common Roots and Combining Forms—continued**

Word Part	Meaning	Example
mast/o	breast	mastectomy, mastitis
melan/o	black	melanoma
mening/o	membrane surrounding brain and spinal cord	meningitis, meningocele
mens	moon, month	menses, menstruation
mnem/o	memory	mnemonic
morb/o	sick	morbidity
morph/o	shape, dream	morphology, morphine
muscul/o	mouse, muscle	intramuscular, neuromuscular
myc/o	fungus	onychomycosis
myel/o	bone marrow, spinal cord	myeloid leukemia, myelogram
my/o	muscle	myocardial infarction, myalgia
myx/o, muco	slime	mucous membrane, myxedemic coma
narc/o	sleep	narcotic, narcolepsy
nas/o	nose	nasopharyngitis, nasal spray
nat/i	birth	prenatal
necr/o	dead	necrosis
nephr/o	kidney	nephritis, nephrologist
neur/o	nerve	neurotransmitter
ocul/o	eye	ocular, oculonasal
odont/o	tooth	orthodontics, odontalgia
onc/o	tumor, mass	oncology
onych/o	fingernail, toenail	onychomalacia
ophthalm/o	eye	ophthalmic, ophthalmologist
opi/o	opium	opiate
optic	eye	optician
orchi, orchid/o	testes	orchiditis, orchiectomy
or/o	mouth	oral
orth/o	straight	orthodontia, orthopedics
osm/o,	smell	anosmia
oste/o	bone	osteoporosis, osteopath
ot/o	ear	otic, otoscope
ox/o, oxy	oxygen	hypoxemia, anoxia
ped	child	pediatric
part	parturition, give birth	postpartum
path/o	disease, misery	pathology, nephropathy
pect/o	chest	expectorant, angina pectoris
pod, ped	foot	podiatrist, pedometer
pelvi	pelvis	pelvimetry
phag/o	eat	bacteriophage, dysphagia
pharmac/o	sorcery, poison, drug	pharmacy, pharmacokinetics
phasia	speech	aphasia
phil/o	like, love	hydrophilic, eosinophil
phleb	vein	phlebitis, phlebotomy
phon/o	voice	dysphonia, telephone
phori	carry, bear	diaphoresis
phos, phot/o	light	photosensitivity, phosphorescent
physi	nature, grow	physiological, physical therapy, epiphyseal plate
plasm, plas/o	molded, formation	neoplasm, aplastic anemia

(continues)

Table 3.1   **Common Roots and Combining Forms—continued**

Word Part	Meaning	Example
plegi	stroke, paralysis	paraplegic, ophthalmoplegic
pleur/o	lining surrounding lungs	pleurisy, pleural effusion
pneum/o, pneumat/o	breath,air	pneumonia, pneumatic
prandial	meal	postprandial
proct/o	rectum	proctologist, Procto-Foam
psych/o	spirit, mind	antipsychotic, psychotropic
pty, ptyal/o	spit	hemoptysis
pulm/o, pulmon/o	lung	pulmonary, Pulmicort
pyr, pyr/o	fever, fire	pyrogen, antipyretic
radi/o	radiation, x-ray	radiogram
ren/o	kidney	renal, adrenal gland
retin/o	retina	retinopathy
rhin/o	nose	rhinovirus, rhinitis
sarc/o	flesh	sarcoma
scler/o	hard	atherosclerosis, sclerosing agent
seb/o	fat, oil	sebum, seborrheic dermatitis
sect/o, seg	cut	section, segment, dissect
seps, sept	rot, infection	antiseptic, aseptic technique
sial	saliva	sialolith
soma,	body	psychosomatic, somatropin
spasm/o	drawing tight	antispasmodic
spondyl/o	spine	spondylitis, spondylodesis
sphygm/o	heartbeat, pulse	sphygmomanometer (BP cuff)
spir/o	breathing	spirometer, inspiration
staphyl/o	cluster of grapes	staphylococcus
stern/o	breastbone	sternum
stom/o, stomy	mouth, surgical opening	stomatitis, colostomy
strept/o	wavy, twisted chain	streptomycin, streptococcus
ten/o, tend/o	stretch	tendonitis, tenosynovitis
thorac/o	chest	pneumothorax, thoracic
thromb/o	blood clot	thrombolysis, thrombosis
thyr/o	thyroid	hypothyroidism, thyroiditis
tom, tome	cut, instrument to cut	lobotomy, craniotome
tox, toxo	poisonous	toxic, toxicology
troph, trop/o	growing, nourish, develop	atrophy, somatotropin
tympan/o	eardrum	tympanocentesis
ur/o	urine	urology
uter/o	uterus, womb	intrauterine
vas/o	blood vessel	vasodilation
ven/o, phleb/o	vein (as opposed to artery)	venule, phlebotomy
vert	turn	vertigo, divert
viscer/o	internal organs	viscera, visceromegaly
xer/o	dry	xeroderma, xerostomia

Table 3.2   **Common Prefixes**

Word Part	Meaning	Example
acu-	sharp, abrupt, sudden	acupuncture, acute
a-, ad-	towards	adsorbent, adsternal

Table 3.2   Common Prefixes—continued

Word Part	Meaning	Example
a-, an-	without	anesthesia, apathy, anemia
ab-	from, away from	abaxial, abnormal, abscess
allo-	other, another	allopathy, AlloDerm
ana-	up to, back, again, apart	anaplastic, anabolic
ante-	before, forwards	antecubital, ante-cibum
anti-	against, opposite	antitoxin, antiseptic, antidepressant
auto-	self	autoimmune
bi-	twice, double	biceps, bisulfite
brady-	slow	bradycardia, bradytaxia
cata-	down	catabolism
circum-	around	circumoral, circumcision
con-	together	congestion, concurrent
contra-	against	contraindication
cuti-	skin	cuticle
de-	from, away from, down from	decongestant
deci-	ten	decimal
di-, dis-	two	distillation, dissect
dia-	through, complete	dialysis, diarrhea
dipl-, diplo-	double	diplococci, diplopia
dis-	separation	distended
dur-	hard, firm	durable
dys-	bad, abnormal	dystrophy, dyspepsia
e-, ec-, ecto-	out, from out of	ectopic
en-, endo-	into	endoarteritis, endometriosis
epi-	on, up, against, high	epidermis, epidural
eu-	well, normal, abundant	eupnea, euphoria
ex-, exo-	out, from out of	exotropia, excision
extra-	outside, beyond, in addition	extraoral, extrahepatic
hemi-	half	hemiplegia
hetero-	different	heterophilic
homo-	same	homeopathy, homogenous
hyper-	above, excessive	hyperalimentation, hypertension
hypo-	below, deficient	hypodermic, hypovolemic
im-, in-	not	impotence, inaccurate
in-	into	invasive
infra-	below, underneath	infracardiac
inter-	among, between	intercostal
intra-	within, inside, during	intravenous, intrauterine
iso-	equal, same	isomorphic, isotonic
macro-	large	macrocytic, macrophage
mal-	bad	malnutrition, malaise
mega-	large	megavitamin
megalo-	large	megalomania
meta-	change, between	metastasize, metacarpal
micro-	small	micron, microscope
mono	one	mononucleosis, monocyte
neo-	new	antineoplastic, neonate
non-	not	nontoxic, nonsteroidal
pan-	all, across, throughout	pandemic, panacea
para-	beside, to the side of, wrong	paranasal, parasympathetic

(continues)

Table 3.2   Common Prefixes—continued

Word Part	Meaning	Example
per-	by, through, throughout	percutaneous
peri-	around	pericardium
poly-	many	polymorphonuclear, polypharmacy
post-	behind, after	postpartum, postoperative
pre-	before, in front	prenatal, premature infant
primi-	first	primigravida
pro-	before, in front	proptosis
pros-	besides, in addition	prosthesis
pseudo-	false	pseudoplegia
quadri-	four	quadriplegia
re-, red-	back, again	reconstitute, reduce
retro-	backwards, behind	retrovirus, retrocardiac
semi-	half	semiconscious
sub-	under, beneath	subcutaneous
super-	above, in addition, over, excessive	supersensitive
supra-	above, on upper side, excessive	suprarenal
syn-	together, with	syndrome
tachy-	rapid	tachypnea
tetra-	four	tetracycline
trans-	across, beyond, through	transocular, transfusion
tri-	three	triceps, tricyclic
uni-	one	unicellular
ultra-	beyond, excess, more	ultrasound, ultrasensitive

Table 3.3   Common Suffixes

Word Part	Meaning	Example
-ac	pertaining to	cardiac
-al	pertaining to	myocardial
-algia, -algesia	pain	cephalgia, neuralgia, analgesia
-ar	pertaining to	lumbar
-ase	enzyme (makes a noun)	amylase
-ate	(makes a verb)	expectorate
-cele	herniation, prolapse	rectocele, cystocele
-cide	killer	spermicide
-centesis	surgical puncture to remove fluid	arthrocentesis, amniocentesis
-coccus	berry	staphylococcus
-clasis	break	osteoclasis
-cyte	cell	osteocyte, hepatocyte
-desis	binding, fixation	arthrodesis
-dipsia	thirst	polydipsia
-dynia	pain	lumbodynia, myodynia
-ectomy	removal of, cut out	appendectomy
-emesis	vomiting	hematemesis, antiemetic

Table 3.3	Common Suffixes—continued	
Word Part	**Meaning**	**Example**
-emia	condition of the blood	anemia, drepanocytemia, hypoglycemia
-genic	producing	carcinogenic, iatrogenic
-gram	a record	angiogram, myelogram
-graph	a device which records	electrocardiograph
-graphy	the process of recording	radiography
-iasis	abnormal condition	nephrolithiasis
-iatry	treatment	podiatry, psychiatry
-ism	condition, state	alcoholism
-ist	specialist	podiatrist
-itis	inflammation	colitis, rhinitis
-ium	tissue	pericardium
-ize	(makes a verb)	immunize
-lepsy	seizure	narcolepsy
-logy	study of, reasoning about	etiology, biology
-lysis	to break apart	urinalysis, hemolysis
-malacia	softening	osteomalacia
-meter	to measure	pelvimeter
-oid	resembling	ovoid, adenoid
-ol	alcohol	ethanol
-oma	tumor	melanoma
-opia	vision	myopia
-ose	carbohydrate	glucose
-ose	full of	adipose tissue
-osis	abnormal condition	halitosis, nephrosis
-path, -pathy	disease, suffering	homeopathy, cardiomyopathy
-pepsia	digestion	dyspepsia
-philia	attraction to, liking for	hydrophilia
-plasty	reshaping, repair of	rhinoplasty, tympanoplasty
-rhea	discharge, flow	diarrhea, leukorrhea
-rrha, -rrhag	discharge, flow, burst forth	hemorrhage
-sclerosis	hardening	arteriosclerosis, otosclerosis
-scope	device to view with one's eye	microscope, otoscope
-scopy	the process of viewing with the eye	endoscopy, ophthalmoscope
-sis	process, state of	diagnosis
-stasis	stopping, controlling, stand	hemostasis, metastasis
-stat	stop	bacteriostat, hemostat
-stomy	surgical opening	colostomy
-tomy	cut	nephrotomy
-ule	little, minute	venule
-uria	urinary condition	dysuria

DRUG NOMENCLATURE

Drugs are named according to a protocol developed by scientists that applies to the chemical name and the generic name. The chemical name is dictated by the chemical components in the drug and the generic name is given when a compound is classified into a particular drug class. Drugs can often be identified by class when looking at the generic name. Table 3.4 contains a few of the more common word parts that are used in generic names of drugs.

One of the most serious events that can occur in pharmacy practice is the accidental substitution of one drug or pharmaceutical ingredient for another. At all times, great caution must be taken to make sure that such substitution does not occur. In one infamous case, *Toppi v. Scarf, 1971,* a pharmacist accidentally dispensed Nardil, an antidepressant, instead of Norinyl, a contraceptive. The woman who received the wrong drug gave birth to a child, and the Michigan Court of Appeals held the pharmacist liable not only for the medical expenses incurred in the woman's pregnancy but also for the costs of raising the child. Given the potency and potential toxicity of drugs and the danger of not receiving the drug prescribed for treatment or prevention, one must be extremely careful not to substitute drugs that have similar names. Table 3.5 lists the names of some drugs that are near homonyms (words that sound alike) or homographs (words that are similar in spelling). This is by no means a complete list of names of drugs that sound and/or look alike. The highest degree of caution must be exercised at all times to avoid accidental substitution of one drug or pharmaceutical product for another.

Table 3.4   Drug Nomenclature

Word Part	Drug Class	Example
-azepam	benzodiazepine	diazepam
-azosin	vasodilator	terazosin
barb	barbiturate	phenobarbital
-caine	local anesthetic	lidocaine
cef, cefp, ceph	cephalosporin antibiotic	cefprozil, cephalexin
-cillin	penicillin	amoxicillin
cod	narcotic analgesic	hydrocodone
-conazole	antifungal	miconazole
cort	steroid anti-inflammatory	hydrocortisone
-cycline	tetracycline antibiotic	minocycline
estro	estrogen hormone	estropipate
flox	quinolone antibiotic	ciprofloxacin
-mycin	macrolide antibiotic	azithromycin
nitr	coronary vasodilator	isosorbide dinitrate, nitroglycerin
-olol	beta blocker	atenolol
-olone	steroid anti-inflammatory	triamcinolone
-pril	ACE inhibitor	lisinopril
-profen	steroid anti-inflammatory	ketoprofen
-semide	loop diuretic	furosemide
-statin	cholesterol lowering drug	lovastatin
sulfa	sulfonamide antibacterial	sulfasalazine
-tidine	H_2 blocker	ranitidine
-triptan	migraine drug	zolmitriptan
-triptyline	tricyclic antidepressant	nortriptyline
vir	antiviral	acyclovir
-vudine	antiviral	zidovudine

Table 3.5 Near Homonyms and Homographs among Drug Names

acetazolamide	acetohexamide	diphenhydramine	dimenhydrinate
Adderall	Inderal	enalapril	Anafranil
albuterol	atenolol	Fioricet	Fiorinal
Aldomet	Aldoril	glipizide	glyburide
Allegra	Viagra	hydralazine	hydroxyzine
alprazolam	lorazepam	Inderal	Isordil
amitriptyline	imipramine	Lamictal	Lamisil
amitriptyline	nortriptyline	lamotrigine	lamivudine
azithromycin	erythromycin	Lanoxin	Levoxyl
Apresazide	Apresoline	Lioresal	lisinopril
Catapres	captopril	Lithotabs	Lithobid
Catapres	Combipres	Levoxine	Lanoxin
chlorpromazine	chlorpropamide	Norvasc	Navane
chlorpromazine	promethazine	Orinase	Ornade
clonidine	Klonopin	Pravachol	propranolol
Celebrex	Celexa, Cerebyx	Prevacid	Pravachol,
Celexa	Celebrex, Cerebyx	Prinivil	
Celexa	Zyprexa	Prilosec	Plendil
Cytotec	Cytomel	quinine	quinidine
Cytotec	Cytovene	Sinequan	saquinavir
Darvocet–N	Darvon–N	tolazamide	tolbutamide
desipramine	imipramine	Xanax	Zantac
desipramine	diphenhydramine	Zyprexa	Zyrtec
digitoxin	digoxin	Zyrtec	Xanax, Zantac

IMPORTANT TERMINOLOGY

The *United States Pharmacopeia* defines the term *drug* as "an agent intended for use in the diagnosis, mitigation, treatment, cure, or prevention of disease in man or animals." Let us examine this definition closely.

Diagnosis is the process by which a physician or other healthcare professional determines the nature of a disease condition by examination of a patient's signs and symptoms.

If the definition in the *United States Pharmacopeia* is to cover all legitimate uses of drugs, then the term *disease* in the definition must be taken in its root sense of "not at ease," referring to any adverse condition. Ordinarily, however, people use the term with a more narrow meaning, to refer to any particular destructive physical process in an organ or organism with a specific cause, or causes, and characteristic symptoms. Of course, drugs are used to treat not only disease but also other abnormal or adverse conditions, including fractures, cuts, abrasions, wounds, and other such traumas, as well as various physical and mental disorders, which are congenital (inborn) or acquired abnormalities that are less than optimal, including physical disorders such as scoliosis, or curvature of the spine, and psychological disorders such as depression. Of course, the lines between diseases, traumas, and disorders are rarely clear-cut. A trauma can lead to an infection and thus the beginning of a disease process, a disease can cause a physical or psychological disorder, and a disorder, if it is destructive, may itself be considered a disease. A disease, trauma, or disorder is called acute if it is of short duration or is especially severe, sharp, or immediate in impact. This would be said, for example, of most traumas. A disease, trauma, or disorder is called chronic if it is of extended duration. Chronic asthma, for example, is asthma present over a long period of time.

In all cases, for the disease, trauma, or disorder to become known, it must present symptoms. A symptom is any condition accompanying or resulting from a disease, disorder, or other abnormality that provides evidence for its existence. Sometimes, symptoms are obvious upon examination and can lead to a ready diagnosis, or identification of the disease or disorder. Symptoms are generally referred to as the patient's description of the physical sensation experienced. For example a patient may indicate that he feels nauseous and has abdominal pain. Signs are the outward physical changes that a healthcare provider can see or easily measure. For example, the patient may appear flushed and have a temperature of 101 degrees. At other times, extensive examination using special instruments or testing may be necessary to reveal the telltale signs of a given disease or disorder.

A set of signs and symptoms that occur together and characterize a particular disease or disorder is known as a syndrome. It is usually the identification of a set of related symptoms that leads to a particular diagnosis.

Mitigation is the process of making something less severe or painful. An example of mitigation is the use of the drug morphine to relieve the pain of a cancer patient. Drugs can be used to mitigate symptoms without a particular diagnosis having been determined; however, in most cases, mitigation, treatment, and cure take place as a result of a plan of action based upon a particular diagnosis.

Treatment is the taking of action against a disease or other abnormality. Treatment may include a particular therapy, or extended treatment, such as physical therapy or drug therapy.

A cure is the effective elimination of a disease condition.

Prevention or prophylaxis is taking steps before a disease or other abnormality occurs to keep it from occurring.

Drugs can be used to diagnose, mitigate, treat, cure, or prevent disease. To accomplish these purposes, a great variety of types of drugs, with particular kinds of effects, have been identified or created. Appendix B lists some of the most common categories of drugs, along with examples and specific purposes for which the drugs are used.

As was noted in Chapter 1, the word *pharmacy* derives from the Greek *pharmakon*, meaning "drug." As the term was used in the time of the Greek poet Homer, it meant, alternately, drug, poison, sorcerer's charm, or potion. Today, the same root has given us many terms related to pharmacy practice, as described here.

Also, www.drugtopics.com is an online news magazine for pharmacists. As defined by the American Pharmaceutical Association, the word *pharmacy* means "the health profession that concerns itself with the knowledge system that results in the discovery, development, and use of medications and medication information in the care of patients. It encompasses the clinical, scientific, economic, and educational aspects of the profession's knowledge base and its communication to others in the healthcare system." The word *pharmacy* also applies to the physical place where drugs are stored and dispensed, as a hospital pharmacy or community pharmacy.

Clinical pharmacology is that area of pharmacology that applies knowledge of pharmacological principles related to the effects of drugs on the body to particular drug therapies and to institutional practices and procedures, through counseling of customers, patients, or healthcare providers; through review of prescriptions, patient profiles, and drug therapies; through participation in drug utilization reviews (DURs); through establishment of formularies, or lists of drugs and dosage forms in stock; through monitoring of drug regimens; and through other means related to patient or customer care.

Clinical pharmacy is that area of pharmacy that applies the pharmacist's knowledge and expertise to counseling related to drug therapies and to participating, as part of a total healthcare team, in the provision of clinical services to patients.

Web Link

Visit Pharmacy Times at www.pharmacytimes.com for a list of the top 200 drugs. Also visit www.drugtopics.com, an online news magazine for pharmacists.

Nuclear pharmacy is that branch of the pharmacy profession that deals with the provisions of services related to radiopharmaceuticals. This branch of study often aids in treatment of cancer patients.

A pharmaceutical is any drug manufactured or compounded to be used for the mitigation, treatment, cure, or prevention of a disease or other abnormal condition.

A pharmacist is a licensed professional, skilled in the procurement, compounding, and dispensing of drugs; knowledgeable in a wide range of areas related to drug formulation, dosage forms, use, and effects; skilled in the management of institutional or retail pharmacy operations; and dedicated to providing the service of dispensing drugs, drug information, and drug-related clinical services to customers, patients, and other healthcare professionals. As defined by the American Association of Pharmacy Technicians (AAPT), pharmacy technicians "are healthcare professionals who assist pharmacists in providing the best possible care for patients."

Pharmacodynamics is that branch of pharmacology that deals with the effects and reactions of drugs within the body, including their mechanisms of action. Pharmacoeconomics is the study of the economic aspects of drugs. It includes study of the production, distribution, and consumption of drugs and of related costs and benefits. Aspects of pharmacoeconomics of particular interest include the

- ⬦ costs of drug development and therapy as weighed against therapeutic benefits
- ⬦ economic cost of drug abuse, misuse, diversion, misbranding, and adulteration
- ⬦ economic forces and factors underlying drug distribution systems
- ⬦ effective control of drug costs at the development, federal, state, individual, institutional, wholesale, and retail levels
- ⬦ factors influencing the formulation, dosage forms, packaging, and marketing of drugs
- ⬦ management of pharmaceutical development, institutional pharmaceutical operations, and community or retail operations
- ⬦ study of drug utilization by consumers, within institutions, and by specific demographic groups by age, gender, race, and ethnicity
- ⬦ tensions among for-profit production, use of drugs, and societal needs

Pharmacogenetics is the study of genetic variation as revealed by reactions to drugs. There is a growing specialty within this field that involves the use of drugs involved in gene therapy.

Pharmacognosy is the science that deals with medicinal products of plant, animal, or mineral origin in their crude or unprepared state. The development of modern-day pharmaceuticals has, of course, dramatically decreased the importance of pharmacognosy to the practice of pharmacy.

Pharmacokinetics is that branch of pharmacology that deals with the scientific study of the absorption, distribution, metabolism, and excretion (ADME) of drugs over time.

- ⬦ Absorption is the process by which a substance is taken up from the site of administration by the system.
- ⬦ Distribution is the process of movement of the drug through the blood and transfer from the blood to other bodily fluids and tissues.
- ⬦ Metabolism of a drug is the transformation of the drug by the physiological processes of the body into other forms, usually less potent or toxic than the original form, that can then be eliminated.
- ⬦ Excretion is the elimination of the drug from the body, primarily through urination, defecation, perspiration, respiration, salivation, and, in lactating women, lactation.

Pharmacology is the scientific study of the nature of drugs and of their interactions with food and drink, other drugs, and the biochemical processes of the body, including the therapeutic uses of drugs for treating conditions of disease or other abnormality, with special reference to the pharmacokinetics and toxicology, or adverse consequences, of drugs.

A pharmacopeia is an authoritative reference containing a list and descriptions of drugs, pharmaceutical ingredients, and dosage forms, together with standards established under law for their production, dispensation, and use. The *United States Pharmacopeia (USP),* published by the United States Pharmacopeial Convention, is the official pharmacopeia of the United States.

A pharmacy fellowship is a directed, highly individualized postgraduate program designed to prepare a graduate pharmacist to become an independent researcher in a scientific area related to pharmacy.

A pharmacy residency is an organized, directed training program undertaken by a graduate of a pharmacy training program for the purpose of learning more about a defined area of practice. Some states also call these programs pharmacy externships.

Web Link

Visit the United States Pharmacopeia at www.usp.org

THE LANGUAGE OF PRESCRIPTIONS AND MEDICATION ORDERS

Under the law in most states, a pharmacist may not prescribe or engage in the manufacture of medications, although he or she can fill prescriptions and do small-scale extemporaneous (as needed) compounding (mixing and assembling) of medications in response to or in anticipation of prescriptions. In some states, registered pharmacists have been granted prescriptive authority. A prescription, or order for medication, must be written by a physician or by another licensed healthcare professional granted the right to prescribe under the applicable law (state, military, maritime, etc.). In a hospital, long-term care facility, or other institutional setting, a prescription is called a medication order or physician's order.

The forms of prescriptions and medication orders differ somewhat. Figure 3.1 shows a typical prescription. Figure 3.2 shows a typical institutional medication order. Sometimes a prescription or medication order calls for the pharmacist to dispense prefilled or prefabricated medications or dosage forms, such as a given number of capsules, tablets, patches, or prefabricated, prefilled syringes. At other times, the order requires that the pharmacist compound a medication, preparing a powder, for example, and filling capsules with it, or preparing a solution for intravenous infusion. The precise nature of these operations will be treated in subsequent chapters.

Forms used by institutions for medication orders vary, but they typically include patient information (name, address, age, sex, etc.); the name of the physician; the patient's room number; and lines for physician's orders, including spaces for the date, time, and the orders themselves. Both prescriptions and medication orders are generally handwritten in ink on preprinted forms. Prescriptions typically make use of metric measurements, although other measurement systems are used. (See Chapter 6 for more information on pharmaceutical calculations and measurements.) On a prescription form, decimal points used to express quantities and measurements may be replaced by handwritten or preprinted vertical lines, as follows:

$$1.94 \text{ mg} = 1|94 \text{ mg}$$

Figure 3.1

A Prescription

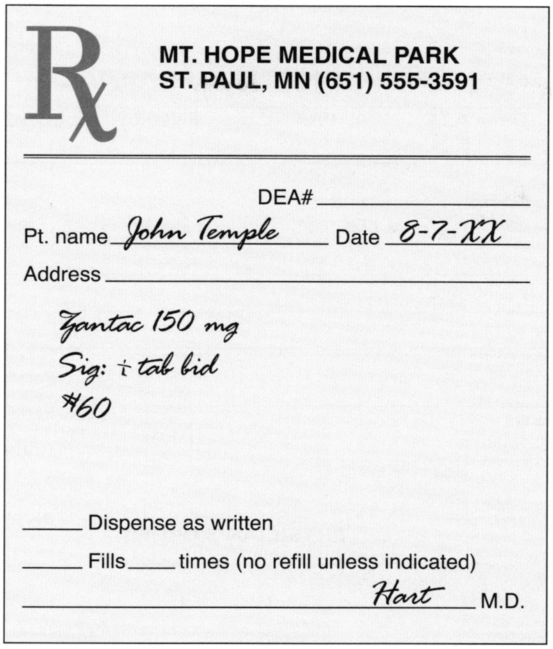

R̠x

**MT. HOPE MEDICAL PARK
ST. PAUL, MN (651) 555-3591**

DEA# _____

Pt. name _John Temple_ Date _8-7-XX_

Address _____

Zantac 150 mg
Sig: ī tab bid
_#60_

_____ Dispense as written

_____ Fills _____ times (no refill unless indicated)

_____ _Hart_ ____ M.D.

Prescriptions also make use of both Arabic (1, 2, 3, etc.) and Roman (ī, īī, īīī) numerals, as well as a great variety of special abbreviations and symbols. Roman numerals are adapted by writing in lowercase and placing a line over the number. Information on Roman numerals is provided in Chapter 6.

To the uninitiated, a prescription often reads like gobbledygook, and not just because of the famed illegibility of physicians' handwriting. Consider this example:

Sig: ī cap po c aq qid pc hs

Translated, the example means, "Write on the label, 'Take one capsule by mouth, with water, four times daily, after meals and at bedtime.'" If these abbreviations and symbols seem at first like a foreign language, well, they are. For the most part, they are abbreviations of Latin terms.

Chapter 7 deals in detail with receiving prescriptions and preparing orders based on them, but you can begin now to learn the abbreviations used in prescriptions and physician orders by studying the information provided in Tables 3.6 through 3.12. Individual prescriptions/medication orders will vary regarding whether abbreviations are given in uppercase or lowercase letters and with or without periods (e.g., gram 5 g, g., gm., gm, G., G, GM., GM). For consistency, this text follows a lowercase, no period style for most abbreviations. Hospital pharmacies will often have a list of acceptable abbreviations to help guide individuals writing prescriptions to be filled at the pharmacy.

Occasionally, prescriptions and medication orders make use of older systems of measurement such as the apothecary and avoirdupois systems. These systems are treated in Chapter 6. The related symbols are described in Table 3.13.

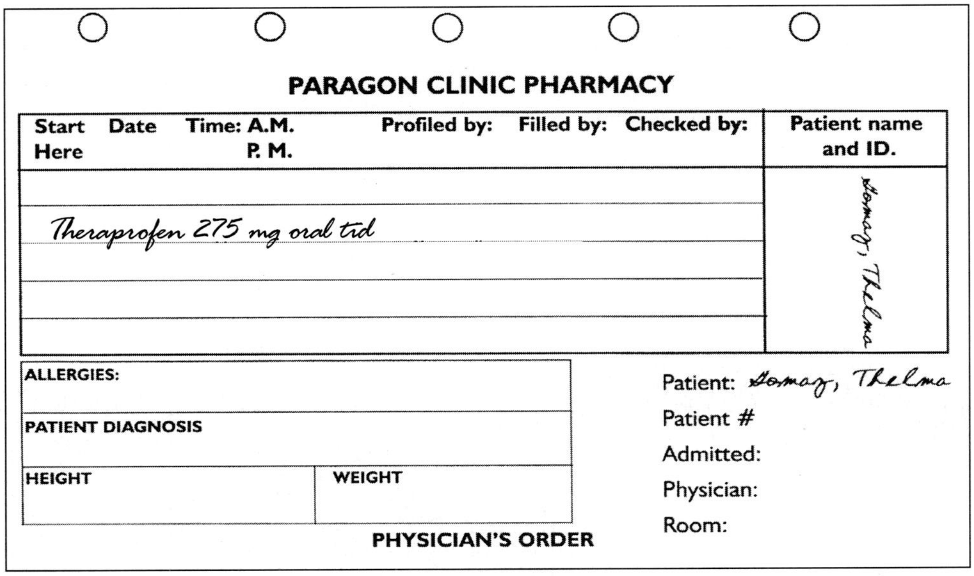

Figure 3.2

A Typical
Institutional
Medication Order

PARAGON CLINIC PHARMACY

| Start Date | Time: A.M. | Profiled by: | Filled by: | Checked by: | Patient name |
| Here | P. M. | | | | and ID. |

Theraprofen 275 mg oral tid

Domay, Thelma

ALLERGIES:

PATIENT DIAGNOSIS

| HEIGHT | WEIGHT |

PHYSICIAN'S ORDER

Patient: *Domay, Thelma*

Patient #

Admitted:

Physician:

Room:

Table 3.6   Amounts

Abbreviation	Derivation	Meaning
aa	*ana*	of each
ad	*ad*	up to, so as to make
C	—	Celsius
cc	—	cubic centimeter (mL)
dtd	*datur talis dosis*	dispense such doses
F	—	Fahrenheit
g	*gramma*	gram
gr	*granum*	grain
gtt	*guttae**	drop(s)
h, hr	*hora*	hour
lb	*libra*	pound
m²	—	square meter
mcg, μg	—	microgram
mEq	—	milliequivalent
mg	—	milligram
mg/kg	—	milligrams of drug per kilogram of body weight
mg/m²	—	milligrams of drug per square meter of body surface area
ℳ	—	minim
mL	—	milliliter
#	*numerus*	number
qs	*quantum sufficiat*	a sufficient quantity
qsad	*quantum sufficiat ad*	a sufficient quantity to make, up to
s̄s̄	*semis*	one-half
stat	*statim*	immediately
T	—	temperature
tbsp	—	tablespoonful
tsp	—	teaspoonful
unit	*unitas*	unit
w/v	—	weight to volume ratio
&	—	and
+	—	and

* Middle English

Table 3.7 Bodily Functions or Conditions

Abbreviation	Meaning
BM	bowel movement
BP	blood pressure
BS	blood sugar
CA	cancer
CHF	congestive heart failure
DT	delirium tremens
GT	gastrostomy tube
HA	headache
HBP	high blood pressure
HT, HTN	hypertension
NKA	no known allergies
N&V, N/V	nausea and vomiting
SCT	sickle-cell trait
SOB	shortness of breath
URI	upper respiratory infection,
UTI	urinary tract infection
VS	vital signs
WBC	white blood cell (count)

Table 3.8 Dosage Forms, Solutions, and Delivery Systems

Abbreviation	Derivation	Meaning
amp	*ampulla*	ampule
aq	*aqua*	water
cap	*capsula*	capsule
D_5LR	—	5% dextrose in lactated Ringer's solution
D_5NS	—	5% dextrose in normal saline solution
DW	—	distilled water
D_5W	—	5% dextrose in water
$D_{10}W$	—	10% dextrose in water
ECT	—	enteric-coated tablet
elix	*elixir*	elixir
fl	*fluidus*	fluid
fl oz	—	fluid ounce
inj	*injectio*	injection
IV	*intra venosus*	intravenous
IVP	—	intravenous push
IVPB	—	intravenous piggyback
KVO	—	keep vein open
NS	—	normal saline (0.9% sodium chloride)
½NS	—	half-strength normal saline (0.45%)
NTG	—	nitroglycerin
MDI	—	metered dose inhaler
oint	—	ointment
O/W	—	oil-in-water
RL, R/L	—	Ringer's lactate (solution)
sol	*solutio*	solution
supp	*suppositorium*	suppository
susp	*suspensus*	suspension
SWFI	—	sterile water for injection
syr	*syrupus*	syrup
tab	*tabella*	tablet

(continues)

Table 3.8 Dosage Forms, Solutions, and Delivery Systems—continued

Abbreviation	Derivation	Meaning
TDS	—	transdermal delivery system
TPN	—	total parenteral nutrition
ung	*unguentum*	ointment
W/O	—	water-in-oil

Table 3.9 Drugs and Drug References

Abbreviation	Derivation	Meaning
Drugs		
APAP		acetaminophen
ASA	acetylsalicylic acid*	aspirin
HC		hydrocortisone
HCTZ		hydrochlorothiazide
LCD	*liquor carbonis detergens*	coal tar solution
MS	—	morphine sulfate
NTG	—	nitroglycerin
PCN		penicillin
SMZ/TMP		sulfamethoxazole/trimethoprim
TCN		tetracycline
ZnO	—	zinc oxide
References		
NF	—	*National Formulary*
PDR		*Physician's Desk Reference*
USP	—	*United States Pharmacopeia*

* English

Table 3.10 Time and Time of Administration

Abbreviation	Derivation	Meaning
ā	*ante*	before
ac	*ante cibum*	before meals
ad lib	*ad libitum*	at pleasure, freely
am	*ante meridiam*	morning, before noon
ATC	—	around the clock
bid	*bis in die*	twice a day
h, hr	*hora*	hour
hs	*hora somni*	at bedtime
noct	*nocte*	at night
p	*post*	after
pc	*post cibum*	after meals
pm	*post meridiem*	evening, after noon
post-op	—	postoperative
pp	*postprandial*	after meals
prn	*pro re nata*	as needed
q	*quaque*	each, every

Table 3.10 **Time and Time of Administration—continued**

Abbreviation	Derivation	Meaning
qd	*quaque die*	every day
qh	*quaque hora*	every hour
q3h	*quaque 3 hora*	every three hours
qid	*quater in die*	four times a day
qod	*quaque alternis die*	every other day
tid	*ter in die*	three times a day
tiw	—	three times a week
wk	—	week

Table 3.11 **Sites of Administration/Parts of the Body**

Abbreviation	Derivation	Meaning
ad	*auris dextra*	right ear
as	*auris sinistra*	left ear
au	*auris uterque*	each ear
BSA	—	body surface area
GI	—	gastrointestinal
GU	—	genitourinary
IA	—	intra-arterial
ID	—	intradermal
IM	—	intramuscular
IT	—	intrathecal
npo	*non per os*	nothing by mouth
od	*oculus dexter*	right eye
os	*oculus sinister*	left eye
ou	*oculus uterque*	each eye
per	—	by or through
po	*per os*	by mouth
R	*rectum*	by rectum, rectal
SC, SQ, or subq	*sub cutis*	subcutaneous
SL	*sub lingua*	sublingual
top	*topikos*	topical
vag		vaginally

Table 3.12 **Pharmacy and Provider Instructions**

Abbreviation	Derivation	Meaning
c̄	*cum*	with
comp	*compositus*	compound
DAW		dispense as written
D/C	*discontinuare*	discontinue, discharge
dil	*diluere*	dilute, dissolve
disp	*dispensare*	dispense
div	*dividere*	divide
DT	—	discharge tomorrow
ECT	—	electroconvulsive therapy

(continues)

Table 3.12 Pharmacy and Provider Instructions—continued

Abbreviation	Derivation	Meaning
m ft	*misce et fiat*	mix and make
non rep, NR	*non repetatur*	do not repeat
O_2	—	oxygen
PBO		prescribe brand only
℞	*recipe*	take
s̄	*sine*	without
sig	*signa, signetur*	write on label
sos	*si opus sit*	if there is need
TAb	—	therapeutic abortion
TT, PTT	—	thrombin time (prothrombin time)
ut dict, ud	*ut dictum*	as directed
w/	—	with
w/o	—	without
y/o	—	years old
Δ	—	change

Table 3.13 Common Symbols from the Apothecary and Avoirdupois Measurement Systems

Symbol	Name	Equivalent in Metric System
Fluid Measure		
♏	minim*	0.06 mL
f ʒ	fluid drachm, fluidram*	3.69 mL
f ℥	fluidounce*	29.57 mL
pt	pint*	473 mL
qt	quart*	946 mL
gal	gallon*	3785 mL
Dry Measure		
gr	grain* **	65 mg
℈	scruple*	1.3 g
ʒ	drachm, dram*	3.9 g
℥	ounce*	31.2 g
#	pound*	374.4 g
oz	ounce**	437.5 gr

* Apothecary
** Avoirdupois

Chapter Summary

In order to communicate precisely with other professionals, specialists in various fields of endeavor, including pharmacists, create unique terminology, abbreviations, and symbols to describe the elements of their disciplines. Medical terminology commonly encountered in the practice of pharmacy makes extensive use of Greek and Latin roots, prefixes, and suffixes.

Pharmacy, of course, is the practice of dispensing drugs and information about drugs. A clear understanding of what, exactly, a drug is involves an understanding of its uses and of terms related to drug uses, including diagnosis, disease, trauma, disorder, acute, chronic, symptom, syndrome, mitigation, treatment, cure, prevention, generic name, and brand name. A wide variety of drugs is currently used, from absorbents to take up toxic chemicals in the body to vitamins to aid metabolism.

The Greek word from which the word *pharmacy* derives also provides the root of words to describe many fields of study and activity within pharmacy, including clinical pharmacy, pharmacology, clinical pharmacology, pharmacodynamics, pharmacokinetics, nuclear pharmacy, pharmacoeconomics, pharmacogenetics, and pharmacognosy.

Persons practicing pharmacy must be familiar with a great many abbreviations used on prescriptions and medication orders, including ones used to name amounts, bodily functions and conditions, dosage forms and delivery systems, drugs, drug references, time, time of administration, sites of administration, and parts of the body. A pharmacist or pharmacy technician must also be familiar with common symbols for weights and measures and with sound-alike and look-alike names of drugs which have the potential for leading to severe medication errors.

Chapter Review

Knowledge Inventory

Choose the best answer from those provided.

1. The word part *sub* in "sublingual" is a
   a. suffix meaning "above."
   b. prefix meaning "above."
   c. suffix meaning "below."
   d. prefix meaning "below."

2. The determination of the nature of a disease condition by examining a patient's symptoms is known as a
   a. disease.
   b. prognosis.
   c. syndrome.
   d. diagnosis.

3. An abnormality with which a person is born (that is, one that is not caused by environmental factors after birth), such as a cleft palate, is described as
   a. acute.
   b. congenital.
   c. mitigated.
   d. traumatic.

4. A group of symptoms that together characterize a particular abnormal condition is known as a
   a. disorder.
   b. disease.
   c. syndrome.
   d. treatment.

5. Tylenol is a
   a. generic drug name.
   b. nonproprietary drug name.
   c. brand name.
   d. chemical name.

6. The practice of counseling people about drug therapies and participating, as part of a total healthcare team, in the provision of services to patients is known as
   a. pharmacology.
   b. clinical pharmacy.
   c. pharmacokinetics.
   d. pharmacodynamics.

7. Drugs may be eliminated from the body via
   a. urination.
   b. perspiration.
   c. respiration.
   d. All of the above

8. The equivalent of a prescription, in a hospital or other institutional setting, is the
   a. medication order.
   b. drug list, or formulary.
   c. dispensatory.
   d. materia medica.

9. An abbreviation that does not describe an amount of a medication to be taken is
   a. g.
   b. mL.
   c. N&V.
   d. s̄s̄.

10. In the case of *Toppi vs. Scarf,* a pharmacist accidentally substituted Nardil, an antidepressant, for Norinyl,
   a. an antiemetic.
   b. a contraceptive.
   c. an antipsychotic.
   d. a vasoconstrictor.

Pharmacy in Practice

1. Rewrite each of the following prescriptions or medication orders in standard English
   a.   ī bid ac and īī hs
   b.   one cap qid q4h prn pain
   c.   ī tab qd am
   d.   4 tabs stat
   e.   2 tabs bid
   f.   tab iv stat
   g.   tab īī qid
   h.   1 & ½ tab qid
   i.   1 fl oz q3–4h prn
   j.   2 caps tid pc
   k.   v gtts tid

2. The following is a passage from a package insert included with Albuterol, USP Inhalation Aerosol. Read the passage and define the underlined medical terms. For these words, list the terms and their prefixes, suffixes, and/or root(s) with their definitions.

   ### PRECAUTIONS

   General: Albuterol, as with all <u>sympathomimetic</u> amines, should be used with caution in patients with <u>cardiovascular</u> disorders, especially <u>coronary</u> insufficiency, cardiac <u>arrhythmias</u>, and <u>hypertension</u>; in patients with <u>convulsive</u> disorders, <u>hyperthyroidism</u>, or <u>diabetes mellitus</u>; and in patients who are unusually responsive to sympathomimetic amines.

Large doses of <u>intravenous</u> albuterol have been reported to aggravate pre-existing diabetes and <u>ketoacidosis</u>. Additionally, beta-agonists, including albuterol, when given intravenously may cause a decrease in serum potassium, possibly through <u>intracellular</u> shunting. The relevance of this observation to the use of Albuterol Inhalation Aerosol is unknown, since the aerosol dose is much lower than the doses given intravenously. Although there have been no reports concerning the use of Albuterol Inhalation Aerosol during labor and delivery, it has been reported that high doses of albuterol administered intravenously inhibit <u>uterine</u> contractions. Although this effect is extremely unlikely as a consequence of aerosol use, it should be kept in mind. . . .

ADVERSE REACTIONS

The adverse reactions of albuterol are similar in nature to those of other sympathomimetic agents, although the incidence of certain cardiovascular effects is less with albuterol. A 13-week double-blind study compared albuterol and isoproterenol aerosols in 147 <u>asthmatic</u> patients. The results of this study showed that the incidence of cardiovascular effects was: <u>palpitations</u>, less than 10 per 100 with albuterol and less than 15 per 100 with isoproterenol; <u>tachycardia</u>, 10 per 100 with both albuterol and isoproterenol; and increased blood pressure, less than 5 per 100 with both albuterol and isoproterenol. In the same study, both drugs caused tremor or nausea in less than 15 patients per 100; dizziness or heartburn in less than 5 per 100 patients. Nervousness occurred in less than 10 per 100 patients receiving albuterol and in less than 15 per 100 patients receiving isoterenol. Rare cases of <u>urticaria</u>, <u>angioedema</u>, rash, <u>bronchospasm</u>, and <u>oropharyngeal</u> edema have been reported after the use of inhaled albuterol. In addition, albuterol, like other sympathomimetic agents, can cause adverse reactions such as hypertension, <u>angina</u>, vomiting, <u>vertigo</u>, central nervous system stimulation, <u>insomnia</u>, headache, unusual taste, and drying or irritation of the <u>oropharynx</u>.

3. Choose one of the following subfields of pharmacy in which you are particularly interested, research on the Internet and/or by contacting specialists in the field, and prepare a written or oral report explaining to other pharmacy technician students the subjects of interest to practitioners in this field. The resource *Remington: The Science and Practice of Pharmacy* is an excellent resource that may be found in the college library.
    a.   clinical pharmacy
    b.   pharmacology
    c.   clinical pharmacology
    d.   pharmacokinetics
    e.   nuclear pharmacy
    f.   pharmacoeconomics
    g.   pharmacogenetics
    h.   pharmacognosy

4. Choose four of the pairs of drugs listed in Table 3.5. Do some research on each drug by looking it up in the *Drug Facts and Comparisons* or *Physician's Desk Reference* or another standard reference work. (See Appendix D, "Resources.") Explain the use or indication for each drug and then list and define some of the unfamiliar side effects.

Improving Communication Skills

1. Using a medical dictionary, write the meaning for each of the following terms and then determine what the common lay person term or phrase is for the following medical terms.

rhinorrhea	photophobia
dysphagia	diplopia
otalgia	gastritis
cephalgia	coryza
pyrexia	cystitis

   (For example, rhinorrhea means a discharge from the nose, and the patient would refer to this as a "runny nose.")

2. Make a list of ten lay person or slang terms for diseases, conditions, or symptoms and share them with the class. Determine the medical term for each slang term you list.

Internet Research

1. Use the Merck Manual online, at www.merck.com to look up a disease condition or disorder in which you are interested. Explain whether the condition is an acute or chronic condition. List its symptoms and describe its normal treatment. Make use of both medical terms and lay person terminology in your description.

2. Test your medical knowledge online at www.drugfacts.com. This site has a trivia game on various health related topics. Begin with "medical terminology." Print out your results. List at least five new things you learned from the online trivia game.

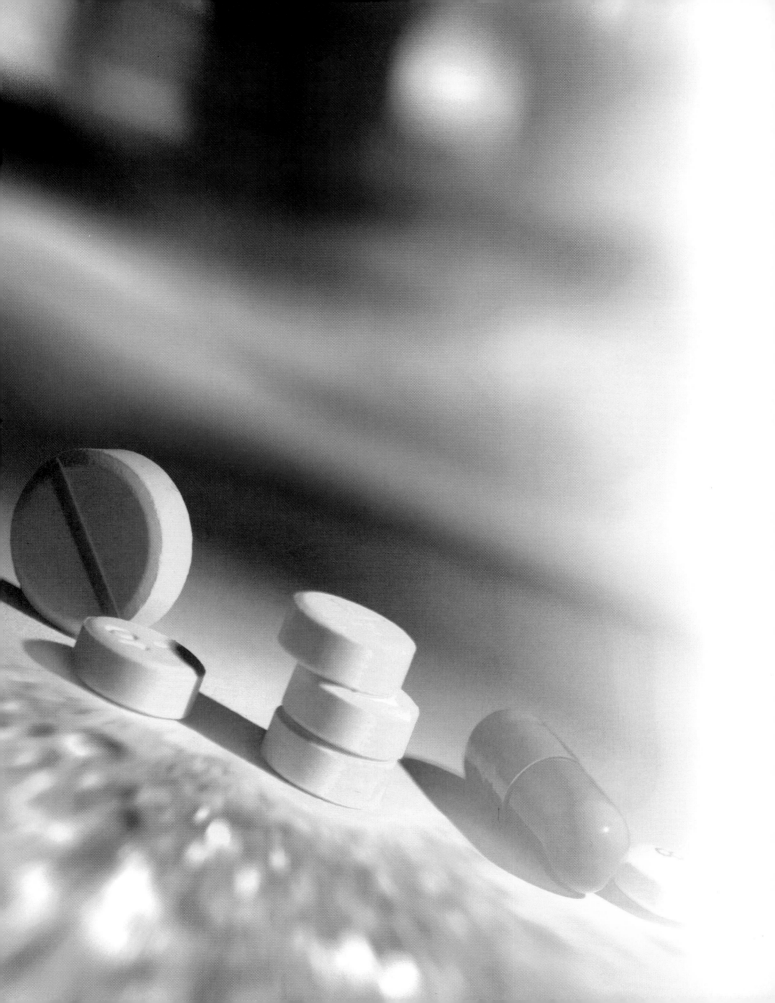

Drugs, Dosage Forms, and Delivery Systems

Learning Objectives

◇ Define the term *drug*.

◇ Distinguish between over-the-counter and legend drugs.

◇ Explain the parts of a National Drug Code number.

◇ Categorize drugs by source as natural, synthetic, synthesized, or semisynthetic.

◇ Explain the uses of drugs as therapeutic, pharmacodynamic, diagnostic, prophylactic, and destructive agents.

◇ Define and differentiate between the terms *dosage form* and *delivery system*.

◇ Enumerate and explain the properties of the major dosage forms and delivery systems for drugs.

◇ Identify advantages and disadvantages of the major dosage forms and delivery systems.

In no area of modern life, with the possible exception of computing, has technology so transformed everyday lives as in the area of pharmaceuticals. Modern pharmaceutical science has given us a vast array of medicines used for a wide variety of purposes and administered in an equally wide variety of forms. In this chapter, you will learn the uses of the modern pharmaceutical arsenal and about the many different forms—the dosage forms and delivery systems—that pharmaceutical scientists have created.

PHARMACEUTICALS

A drug is any substance taken into or applied to the body for the purpose of altering the body's biochemical functions and thus its physiological processes. In years past, the pharmacist and the physician used drugs in a more crude state, often powders, extracts, and tinctures containing herbal remedies. Modern science has led to the development of highly researched and standardized medications. Drugs are no longer just the "drug," they are products designed with a specific use in mind and contain many other components besides the "drug." The drug is now often referred to as the active ingredients. The biochemically reactive component or components of the drug, the active ingredient or ingredients, are rarely given in pure (i.e., in undiluted or uncut) form. Instead, one or more active ingredients are combined with one or more inert ingredients that have little or no physiological consequences. Most drugs contain one or more active ingredients commingled, dispersed, or in solution or suspension within an inert primary base, or vehicle, that may contain other ingredients, such as antimicrobial preservatives, colorings, and flavorings.

Drug References

Two reference works published by the United States Pharmacopeial Convention establish the official legal standards for drugs in the United States: the *United States Pharmacopeia (USP)* and the *National Formulary (NF)*. The *USP* describes drug

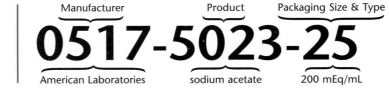

Pharmacists will use the *Drug Facts and Comparisons* and computerized databases for up-to-date drug information.

substances and dosage forms. The *NF* describes pharmaceutical ingredients. Both are revised every five years, and supplements are published in the interim between revisions. Useful to practitioners is the three-volume work *USP Drug Information (USP DI)*, available in print and computer database form, which includes *Drug Information for the Health Care Professional* (Vol. 1), *Advice for the Patient* (Vol. 2), and *Approved Drug Products and Legal Requirements* (Vol. 3). Also useful is the *Physician's Desk Reference*, published annually, a reference work that reprints package inserts for commonly used drugs. (For more information on drug literature, see Appendix D.) A reference commonly used in the pharmacy is *Drug Facts and Comparisons*. It is available as a resource that is updated with new inserts monthly.

National Drug Code (NDC)

Under the Drug Listing Act of 1972, a unique National Drug Code (NDC) number appears on all drug labels, including labels of prescription containers. The 10-character NDC includes a 4-number Labeler Code, identifying the manufacturer or distributor of the drug; a 3- or 4-number Product Code, identifying the drug (active ingredient and its dosage form); and a 2- or 3-number Package Code, identifying the packaging size and type. Figure 4.1 illustrates the parts of the NDC number.

Classes of Drugs

Drugs are classified as over-the-counter (OTC) or legend. An OTC drug is one that can be dispensed without a prescription. A legend drug can be dispensed only with a prescription and must bear on its label the legend "Caution: Federal law prohibits dispensing without prescription" (see Figure 4.2). Therefore, such drugs are known as legend drugs. (However, now many have only the symbol ℞.) Drugs with potential for abuse are classified, under the Comprehensive Drug Abuse Prevention and Control Act of 1970, according to five drug schedules, from Schedule I drugs with no accepted medical use and a high potential for abuse to Schedule V drugs with accepted medical uses, low potential for abuse, and limited potential for creating physical or psychological dependence. (Drug schedules were covered in more detail in Chapter 2.)

SOURCES OF DRUGS

Drugs come from various sources and can be classified as natural (taken from prokaryotic, eukaryotic, animal, plant, fungal, or mineral sources), synthetic (created

Web Link

Visit the NDC Directory at www.fda.gov/cder/ndc.

Figure 4.1

Parts of a National Drug Code (NDC) Number

Manufacturer	Product	Packaging Size & Type
0517-	**5023**-	**25**
American Laboratories	sodium acetate	200 mEq/mL

Figure 4.2

**Drug Caution
Legend**

10 mL MULTIPLE DOSE Vial

DIAZEPAM
INJECTION, USP

5 mg/mL

**FOR INTRAMUSCULAR or
INTRAVENOUS USE**

Each mL contains diazepam 5 mg, propylene glycol 0.4 mL, alcohol 0.1 mL, benzyl alcohol 0.015 mL and sodium benzoate/benzoic acid, a total of 50 mg in Water for Injection pH 6.2–6.9

USUAL DOSE: See package insert for complete prescribing information.

NOTE: Solution may appear colorless to light yellow. Store at controlled room temperature 15°–30° C (59°–86° F).

Caution: Federal law prohibits dispensing without prescription.

Product Code
LOT
EXP.

artificially), synthesized (created artificially but in imitation of naturally occurring substances), and semisynthetic (containing both natural and synthetic components). Radiopharmaceuticals are diagnostic or therapeutic drugs containing radioactive isotopes.

Drugs from Natural Sources

Some drugs are naturally occurring biological products, made or taken from single-celled organisms, plants, animals, people, or fungi. Both Vitamin B_{12} and the antibiotic streptomycin are produced from cultures of the bacterium *Streptomyces griseus*. Opium, the narcotic, comes from poppies; quinine, used to treat malaria, comes from cinchona bark. Thousands of years ago, people learned that they could combat pain by chewing or drinking concoctions made from white willow bark. Today, we know that white willow bark contains salicylic acid. In the drug form of acetylsalicylic acid, it is commonly called aspirin. Insulin for the treatment of diabetes mellitus can be extracted from the pancreas of sheep or oxen. The human growth hormone somatotropin comes, as its name suggests, from human bodies, where it is produced by the anterior pituitary. The naturally occurring forms of the antibiotic penicillin are extracted from certain molds. Some drugs are minerals. One example is magnesia (magnesium oxide or hydrated magnesium carbonate), which is used as an antacid and laxative.

Synthetic, Synthesized, and Semisynthetic Drugs

In the modern era, many naturally occurring chemicals, such as adrenaline, have been synthesized, or artificially created in the laboratory, and used as drugs. Other drugs, such as barbiturates, are completely synthetic. Still others are semisynthetic, and contain both natural and synthetic molecules; an example would be some forms of penicillin. This widely used antibiotic, derived from the molds *Penicillium notatum* and *P. chrysogenum*, was discovered by Alexander Fleming in 1928. Today, natural penicillins are still manufactured from molds, but new semisynthetic penicillins have also been developed. These penicillins combine artificially created molecules with naturally occurring ones

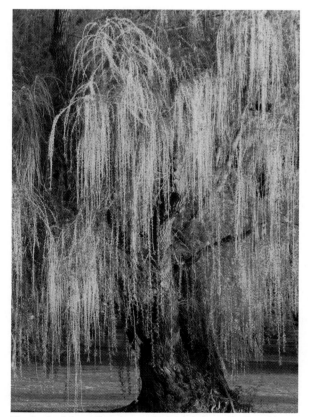

The bark of the willow tree, which contains salicylic acid, has been used for centuries to treat toothache.

and are effective against bacteria that have developed resistance to the natural penicillins.

Synthetic drugs can be created by means of the recombinant DNA techniques of genetic engineering. DNA, or deoxyribonucleic acid, is the complex, helically shaped molecule that carries the genetic code (see Figure 4.3). This molecule contains the instructions, or recipe, for creating messenger RNA, or ribonucleic acid, which in turn contains the recipe for creating amino acids, the building blocks of proteins and thus of the bodies of organisms. Recombinant DNA is DNA constructed of segments taken from different sources, as, for example, from a human being and a sheep. By transferring a segment of recombined DNA into a host cell, scientists can change what proteins the cell produces. In effect, this converts the cell into a small-scale protein factory to produce chemical substances that can be used in drugs or as drugs. For example, using the bacterium *Escherchia coli*, microbiologists and geneticists can induce the production of human insulin or human growth hormone.

Another biotechnological method of drug production is the use of cells from inoculated animals to produce, in the laboratory, hybrid cells that create substances known as monoclonal antibodies. Antibodies are created by the immune system in response to foreign substances in the body known as antigens. Laboratory-produced monoclonal antibodies can be used to attack tumors and to diagnose a great variety of conditions, from pregnancy to anemia to syphilis. Genetic engineering, the hybridization techniques for creating monoclonal antibodies, and other biotechnologies are already used to create a great variety of drugs, such as clotting factors for treating hemophiliacs and interferons for combating viral infection and some cancers. Such technologies promise to bring many new drugs to the market and to decrease the difficulty and cost of producing drugs already known.

Numerous drugs in various stages of research utilize technology evolved with the mapping of the human genome. The Human Genome Project has been under way since the 1980s and is best described as the mapping of the biochemical instructions that make up the human body in health and disease. As more of the genome is mapped and understood and more disease states are located, new treatments can be specifically designed to treat the identified biochemical errors located in the human genome.

Web Link

Learn more about the Human Genome Project at www. ornl.gov/hgmis

Figure 4.3

Modeling DNA
(a) A single nucleotide. (b) A short section of a DNA molecule consisting of two rows of nucleotides connected by weak bonds between the bases adenine (A) and thymine (T), guanine (G), and cytosine (C). (c) Long strands of DNA twisted to form a double helix.

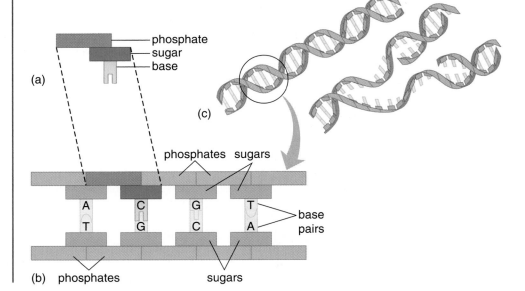

Radiopharmaceuticals

Chemicals containing radioactive isotopes, used diagnostically or therapeutically, are known as radiopharmaceuticals. (Isotopes are forms of an element that contain the same number of protons but differing numbers of neutrons.) Unstable, radioactive isotopes give off energy in the form of radiation, measured in rads. One rad is equal to 100 ergs of energy absorbed by 1 g of body tissue. Nuclear medicine uses radioactive isotopes such as technetium, ^{99m}Tc and iodine, ^{131}I for imaging regional function and biochemistry in the body, as in a PET (Positron Emission Tomography) or SPECT (Single Photon Emission Computed Tomography) scan, and for therapeutic irradiation and destruction of tissue, as in the treatment of hyperthyroidism or, more recently, ovarian and prostate cancer. Nuclear pharmacy involves the procuring, storage, compounding, dispensing, and provision of information about radiopharmaceuticals, and it is one possible area of specialization for both pharmacists and pharmacy technicians.

USES OF DRUGS

Medications today are being used not just to treat and cure illness, but to do a wide variety of other things, such as aid in diagnosis and even prevent illnesses. Healthcare providers have at their disposal numerous agents and dosage forms to customize medicinal treatment of a patient. Pharmaceutical manufacturers have provided various dosage forms for many different medications. The dosage forms give the physician several options to choose from, taking into account the advantages and disadvantages of the various products. It is essential to understand the inherent differences in the different dosage forms utilized today, as the patient outcome may depend on choosing and dispensing the most appropriate medication and dosage form to meet the patient's needs. The action of a medication can not be taken into account without also considering the dosage form selected.

The following categories of drugs are not mutually exclusive. For example, in the eighteenth century, William Withering discovered the effective ingredient in certain folk concoctions for treating people with heart conditions to be leaves of the foxglove plant. We now know the active ingredient in foxglove as the drug digitalis. Digitalis is pharmacodynamic in that it increases heart muscle contractions. It is therapeutic in that it can be used to treat congestive heart failure and irregular heartbeat. A bactericidal ointment is both a destructive agent that kills bacteria and a prophylactic agent that prevents infection. Radioiodine is a diagnostic agent when it is used in imaging and both a destructive and therapeutic agent when used to treat hyperthyroidism.

Therapeutic Agents

A therapeutic agent helps to maintain health, relieve symptoms, combat illness, and reverse disease processes. Examples of such drugs include vitamins to regulate metabolism and otherwise contribute to the normal growth and functioning of the body, electrolytes, enzymes, hormones, anti-inflammatories, antibiotics, sulfa drugs, laxatives, painkillers, antidepressants, insulin, and antiviral or antifungal agents.

Pharmacodynamic Agents

A pharmacodynamic agent alters bodily functioning in a desired way. Drugs can be used, for example, to stimulate or relax muscles, to dilate or constrict pupils, or to make blood more or less coagulable. Examples of pharmacodynamic agents include caffeine to forestall sleep, oral contraceptives to prevent pregnancy, expectorants to increase fluid in the respiratory tract, anesthetics to cause numbness or loss of consciousness, and digitalis to increase heart muscle contraction.

Diagnostic Agents

A diagnostic agent facilitates an examination, usually one conducted in order to arrive at a diagnosis, or conclusion as to the nature or extent of a disease condition. Examples of diagnostic agents include barium meals or enemas given to facilitate x-ray observation of the gastrointestinal tract and the radiopharmaceutical thallium chloride given to facilitate a SPECT scan.

Prophylactic Agents

A prophylactic agent prevents illness or disease from occurring. Examples of prophylactic agents include the antiseptic and germicidal liquid iodine used for prevention of infection, emetics given to induce vomiting of previously ingested toxic substances, smallpox vaccine, and the Salk and Sabin vaccines used to prevent the disease poliomyelitis (polio).

Destructive Agents

A destructive agent, as the name suggests, destroys. Examples of destructive agents are antiseptics for killing bacteria and antineoplastic (literally "anti-new-formation") drugs used in chemotherapy to destroy malignant tumors. Another example is radioiodine, which is used to destroy the thyroid gland in patients with hyperthyroidism or thyroid cancer before they are given natural or synthetic thyroid hormone medication.

DOSAGE FORMS AND DELIVERY SYSTEMS

The term *dosage form* refers to the physical manifestation of a drug as a solid, liquid, or gas that can be used in a particular way. Examples of dosage forms include tablets, creams, solutions, injections, and aerosols.

The term *delivery system* encompasses the drug in its particular solid, liquid, or gaseous form; any mechanism used to deliver the drug (such as a teaspoon, hypodermic, IV, or osmotic pump); and any design feature of the dosage form that affects the delivery of the drug (such as the coating on some capsules that resists breakdown by the gastric fluids in the stomach so that the capsule will release medication, instead, into the intestines). Health practitioners use the term *delivery system* to describe the means for transporting a particular amount of a drug at a certain rate to the particular site or sites of action of the drug within the body.

Delivery systems differ in their pharmacological properties, that is, in their sites of action, rate of delivery, and quantities of active ingredient delivered. Consider, for example, the drug nitroglycerin, commonly used to treat angina pectoris (pain in the chest and left arm associated with a sudden decrease in blood supply to the heart). Nitroglycerin dilates blood vessels, thus increasing blood supply to the heart and decreasing blood pressure. Two common delivery systems for nitroglycerin are sublingual tablets, placed under the tongue, and transdermal patches, worn on the skin. Sublingual nitroglycerin tablets are fast acting but deliver their active ingredient for only a short period of time, about 30 minutes. Transdermal patches, in contrast, act slowly, with a delivery onset of about 30 minutes, but they can deliver a steady amount of the drug for up to 24 hours. Another example of differing delivery systems is the use of acetylsalicylic acid (aspirin) in tablet form taken orally (by mouth) for relief of minor aches and pains as opposed to salicylic acid applied topically (locally) in a liquid solvent mixture to remove a corn on the foot. Obviously, the choice of delivery system depends upon many factors, including

- ◇ what active ingredient is to be delivered
- ◇ how much of the active ingredient is to be delivered
- ◇ by what means or by what route the ingredient is to be delivered
- ◇ to what sites
- ◇ at what rate
- ◇ over what period of time
- ◇ and for what purpose

Today, drugs are administered in a wide variety of dosage forms that are part of an even wider variety of delivery systems. Because of the variety and overlap of dosage forms and delivery systems, it is impossible to create a rigid, mutually exclusive taxonomy, or classification, of them.

Solid Dosage Forms

Solid dosage forms are used more frequently than any other form and are safer for the patient to self-administer. Capsules and tablets are the two most common types and are very inexpensive to manufacture. Of course there are a wide variety of capsule types and sizes and several manufacturers have begun to utilize a hybrid of the capsule and tablet, the caplet. Other solid dosage forms are utilized less frequently but are still very important because they enable the physician and pharmacist to more adequately meet the needs of an individual patient.

CAPSULES The capsule is a solid dosage form consisting of a gelatin shell that encloses the drug. Gelatin is a protein substance obtained from vegetable matter and from the skin, white connective tissue, and bones of animals. A capsule may be a placebo, containing no active ingredients. (Placebos in encapsulated or other dosage forms are commonly given as controls in drug tests and experiments.) Generally, however, the capsule contains powder, granules, liquids, or some combination thereof with one or more active ingredients. In most cases, the powder, granules, or liquids in the capsule also contain one or more pharmacologically inert filler substances, or diluents. The capsule may also contain disintegrants (which help to break up the ingredients), solubilizers (which maintain the ingredients in solution or help the ingredients to pass into solution in the body), preservatives (which maintain the integrity of the ingredients), colorings, and other materials. Because a capsule is enclosed, flavorings are not common for this dosage form. The gelatin shell of a capsule, which can be hard or soft, may be transparent, semitransparent, or opaque and may be colored or marked with a code to facilitate

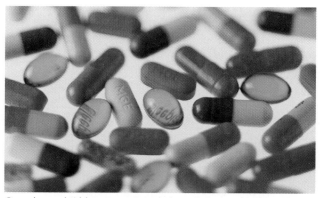
Capsules and tablets come in a variety of sizes and colors. The distinctive markings help patients identify the drug.

identification. In most cases, the capsule is meant to be swallowed whole. Examples of drugs available in capsule form include amoxicillin 250 and 500 mg, indomethacin 25 and 50 mg, and secobarbital sodium 50 mg. Patients often prefer capsules, as they are tasteless and are often easier to swallow than tablets.

Hard gelatin shells are made of gelatin, sugar, and water. Such shells commonly contain powders or granules and are used for extemporaneous (to order) hand-filling operations and for commercial manufacturing. In commercial manufacturing, the body and the cap may be sealed to protect the integrity of the drug within (a practice that has increased since the 1980s, when highly publicized incidents of capsule tampering occurred). Hard shell capsules come in standard sizes indicated by the numbers 000, 00, 0, 1, 2, 3, 4, 5 (from largest to smallest). The largest capsule, size 000, can contain about 1,040 mg of aspirin; the smallest, size 5, about 97 mg (see Figure 4.4).

Most hard shell capsules are meant to be swallowed whole, but a few are meant only as conveyances for granules or powders to be sprinkled on food or in drink. Capsules should not be used in this latter fashion, however, except when specifically intended for this purpose, because opening the capsule can defeat the capsule's controlled release properties. A controlled release dosage form may be used to deliver a drug over a particular period of time (sustained release) or at a particular site (delayed action). Some capsules and tablets, for example, have an enteric coating allowing the dosage form to pass through the gastric fluids of the stomach relatively undisturbed and to then dissolve and release the medication into the intestines. Others are designed to disintegrate at a particular rate, matching that of the metabolism of the drug by the body and so providing a steady replenishment of the medication, over time, in a more or less precise amount. The design of a wide variety of controlled release tablets, capsules, granules, and other dosage forms has proved to be a fertile field for the imaginations of pharmaceutical developers, and the naming of these varieties has provided much diversion to these developers' marketing personnel. Names for controlled release forms include constant release, continuous action, continuous release, controlled release, delayed absorption, depot, extended action, extended release, gradual release, long acting, long lasting, long term release, programmed release, prolonged action, prolonged release, protracted release, rate controlled, repository, retard, slow acting, slow release, sustained action, sustained release, sustained release depot, timed coat, timed disintegration, and timed release.

The specialized capsules now available have a tremendous advantage over some of the older dosage forms. The long acting capsules are taken less often, and patients are more likely to be compliant. It is much easier to remember to take medication once daily than to take several doses throughout the day. A long acting form may also give the patient better control over the disease state or symptoms. Although the units may be initially more expensive, fewer need to be purchased. One drawback to using sustained release capsules involves the longer time it may take for adverse drug reactions to subside.

Soft gelatin shells are spherical, oblong, ovoid, or elliptical dosage forms of sealed, one-piece construction that come prefilled from commercial manufacturers with powders or, more commonly, with liquids, suspensions, pastes, or other materials that could leak from capsules having a two-part, hard shell construction. Soft shell capsules are particularly suited to volatile prepara-

Figure 4.4

Hard Shell Capsule Sizes
The sizes in which hard shell capsules are available range from 5, the smallest, to 000, the largest.

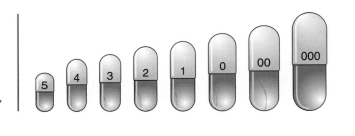

tions, which vaporize or evaporate rapidly in air, and to preparations otherwise subject to deterioration on exposure. Soft capsule shells are made of gelatin and added substances, such as glycerin or sorbitol, that give the gelatin its softness, or plasticity. They generally contain from 1 to 480 minims (from 0.0616 mL to about 30 mL).

EFFERVESCENT SALTS Effervescent salts are granules or coarse powders containing one or more medicinal agents (such as an analgesic), as well as some combination of sodium bicarbonate with citric acid, tartaric acid, or sodium biphosphate. When dissolved in water or some other liquid, effervescent salts release carbon dioxide gas, causing a distinctive bubbling. A common example of an effervescent salt is effervescent sodium phosphate, used as a cathartic, or purgative (a medicine for stimulating evacuation of the bowels).

IMPLANTS OR PELLETS Implants, or pellets, are dosage forms that are placed under the skin by means of minor surgery and/or special injectors. They are used for long term, controlled release of medications, especially hormones. An example of an implant is Norplant, which contains levonorgestrel to prevent pregnancy. The advantages of a product such as this include enhanced patient compliance and convenience.

LOZENGES, TROCHES, OR PASTILLES Lozenges, also known as troches or pastilles, are dosage forms containing active ingredients and flavorings, such as sweeteners, that are administered buccally (dissolved in the mouth). They generally have local effects. Commercial over-the-counter lozenges for relief of sore throat are quite common, although many other drugs, including such prescription drugs as nystatin or clotrimazole, are also available in lozenge form.

PILLS The small, almost perfectly spherical dosage form known as the pill, once very common in pharmacy, has now largely been replaced by tablets and capsules.

PLASTERS Plasters are solid or semisolid, medicated or nonmedicated preparations that adhere to the body and contain a backing material such as paper, cotton, linen, silk, moleskin, or plastic. An example is the salicylic acid plaster used to remove corns.

POWDERS AND GRANULES To a layperson, a powder is any finely ground substance. To a pharmacist, a powder is a finely divided combination, or admixture, of drugs and/or chemicals ranging in size from extremely fine (1 micron or less) to very coarse (about 10 mm). Official definitions of powder size include very coarse (No. 8 powder), coarse (No. 20 powder), moderately coarse (No. 40 powder), fine (No. 60 powder), or very fine (No. 80 powder), according to the amount of the powder that can pass through mechanical sieves made of wire cloth of various dimensions (No. 8 sieves, No. 20 sieves, and so on).

In the past, it was common for the pharmacist/apothecary to prepare medicines in the form of powders. However, powders dispensed in bulk amounts had the disadvantage of leading to inaccuracy in the dosage taken by the patient. Commonly dispensed bulk powders include antacids, brewer's yeast, laxatives, douche powders, dentifrices and dental adhesives, and powders for external application to the skin. In the past, pharmacists often dispensed divided powders, or charts, that were prepared, measured, mixed, divided into separate units, and placed upon pieces of paper that were then folded. Today, dispensing of medicines in the divided powder dosage form is rare, although powders are very widely used as components of such commercially prepared dosage forms as capsules and tablets.

Powders are combined and mixed by a variety of means, including spatulation (blending with a pharmaceutical spatula), trituration (grinding or pulverizing, as with a mortar and pestle), sifting, and tumbling in a container or blending machine. They may also be levigated (formed into a paste employing a small amount of liquid) in preparation for being added to an ointment base. In large-scale commercial manufacturing, powders are milled and pulverized by machines. An example of a medication in the powder dosage form is polymyxin B sulfate and bacitracin zinc topical powder, which is used to prevent infection.

Granules are larger than powders and are formed by adding very small amounts of liquid to powders and then passing the mixture through a screen or a granulating device. Granules are generally of irregular shape, have excellent flow characteristics, are more stable than powders, and are generally better suited than powders for use in solutions because they are not as likely simply to float on the surface of a liquid. Tablets are often prepared by compressing granules, and capsules are often filled with granules. Granules may contain colorings, flavorings, and coatings and may have controlled release characteristics. Some drug products in granular form are combined by the pharmacist with water before dispensing. Some are dispensed as granules and measured, for prescription and dosage, by the teaspoonful or tablespoonful.

SUPPOSITORIES Suppositories are solid dosage forms designed for insertion into bodily orifices, generally the rectum or the vagina or, less commonly, the urethra.

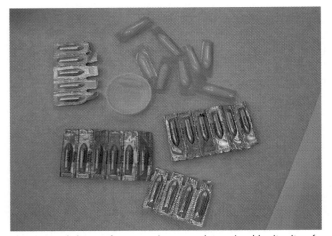

The size and shape of a suppository are determined by its site of administration.

Suppositories vary in size and shape, depending on their site of administration and the age and gender of the patient for whom they are designed. Some are meant for local action. Rectal suppositories, however, are often used as vehicles for systemic drugs because the large numbers of blood and lymphatic vessels in the rectum provide for exceptional absorption. Suppositories may be the preferred dosage form in some cases when the patient has severe nausea and vomiting. However, many patients avoid the use of a suppository when possible because of their discomfort. A variety of bases are used in suppositories, including cocoa butter, hydrogenated vegetable oils, and glycerinated gelatin. Suppositories are produced by molding and by compression.

TABLETS The tablet is a solid dosage form produced by compression (or, in the past, by molding) and containing, as capsules do, one or more active ingredients and, commonly, other pharmacological ingredients, including diluents, binders (to promote adhesion of the materials in the tablet), lubricating agents (to give the tablet a sheen and to aid in the manufacturing process), disintegrants, solubilizers, colorings, and coatings. For obvious reasons, tablets also commonly contain flavorings. Coatings can be used to protect the stability of the ingredients in tablets; to improve appearance, flavor, or ease of swallowing; or to provide for controlled (sustained or delayed) release of medication. Tablets are available in a wide variety of shapes, sizes, and surface markings. Manufacturers also make an oblong tablet, often called a caplet. The caplet is simply a tablet shaped like a capsule, and sometimes coated to look like a capsule. The inside of the caplet is solid, whereas the inside of a capsule is often powder or granular. Tablets are extremely convenient because of the ease with which various doses can be delivered. A patient can take one tablet, several tablets, or a portion of a tablet, as required. Some tablets are scored to facilitate breaking into portions. If a tablet is not scored, it should not be broken. Scoring will equally divide the dose. Several routes of administration are possible for tablets. Most tablets are meant to be swallowed whole and to dissolve in the gastrointestinal tract. However, some tablets are designed to be chewed or to be dissolved in liquid, in the mouth, under the tongue, or in the vagina. Examples of drugs available in tablet form include digoxin 0.125, 0.25, and 0.5 mg; ibuprofen 300, 400, 600, and 800 mg; nitroglycerin 0.15, 0.3, 0.4, and 0.6 mg; and penicillin V potassium 250 and 500 mg.

Almost all tablets produced today are created by punch and die machines that compress the ingredients of each tablet in a single stroke. Compression tablets are the most inexpensive and common dosage form utilized today. Some tablets are produced by multiple compressions and are, in effect, either tablets on top of tablets or tablets within tablets. These are called multiple compression tablets (MCT) (see Figure 4.5). A multiple compression tablet may contain a core and one or two outer shells or two or three different layers, each containing a different medication and colored differently. Multiple compression tablets are created for appearance alone, to combine incompatible substances into a single medication, or to provide for controlled release in successive events, or stages.

Trituration is the process of rubbing, grinding, or pulverizing a substance into fine particles or powder. In the past, tablets were created by placing moist, triturated ingredients into a mold. Today, however, such molded tablets have been almost entirely replaced by ones produced by the compression methods described above.

Tablets can be coated, containing a special outside layer that dissolves or ruptures at the site of application, or uncoated, not containing such a layer. Sugar-coated tablets (SCT) contain an outside layer of sugar that protects the medication and improves both appearance and flavor. If a drug is particularly foul tasting, then sugar coating and other flavoring may be necessary. Of course, in pharmacy, as in life, sugar coating tends to improve compliance, which pharmacy personnel define as the taking of medication in the prescribed amount and at the prescribed times. Unfortunately, sugar coating, both in pharmacy and in life, has disadvantages as well. The sugar coating makes tablets much larger and heavier. Film coated tablets (FCT) contain a thin outer layer of a polymer (a substance containing very large molecules) that can be either soluble or insoluble in water. Film coatings are thinner, lighter in weight, and cheaper to manufacture than sugar coatings and are colored to provide an attractive appearance. Enteric coated tablets (ECT) are used for drugs that are destroyed by gastric acid, that might irritate the esophageal tract or stomach, or that are better absorbed by the intestines if they bypass the stomach. The enteric coating is designed to resist destruction by gastric fluids and to break down once the tablet reaches the intestines.

Containing a base that is flavored and/or colored, chewable tablets are designed to be masticated and are a preferred dosage form for antacids, antiflatulents, commercial vitamins, and tablets for children.

Effervescent tablets are made with granular effervescent salts or other materials that release gas and so dispense active ingredients into solution when placed in water. Most

Figure 4.5

Multiple Compression Tablets
(a) Two layers or compressions. (b) Three layers or compressions.

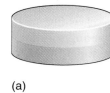

(a)

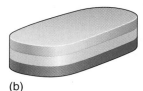

(b)

people are familiar with such tablets in the form of commercial analgesics (pain relievers).

Buccal tablets are meant to be placed in the buccal pouches (between the cheek and the gum) and dissolved and absorbed by the buccal mucosa. (The mucosa, or mucous membrane, is the mucus-secreting lining of bodily cavities and canals which communicate with the exterior. For more information on this, see Chapter 5.)

Sublingual tablets, such as those used to deliver nitroglycerin, are designed to be dissolved under the tongue (sub = "under"; lingua = "tongue") and absorbed. Medication dissolved under the tongue is absorbed very quickly and has the advantage of immediately entering the blood stream.

Also known as vaginal inserts, vaginal tablets are designed to be placed into the vagina by means of an applicator and dissolved and absorbed by the vaginal mucosa.

A controlled release tablet is one designed to regulate the rate at which a drug is released from the tablet and into the body.

Liquid Dosage Forms

Liquid dosage forms consist of one or more active ingredients in a liquid medium, or vehicle. These dosage forms can be divided into two major categories: solutions, in which active ingredients are dissolved in the liquid vehicle, and dispersions, in which undissolved ingredients are dispersed throughout a liquid vehicle.

Liquid dosage forms that are meant for oral consumption have several advantages over solid dosage forms, including ease of swallowing and of adjusting the dose. A liquid dosage can be easily adjusted, whereas tablets or capsules can not always be divided easily. For the patient, taste preference may be either an advantage or disadvantage. For adults this is not usually a concern; however children's medication is often flavored in the most palatable way possible to improve compliance. Liquid dosage forms are often slightly less stable than their solid counterparts, and care should be taken to monitor storage conditions of the liquid dosage forms, rotate stock, and check expiration dates often.

Liquid and semisolid dosage forms meant for topical application often have specific indications for which they are most suited. Creams and lotions, for example, will easily cover a large area, and are vanishing. Ointments however are sticky and will leave the area feeling greasy. An ointment is especially good for extremely dry areas where moisture needs to be retained and for areas prone to friction from clothing or other body parts. Gels are yet another product that may be designed with a specific indication in mind. They apply evenly and leave a dry coat of the medication in contact with the area.

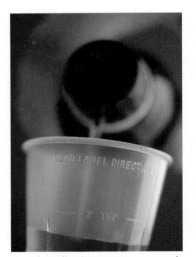

Liquid medications are easy to swallow and the dose can be adjusted.

SOLUTIONS The vehicle that makes up the greater part of a solution is known as a solvent. An ingredient dissolved in a solution is known as a solute. Solutions may be classified by vehicle as aqueous (water-based), alcoholic (alcohol-based), or hydroalcoholic (water- and alcohol-based). They may be classified by contents as aromatic waters, elixirs, syrups, extracts, fluidextracts, irrigating solutions, liniments, ointments, spirits, or tinctures. They may also be classified by site or method of administration as topical (local), systemic (throughout the body), epicutaneous (on the skin), percutaneous (through the skin), peroral (for or through the mouth), otic (for or through the ear), ophthalmic (for the eye), parenteral (for injection or intravenous infusion), rectal (for or through the rectum), urethral (for the urethra), or vaginal (for or through the vagina).

Aromatic waters are solutions of water containing oils or other substances that both have a pungent, and usually pleasing, smell and are volatile, or easily released into the air. Rose water is an example.

Collodions are liquid dosage forms for topical application containing pyroxylin (tiny particles of cellulose derived from cotton) dissolved in a mixture of alcohol and ether, to which medicinal ingredients may be added. On application, the highly volatile alcohol and ether solvent vaporizes, leaving on the skin a film coating containing the medication. Flexible collodion, containing castor oil and camphor, may be applied to bandages or stitches to waterproof them. The product with the brand name Compound W is a collodion containing salicylic acid used to remove corns or warts.

Diluted acids are aqueous dilutions of concentrated acids. An example is 1% acetic acid solution used as a surgical dressing, irrigating solution, and spermicide.

A clear, sweetened, flavored hydroalcoholic solution, containing water and ethanol, is known as an elixir. Such a solution can be medicated or nonmedicated. An example of a drug in this dosage form is phenobarbital elixir, containing phenobarbital, orange oil, propylene glycol, alcohol, sorbitol solution, color, and purified water. Children's Tylenol Elixir, a vehicle for acetaminophen, is another example. Elixirs are similar to syrups but, because they are hydroalcoholic, are preferable as vehicles for medications compounded of both water-soluble or alcohol-soluble ingredients. Additional solvents, such as glycerin and propylene glycol, may be used in elixirs. The choice of sweeteners in an elixir depends on the alcoholic content. If the active ingredients in an elixir are largely water soluble, then a natural sweetener such as sucrose or sorbitol may be used, but if the elixir has high alcohol content, then an artificial sweetener such as saccharin is preferable. In the past, pharmacists often used nonmedicated elixirs as palatable vehicles for unpleasant-tasting drugs.

An enema is a solution administered rectally for cleansing or drug administration. Enemas generally come in disposable plastic squeeze bottles. A retention enema is administered to deliver medication locally or systemically. An evacuation enema is administered to clean the bowels.

Extraction is the process by which desired materials, such as the active ingredients of drugs, are removed from plants or other materials through the application of solvents that place the desired materials in solution. The products of extraction, known as extractives, generally contain several ingredients, since several constituents of the plant will be soluble in a given solvent. The process of creating extractives from plants is a central part of so-called galenical pharmacy (see Chapter 1) and was once a major activity of the pharmacist/apothecary. Solvents used for extraction include water, alcohol, hydroalcoholic solutions, and glycerin.

Two methods of extraction are commonly employed: maceration and percolation. In the maceration method, the crude drug from the plant is comminuted, or pulverized, and then soaked in the solvent. In the percolation method, the solvent is made to pass slowly, or percolate, through a column of the comminuted crude material from which the extraction is being made. Types of extractives include tinctures, fluidextracts, and extracts. Fluidextracts are liquid dosage forms prepared by the percolation method from plant sources. They contain the solvent alcohol and 1 g of the drug for each milliliter of liquid. In current practice, fluidextracts are often flavored and/or sweetened and are not directly dispensed to patients but rather are used in the formulation of syrups and other dosage forms.

Extracts are potent dosage forms, from animal or plant sources, from which most or all the solvent has been evaporated to produce a powder, an ointmentlike form, or a solid. They are produced from fluidextracts and used in the formulation or compounding of medications.

An irrigating solution, or douche, is any solution for cleansing or bathing an area of the body. Some are used topically, some otically, some ophthalmically, and some for irrigation of bodily tissues exposed by wounds or surgical incisions. The term *douche* is most commonly used for liquid solutions, often reconstituted from powders, administered into the vaginal cavity.

Liniments are alcoholic or oleaginous (hydrocarbon-containing) solutions or emulsions containing medications and meant for rubbing on the skin.

Parenteral solutions are sterile solutions, with or without medication, for administration by means of a hollow needle or other device used to place the solution through one or more layers of membrane. There are two major delivery systems for parenteral solutions: intravenous (IV) infusions and injections, which may or may not be intravenous. Parenteral solutions must be stable. In other words, they must remain effective without undergoing chemical degradation, until the time of administration. In addition, parenterals must be sterile, or free from all contaminants, including pyrogens, the fever-inducing products of the metabolic action of microorganisms.

Spirits are alcoholic or hydroalcoholic solutions containing volatile, aromatic ingredients. Examples include camphor spirit and peppermint spirit. Some spirits are used as medicines and some as flavorings.

A syrup is an aqueous solution thickened with a large amount (commonly 60 to 80 percent) of sugar, generally sucrose, or a sugar substitute such as sorbitol or propylene glycol. A simple syrup known as Syrup NF can be made by combining 85 g of sucrose with 100 mL of purified water. Syrups may contain additional flavorings, colors, or aromatic agents. Syrups come in two varieties: medicated syrups containing active ingredients, such as lithium citrate syrup or ipecac syrup; and nonmedicated syrups, such as cherry syrup or cocoa syrup, used as vehicles. Because they do not contain alcohol, syrups are often used as vehicles for pediatric medications. Syrups are also sometimes used for elderly patients who cannot easily swallow the commonly available solid forms of certain drugs.

Alcoholic or hydroalcoholic solutions of pure chemicals or of extractions from plants are known as tinctures. Examples include iodine tincture and belladonna tincture.

DISPERSIONS Unlike a solution, a dispersion is not dissolved in its vehicle. Instead, it is simply distributed throughout. The vehicle for a dispersion is known as the dispersing phase or dispersing medium. The particulate or liquid dispersed within the vehicle is known as the dispersed phase. Dispersions are classified by the size of the dispersed ingredient(s) into suspensions and emulsions, containing relatively large particles, and magmas, gels, and jellies, containing fine particles. If a dispersion contains ultra fine particles, less than a micron in size, it is said to be colloidal. One type of colloidal is the microemulsion. Dispersions of solids in a liquid are known as suspensions. Dispersions of a liquid in a liquid are known as emulsions.

A suspension is a type of dispersion in which small particles of a solid, the suspensoid, are dispersed in a liquid vehicle. Some suspensions come already prepared. Others come in the form of dry powders that are reconstituted (re-liquefied), usually with purified water. Suspensions may be classified by route of administration into oral suspensions (taken by mouth), topical suspensions (such as lotions applied locally, generally to the skin), and injectable suspensions. A well-prepared suspension settles slowly, can be redispersed easily throughout the dispersing phase by a gentle shake, and pours easily. A suspension may be a preferred method for dispensing a solid to a young or elderly patient who would find it difficult to swallow a solid dosage form. Examples of suspensions include antacids like the magnesia and alumina oral suspension with the brand name Maalox and the antifungal nystatin oral suspension.

An emulsion is a type of dispersion in which one liquid is dispersed in another, immiscible liquid (one with which it does not readily mix). Common types of emulsions are of oil-in-water (O/W) or water-in-oil (W/O). For example, O/W emulsions contain a small amount of oil dispersed in water. Emulsions contain a third phase, the emulsifying agent, to render the emulsion stable and less prone to separation. Emulsions vary in their viscosity, or rate of flow, from free-flowing liquids such as lotions to semisolid preparations such as ointments and creams.

A lotion is a liquid for topical application containing insoluble dispersed solids or immiscible liquids. Examples include calamine lotion, used for relief of itching, and benzoyl peroxide lotion, used to control acne.

Like suspensions, gels contain solid particles in liquid, but the particles are ultra fine, of colloidal dimensions, and sufficient in number and so linked as to form a semisolid. Examples of gels include lidocaine gel and the antacid aluminum hydroxide gel. A jelly is a gel that contains a high proportion of water, usually formed from a combination of water, a drug substance, and a thickening agent. Antiseptic, antifungal, contraceptive, and lubricant jellies are examples. Jellies are often used as lubricants for examination of body orifices. Because of their high water content, jellies are subject to contamination and therefore they usually contain preservatives.

Glycerogelatins are topical preparations made with gelatin, glycerin, water, and medicinal substances. The hard substance is melted and brushed onto the skin, where it hardens again and is generally covered with a bandage. An example is zinc gelatin, used as a pressure bandage to treat varicose ulcers.

A magma, or milk, is similar to a gel in that it contains colloidal particles in liquid, but the particles remain distinct, in a two-phase system. An example is Milk of Magnesia, containing magnesium hydroxide, used to neutralize gastric acid.

A microemulsion, like other emulsions, contains one liquid dispersed in another, but unlike other emulsions, is clear because of the extremely fine size of the droplets of the dispersed phase. An example of a microemulsion is Haley's M-O.

Ointments, or unguents, are semisolid dosage forms meant for topical application. Ointments may be medicated or nonmedicated and may contain various kinds of bases: oleaginous, or greasy, bases made from hydrocarbons such as mineral oil or petroleum jelly; W/O emulsions such as anhydrous lanolin, lanolin, or cold cream; O/W emulsions such as hydrophilic ointment; and water-soluble or greaseless bases such as polyethylene glycol ointment. Ointments are packaged in jars or tubes.

Pastes are like ointments but contain more solid materials and consequently are stiffer and apply more thickly. Examples are zinc oxide paste, an astringent, and acetonide dental paste, an anti-inflammatory preparation.

Creams are considered O/W emulsions. They apply smoothly to the skin and leave a very thin film. Most creams are considered vanishing, which means they are invisible once applied. Like ointments, they are packaged in jars or tubes.

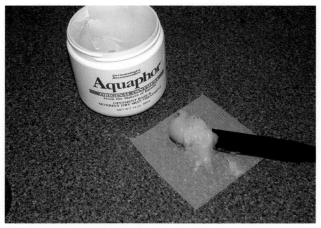

Ointments are referred to as water-in-oil (W/O) preparations. They contain a small amount of water dispersed throughout an oil. They will apply smoothly to the skin, but will often leave the skin with a greasy feeling. Ointments are often yellowish and opaque.

Gas, Vapor, and Other Dosage Forms

Gases, vapors, solutions, or suspensions intended to be inhaled via the nasal or oral respiratory routes are known as inhalations.

A spray is a dosage form that consists of a container with a valve assembly that, when activated, emits a fine dispersion of liquid, solid, and/or gaseous material. An aerosol is a spray in a pressurized container that contains a propellant, an inert liquid or gas under pressure meant to carry the active ingredient to its location of application. Depending on the formulation of the product and on the design of the valve, an aerosol may emit a fine mist, a coarse liquid spray, or a foam. One type of aerosol is the foam spray aerosol, which produces a water-in-oil emulsion when the liquid dispersed phase within the spray container vaporizes into the air.

Most sprays and aerosols are for topical application to the skin or to mucous membranes, but some are inhalation aerosols, meant to be breathed in through the nose or mouth. Sprays and aerosols are commonly used to deliver over-the-counter local anesthetics, antiseptics, deodorants, and, in the case of breath sprays, flavorings. They are also used to deliver prescription drugs. Sprays and aerosols are often used for decongestants and for antiasthmatic and antiallergic drugs.

Delivery Systems

Modern prescription drugs often are created using a high level of technology and in some cases the technology is carrying over to the way a medication is delivered to the patient. Delivery systems used to deliver specific medications are often manufactured and packaged as a unit and then dispensed as a unit for the patient. They contain not only the medication but a specialized delivery mechanism. The wide variety of delivery systems available offer patients a welcome alternative to traditional administration.

INHALATION DELIVERY SYSTEMS Gases such as oxygen and ether are administered by inhalation. Medicated inhalations are often administered via devices such as handheld, breath-activated, propellant-driven inhalers or atomizing machines known as nebulizers, which deliver mists containing extremely small, or micronized, powders. These devices are effective at getting the medication directly to the area intended in the lungs. In some cases the medication is intended to be applied "topically" to the surface of the bronchi and lungs, such as with asthma medications. And in other cases the medication is intended to be absorbed rapidly and put into the blood stream. In fact this method of administration is the most rapid method of administering any medication. For example, general anesthetics used during surgical procedures utilize this route and dosage form. Common vehicles for inhalation solutions include Sterile Water for Inhalation (USP) and sodium chloride inhalation. The solution is placed in a device that will aerosolize both the medication and the vehicle. An example of a medication delivered by inhalation is albuterol for relief of spasms caused by bronchial asthma and amyl nitrite as a vasodilator (a blood vessel expander). Vaporizers and humidifiers are machines commonly used to deliver moisture to the air for relief of cold symptoms. Volatile medications can be used with some vaporizers.

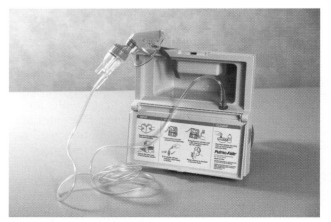
Nebulizers, also called atomizing machines, are effective for delivering mists or micronized powders to the lungs.

SYRINGE, INJECTION, AND INFUSION DELIVERY SYSTEMS Injections, also known as bolus or intravenous push delivery systems, make use of syringes, calibrated devices used to accurately draw up and measure medication and then deliver it to a patient through a needle. The parts of a syringe and needle will be explained in more detail in Chapter 10. The thickness of the needle and size of its lumen are referred to as the gauge, ranging from 30 gauge (the smallest) to 13 gauge (the largest). Because injections introduce medication into the body, they must be sterile. Injections should be given only by trained professionals and healthcare providers, and some risk to the patient is always present. Some medications are in an injection form only, such as insulin. Morphine is available in a tablet form and in an injectable form. Both are effective, however, the injectable form acts more rapidly and controls acute pain effectively. Two types of syringes commonly used for injections are glass and plastic. Glass syringes are fairly expensive and must be sterilized between uses, whereas plastic syringes are easy to handle, disposable, and come from the manufacturer in sterile packaging.

Common types of syringes (see Figure 4.6) include the insulin syringe, used by healthcare professionals and in self-administration of insulin. The tuberculin syringe has a cannula that contains 0.01 to 1.0 mL of liquid. The larger hypodermic syringes have cannulas that range from 3 to 60 mL of liquid.

Unit dose disposable syringes are prefilled syringes that contain a single premeasured dose of medication and are thrown away after use. Syringes used without

Figure 4.6

Typical Syringes
(a) Hypodermic syringes in 6 cc and 3 cc sizes. (b) Insulin syringes in 100 unit and 50 unit sizes. (c) A tuberculin syringe marked with both metric and apothecary measures.

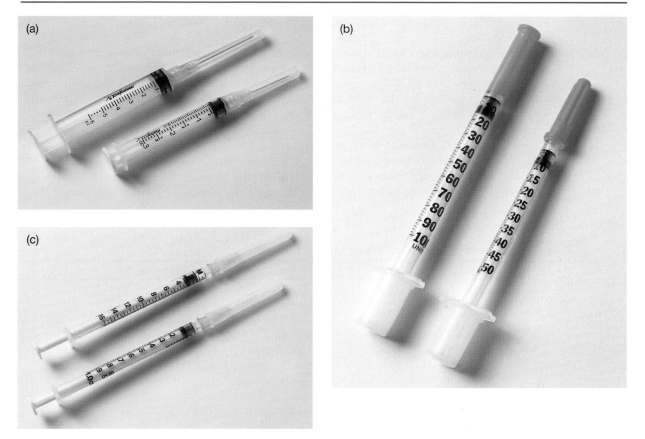

needles include the oral syringe, for oral solutions, and the bulb syringe, for topical solutions (such as irrigation). Injections may be administered to almost any organ or part of the body.

The most common route is intravenous (IV) injection, made into a vein. Also common are intradermal (ID), or intracutaneous, injections made into the skin; subcutaneous (SC, subq., SQ, hypodermic, or hypo) injections made under the skin; and intramuscular (IM) injections made into a muscle. Table 4.1 lists the common routes for parenteral injection and infusion.

In addition to syringes, devices available for injection include patient-controlled analgesia (PCA) devices, which are programmable machines that deliver small doses of pain killers on demand; jet injectors, which use pressure rather than a needle to deliver the medication; and ambulatory injection devices that the patient can wear while moving about. Some injection devices make use of pumps that regulate the amount, rate, and/or timing of injections. Injectables come prefilled or are filled at the time of injection from, most commonly, single- or multi-dose vials, small glass or plastic bottles. Sometimes the medication comes in ampules, small glass containers that are opened by breaking off the neck of the container. Because of the danger of contaminating the medication with glass particles, medication that comes in ampules must be filtered before it is injected. (For more information on injections, see Chapter 10.)

Intravenous infusion is a method for delivering a large amount of liquid over a prolonged period of time and at a slow, steady rate into the blood system. Infusions are used to deliver blood, water, other fluids, nutrients such as lipids and sugars, electrolytes, and drugs. When drugs, in a separate container, are added to an intravenous infusion, they are said to be piggybacked. Typical uses of infusions are to deliver pain-killing medications, or analgesics; to replenish body fluids; and to deliver nutrients to patients who cannot or will not feed themselves.

INTRAUTERINE AND CERVICAL DELIVERY SYSTEMS An intrauterine delivery system is a drug-releasing device placed into the uterus. One such device is used to release progesterone to prevent pregnancy. There are also devices that remain in the vagina and are placed as a ring surrounding the cervix and slowly release medication. They are replaced monthly by the patient and used as contraceptive aids.

TRANSDERMAL DELIVERY SYSTEMS (TDSs) A transdermal delivery system, or patch, is a dosage form meant for delivery percutaneously (through the skin) and consists of a backing, a drug reservoir, a control membrane, an adhesive layer, and a protective strip. The strip is removed, and the adhesive layer is attached to the skin. Drug

Table 4.1	Routes for Parenteral Injection and Infusion
Type	**Site of Delivery of Parenteral Solution**
intra-arterial (IA)	into artery
intra-articular	into joints
intracardiac	into heart
intradermal (intracutaneous) (ID)	into skin
intramuscular (IM)	into muscle
intraspinal	into spinal column
intrathecal (IT)	into spinal fluid
intravenous (IV)	into vein
subcutaneous (SC)	under skin

movement is by osmosis through the control membrane, delivering medication systemically, rather than locally. In some patches, the rate of drug delivery is controlled by the membrane. Whereas in others it is controlled by the skin itself. Medications given with this dosage form can be controlled over 24 hours or longer. Patient convenience and compliance are improved with the use of transdermal patches. Occasionally, patients develop allergies to the adhesives and chemicals in the drug matrix of the patch and thus requires discontinuation of use. The patient may try an alternate brand if one is available. Examples of drugs administered using transdermal delivery systems include nitroglycerin for relief of angina, clonidine for control of hypertension, estrogen for treatment of menopausal symptoms, testosterone for treatment of testosterone deficiency, and nicotine for relief of tobacco cravings.

Transdermal patches should always be disposed of properly after use. Even after the specified time of use, enough medication remains in the patch to harm a small child or pet if it were to be applied or ingested.

OTHER DELIVERY SYSTEMS An oral syringe is a calibrated device consisting of a plunger and a cannula, or barrel, used without a needle for administration of precisely measured amounts of medication by mouth.

A bulb syringe, consisting of a bulb and a tapering funnel with a hollow end, is used to administer liquids topically, as for irrigation. The bulb is first depressed to expel the air that it contains, and the tip is then inserted into the liquid to be administered. The bulb is released while the end is in the liquid, and liquid rises to fill the vacuum thus created. The end of the bulb is then removed from the liquid, and the liquid is administered by depressing the bulb again.

Like a bulb syringe, a dropper uses a bulb to create a vacuum for drawing up a liquid. A dropper contains a small, squeezable bulb at one end and a hollow glass or plastic tube with a tapering point. The dropper may be incorporated into the cap of a vial or other container. As a unit of pharmaceutical measurement for droppers or for intravenous infusions, drop is abbreviated gtt. Because of the differing viscosities (the thicknesses and flow characteristics) of differing fluids, the size of a drop varies considerably from medication to medication. Droppers are often used for otic or ophthalmic administration of medications.

A mucilage is a viscous, adhesive, semisolid, or semiliquid containing a sticky vegetable extractive, with or without additional active ingredients.

Ocular inserts are small, transparent membranes containing medications that are placed between the eye and the lower conjunctiva (the mucous membrane on the inside of the eyelid). An example is the product with the brand name Ocusert, used to deliver pilocarpine for the treatment of glaucoma.

Some hospices and long-term care facilities make use of straws (long, hollow tubes) prefilled with medications.

One contraceptive commonly used in the past consisted of a polyurethane sponge containing a spermicide, nonoxynol 9.

Chapter Summary

Drugs are natural, synthetic, synthesized, or semisynthetic substances, generally compounded and generally taken into or applied to the body to alter biochemical functions and thus to achieve therapeutic, pharmacodynamic, or prophylactic results. Some drugs are also used as diagnostic or destructive agents. Drugs combine active with inert ingredients and can be classified as over-the-counter or legend. Drugs are administered in many dosage forms and using many delivery systems. The choice of dosage form/delivery system is based upon what active ingredient is to be delivered, how much is to be delivered, by what means or route, to what sites, at what rate, over what period of time, and for what purpose.

Solid dosage forms include hard and soft shell capsules, effervescent salts, implants or pellets, lozenges, pills, plasters, powders and granules, suppositories, and tablets. Tablets may be single compression, multiple compression, molded, coated, chewable, controlled release, effervescent, and/or formulated for buccal, sublingual, or vaginal use. Tablets used in compounding include tablet triturates, hypodermic tablets, and dispensing tablets. Liquid dosage forms include such solutions as aromatic waters, collodions, diluted acids, elixirs, enemas, extractives such as tinctures and fluidextracts, irrigating solutions or douches, liniments, parenteral solutions, spirits, or syrups, as well as such dispersions as suspensions and emulsions, including gels, jellies, magmas or milks, and microemulsions. Topical solutions include creams, lotions, ointments, and pastes. Delivery systems include syringe, injection, and infusion devices; intrauterine and cervical systems; transdermal delivery systems; droppers and oral syringes; mucilages; ocular inserts; prefilled straws, and sponges.

Chapter Review

Knowledge Inventory

Choose the best answer from those provided.

1. A biochemically reactive component in a drug is known as
   a. an inert ingredient.
   b. an active ingredient.
   c. a diluent.
   d. a vehicle.

2. A National Drug Code number does not identify the
   a. product manufacturer.
   b. drug.
   c. packaging size and type.
   d. schedule of the drug.

3. A radiopharmaceutical used for imaging is an example of a
   a. therapeutic agent.
   b. pharmacodynamic agent.
   c. diagnostic agent
   d. prophylactic agent.

4. When people use the term *delivery system*, they generally intend, in addition to the dosage form, to refer to the
   a. physical characteristics of the dosage form that determine the method of administration and the site of action of the drug.
   b. restrictions placed upon the ordering, storage, and dispensing of the drug due to its classification under the Comprehensive Drug Abuse Prevention and Control Act.
   c. chemical composition of the drug, including its active ingredients, inert ingredients, and any colorings, flavorings, preservatives, disintegrants, solubilizers, and emulsifying agents.
   d. use of the drug as a therapeutic, pharmacodynamic, diagnostic, prophylactic, or destructive agent.

5. A dosage form used in the rectum, vagina, and urethra is the
   a. inhalation aerosol.
   b. suppository.
   c. elixir.
   d. fluidextract.

6. Enteric coatings
   a. dissolve in the stomach.
   b. dissolve in the intestines.
   c. are comprised of sugar for palatability.
   d. are made of polymers and form a protective film.

7. A solution containing water and ethanol would be described as
   a. hydroalcoholic.
   b. aqueous.
   c. extractive.
   d. immiscible.

8. Some examples of dispersions are
   a. suspensions and emulsions.
   b. tinctures, fluidextracts, and extracts.
   c. aromatic waters and diluted acids.
   d. elixirs and syrups.

9. Dosage forms that are often or always sweetened include
   a. parenteral solutions, spirits, and tinctures.
   b. medicated syrups, elixirs, and fluidextracts.
   c. collodions, microemulsions, and unguents.
   d. liniments, diluted acids, and extracts.

10. Most emulsions are considered dual-phase systems, but one kind of emulsion that is considered single phase is
    a. milk.
    b. gel.
    c. jelly.
    d. magma.

Pharmacy in Practice

1. Recombinant DNA will, in the future, play a great role in gene therapies, in which recombinant DNA is used to supply the body with genes to supplement or replace the action of the existing genes with which the body is endowed. Do some research on gene therapy for the treatment of cystic fibrosis, the most common of all fatal genetic diseases. Such therapy uses a cold virus containing recombinant DNA that carries a gene called the cystic fibrosis transmembrane regulator. Prepare a brief report explaining how such therapy works. In your report, give particular attention to the pharmaceutical implications of gene therapy. If a missing gene is supplied by means of a virus containing recombinant DNA, what dosage form might be used to deliver this virus?

2. Determine the dosage form and indication for the following gene therapy or biotechnology based medications:
   a. epoetin alpha
   b. enfavirenz
   c. infliximab
   d. somatropin
   e. trastuzumab
   f. becaplermin
   g. palivizumab

3. A tree diagram is a chart that shows a classification system. A single characteristic is used to differentiate the items classified under each node on the chart. For example, a tree chart might classify animals in this way:

ANIMALS

Vertebrates (with backbones)
- mammals
- reptiles
- fish
- birds
- amphibians

Invertebrates (without backbones)
- flatworms
- roundworms
- insects
- arachnids
- mollusks

Create tree charts to classify
  a. liquid dosage forms
  b. solutions (by vehicle)
  c. solutions (by contents)
  d. solutions (by site or method of administration)
  e. dispersions (by size of the dispersed ingredients)
  f. dispersions (by type of substance in the dispersed phase)

4. Go to a community or retail pharmacy and make a list of five over-the-counter products in as many different dosage forms as you can identify. For each product on your list, give the manufacturer, the brand name, the active ingredient(s), and the dosage form/delivery system.

5. Different dosage forms have different pros and cons. For example, tablets and capsules are premeasured (pro) but may be difficult for some patients to swallow (con). Create a table comparing the ease of administration, dangers of contamination, duration of shelf-life, ease of obtaining patient compliance, suitability for patients of various ages or conditions, uniformity of dosage size, control of dosage rate, and site of application for each dosage form.

Dosage form	Advantages	Disadvantages
a. tablets		
b. capsules		
c. injections (IM and SC)		
d. IV infusions		
e. syrup		
f. sublingual tablet		
g. transdermal patch		
h. suppository		

Improving Communication Skills

1. A prescription has been brought in for a steroid cream (0.25%) to be applied to an infant's eczema on the cheeks. The mother states that she has the same drug at home in an ointment (1%) and wants to know if she should just use what she has at home since the drug is so expensive. Creams and ointments are very different, and in this case the strength is different as well. What will the pharmacist tell this mother about the differences between the two products?

2. A young man has come in to pick up some prescriptions for his asthma. His physician has just changed his prescription from oral prednisone to an inhaled steroid to control an exacerbation of his asthma and bronchitis. The physician told the patient that the inhaled product would be safer for him in the long run. What are the advantages of the inhaled products over the oral tablets?

3. An elderly man has just picked up two prescriptions for nitroglycerin. One was for sublingual tablets and the other was for transdermal patches. Why is the patient using two different forms of the same drug? What are the advantages of each?

Internet Research

1. The Human Genome Project is mapping the entire human gene "pool." What scientists learn from this project about diseases and their cause has the possibility to change forever the manner in which physicians treat many diseases. There are many websites devoted to the human genome, genetic diseases, and the implications this project has on modern medicine. Select a genetic disease to research and visit Web sites to find out what is known. Prepare a two-page report on your findings. Include a description of the disease, the current prognosis, and a description of what has been learned about the mapping of the disease. Include a list of references.

2. The ethical implications of the Human Genome Project are very serious and involve the pharmacy directly. Physicians may someday be able to instantly diagnose a disease based on the patient's genetic makeup. And drug therapies may be designed specifically for a patient based on the genetic makeup of the patient. Physicians, pharmacists, and many members of the healthcare team will need to access a patient's genetic information. Consider some of the ethical implications of this project and prepare for a class discussion by listing some of the considerations involved and your opinion regarding this issue.

Routes of Drug Administration

Learning Objectives

- Define the phrase *route of administration*.
- Enumerate the reasons why a particular route of administration is chosen over the others available.
- Explain the first-pass effect.
- List the major routes of administration and the dosage forms, advantages, and disadvantages associated with each.

Since ancient times, medications have been administered orally and topically. In the modern era, a wide variety of additional ways to get medications into the body have been developed. This chapter describes those ways.

FACTORS INFLUENCING THE ROUTE OF ADMINISTRATION

As the previous chapter on dosage forms explained, drugs come in many different forms. These forms have been designed by pharmaceutical scientists for administration or application to the body in a wide variety of ways. Many factors determine the choice of route, or way of getting a drug onto or into the body.

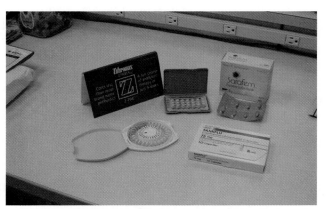

A variety of prepackaged products are now available. Such packaging tremendously improves patient compliance.

Compliance

Compliance is when a patient takes a drug in the amount, on the schedule, and as prescribed. Some drug dosage forms (e.g., flavored and sugared syrups or chewable tablets) are specifically designed to improve compliance by patients.

Ease of Administration

Many people have particular qualities or characteristics that determine to some extent the route of administration chosen. In some situations, patients are unable, because of lack of consciousness, to perform an action such as

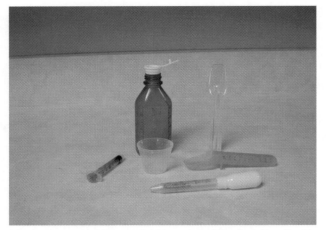

Infants or young children might have less difficulty taking liquid medication that is administered with one of these devices.

swallowing a tablet, capsule, or liquid. A very young or elderly patient might have difficulty swallowing, and in such a case the healthcare provider might have to avoid solid, orally administered dosage forms in favor of oral liquid dosage forms or other, nonoral routes of administration. An oral route of administration might also be inadvisable for a patient experiencing nausea and vomiting, which may expel the drug prematurely from the body.

Site of Action

One obvious factor affecting the choice of route of administration is the desired site of action of the drug. A major distinction can be drawn between drugs intended for local or systemic use. The term *local use* refers to site-specific applications of drugs, for example, when one applies an analgesic ointment to a minor burn or takes an antacid for local relief of excessive gastric acid. The term *systemic use* refers to the application of a drug by means of absorption into the blood and subsequent transportation throughout the body. Of course, even when a drug is meant for systemic administration, it still is usually targeted to specific sites of action. The nature of the disease state being treated and the drugs and dosage forms available aid the physician in determining the route for which a medication is best suited.

Rate of Action

Different routes of administration work more or less quickly. That is, they have different onset rates. In general, the fastest method of administration for action within the body is intravenously. The drug is injected or infused directly into the blood stream and carried immediately throughout the body.

Duration of Action

A route of administration may be chosen on a basis of its action over a long period. For example, a transdermal patch can be used to deliver small amounts of a drug, steadily, over many hours. A similar sustained duration effect can be achieved by means of intravenous infusion.

Quantity of Drug

Sometimes, a route of administration is chosen because of the amount of a drug that must be delivered. A tablet containing a lot of filler, or diluent, might be a preferred method for administering a drug containing a very small amount (e.g., 0.5 mg) of an active ingredient. Intravenous infusion is an excellent method for systemic delivery of large quantities of material, such as blood or glucose.

Susceptibility to Metabolism by the Liver

Drugs differ in their resistance to metabolism by the liver. Some drugs, nitroglycerin for example, are given in very small doses and can then be diluted by gastrointestinal fluids and broken down by the liver in what is known as the first-pass effect. Such drugs have to be given by a means to bypass or overcome metabolism by the liver.

Toxicity

Toxicology is the study of adverse effects of drugs or other substances on the body. Drugs are potent substances, and often their dangers, or toxicity, must be weighed against their therapeutic benefits. Sometimes the toxicity of a drug directly affects the route of administration chosen. For example, a caustic drug that might cause damage if delivered intravenously might be delivered orally instead.

ROUTES OF ADMINISTRATION

A wide variety of routes of administration are currently employed in medicine.

Oral and Peroral

The term *oral* is used to refer to two very different methods of administration—applying topically to the mouth (as for local treatment of a cold sore) and, more commonly, swallowing. The latter route of administration, for local application to parts of the gastrointestinal tract or for absorption along that tract into systemic circulation, is more properly and precisely referred to as peroral.

DOSAGE FORMS Dosage forms for oral or peroral administration include capsules, elixirs, gels, lozenges (also known as troches or pastilles), magmas, powders, solutions, suspensions, syrups, and tablets.

ADVANTAGES AND DISADVANTAGES The peroral route of administration is by far the most common because of the ease and safety of administration. In the case of capsules or tablets, the active ingredient is generally contained in powders or granules. These dissolve or disaggregate in the gastrointestinal tract, and the active ingredient becomes available for absorption into the blood stream. Disadvantages of the peroral route include delayed onset, because the dosage form must disintegrate before it is absorbed; first-pass metabolism by the liver; and destruction or dilution of the drug by gastrointestinal fluids and/or food or drink present in the stomach or intestines. The peroral route is not indicated in patients who are experiencing nausea or vomiting or who are comatose, sedated, or otherwise unable to swallow. Unpleasant taste is another disadvantage of some peroral dosage forms, requiring that the taste be masked by flavorings to promote compliance.

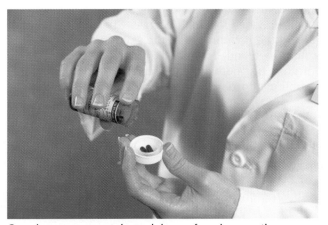

Capsules are a commonly used dosage form because they are easy and safe to dispense.

Sublingual and Buccal

In sublingual administration, the drug is placed under the tongue, where it is absorbed by the sublingual mucosa. In buccal administration, the drug is placed between the gums and the inner lining of the cheek, in the so-called buccal pouch, where it is absorbed by the buccal mucosa. Mucosa, or mucous membranes, are linings of interior surfaces of the body that are rich in blood and lymph vessels and communicate to the exterior.

DOSAGE FORMS Dosage forms for sublingual and buccal administration include tablets and lozenges.

ADVANTAGES AND DISADVANTAGES Sublingual and buccal routes of administration are very rapid in onset (though somewhat slower than intravenous routes) and are thus appropriate for immediate relief, as in use of nitroglycerin for treatment of chest pain due to angina pectoris. However, this route of administration is not appropriate for delivery of medication over an extended period.

Epicutaneous (Topical) or Transdermal

Epicutaneous administration is the application of a drug directly to the surface of the skin. This route of administration is commonly referred to as topical. Drugs applied topically are not designed to be well absorbed into the deeper layers of the skin, and thus they are used most frequently to treat local conditions. Few medications used in this manner are systemically absorbed, however transdermal administration is delivery of a drug via absorption through the skin, especially via a drug-containing patch or disk. The transdermal route is utilized when the drug is intended for systemic absorption.

DOSAGE FORMS Dosage forms for epicutaneous or transdermal administration include aerosols, creams, lotions, ointments, pastes, plasters, powders, and transdermal patches or disks.

ADVANTAGES AND DISADVANTAGES The epicutaneous administration route is superb for local effects. Drugs given epicutaneously for local effects include anesthetics, anti-inflammatories, antifungals, antiseptics, astringents, moisturizers, pediculicides (for killing lice), protectants (e.g., sunscreen), and scabicides (for killing mites). Drugs, such as nicotine, nitroglycerin, and clonidine, are administered epicutaneously for percutaneous (beneath the skin) effects. The skin presents a barrier to ready absorption. However, absorption does occur, slowly, via hair follicles, pores, sebaceous glands, and sweat glands. Relatively small amounts of the drug will be absorbed into the blood vascular system. For percutaneous delivery, the epicutaneous route is slow in onset but relatively long lasting. Transdermal administration of a drug is a convenient way to administer medication intended for systemic use. Chemicals in the patch or disc will force the drug across the membranes of the skin and into the layer of skin where optimal absorption into the blood stream will occur. The site of administration must be rotated and it must be relatively hair free. The transdermal route offers a method of administering medications that will provide a steady level of drug in the system.

Ocular, Conjunctival, Nasal, and Otic

Ocular administration is the application of a drug to the eye. Conjunctival administration is the application of a drug to the conjunctival mucosa, the lining of the inside of the eyelid. Nasal administration is the application of a drug into the passages of the nose. Otic administration is the application of a drug to the ear canal.

Dosage Forms Dosage forms for ocular administration include drug-impregnated contact lenses, solutions, and suspensions. Dosage forms for conjunctival administration include ointments and the Ocusert delivery system, which is an elliptical form for delivery of pilocarpine. Dosage forms for nasal administration include inhalants, ointments, solutions, and sprays. Dosage forms for otic administration include solutions and suspensions.

Advantages and Disadvantages The ocular, conjunctival, nasal, and otic routes of administration are almost always for local effects, to treat conditions of the eye, the nose or sinuses, or the ear. Sprays for inhalation through the nose, however, may be used for systemic effects.

Rectal

Rectal administration is the application of a drug to or within the rectum.

Dosage Forms Dosage forms for rectal administration include ointments, solutions, and suppositories.

Advantages and Disadvantages A major disadvantage of the rectal route of administration is its inconvenience. Another disadvantage is that absorption by the rectal mucosa is erratic and unpredictable. However, such a route is, of course, preferable for local effects (e.g., for cleansing the rectum, administration of laxatives or cathartics, treatment of hemorrhoids, or delivery of barium prior to radiographic examination of the gastrointestinal tract). This may be a preferred method of delivery for systemic drugs in situations in which the drug might be destroyed or diluted by gastrointestinal fluids, in which an oral dosage form is precluded by lack of consciousness or nausea and vomiting, or in which the drug might be too readily metabolized by the liver. Suppositories, solid forms that melt or dissolve in the rectum, may be used to promote discharge of the bowels or to deliver a drug. The large number of blood and lymph vessels lining the walls of the rectum make drug absorption at this administration site quite good, though irregular. Ointments are used for local effects. Rectal solutions, or enemas, are used for cleansing and as laxatives or cathartics.

Vaginal and Urethral

The vaginal route of administration is application of a drug within the vagina. The urethral route of administration is application of a drug to or within the urethra.

Dosage Forms Dosage forms for vaginal administration include emulsion foams, inserts, ointments, solutions, sponges, suppositories, and tablets. Dosage forms for urethral administration include solutions and suppositories and may be effective in treating incontinence or impotence in men.

Advantages and Disadvantages Generally speaking, these routes of administration are for local effects such as cleansing (e.g., douches), contraception, or treatment of infection. Just as with the rectal route, patients often find this route inconvenient.

Intrarespiratory

The intrarespiratory route of administration is application of a drug through inhalation into the lungs. Typically, this inhalation occurs through the mouth.

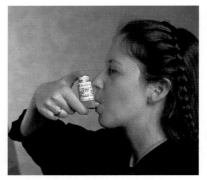
A metered dose inhaler is a common device used to administer a drug through inhalation into the lungs.

DOSAGE FORMS The usual dosage form for intrarespiratory administration is gas or aerosol. However, volatile liquids can also be given in this manner.

ADVANTAGES AND DISADVANTAGES
The lungs are designed for absorption of oxygen into the bloodstream. Therefore, they are an excellent site for absorption of gases or drugs. Entry into the bloodstream is extremely rapid, second only to direct injection or infusion. The intrarespiratory route is used to deliver bronchodilaters to asthma sufferers, to provide oxygen to those suffering from oxygen deprivation, and to deliver general anesthetics.

Parenteral

Parenteral administration is injection or infusion by means of a needle or catheter inserted into the body. The parenteral route, because of its complexity, is discussed in detail in the next section.

DOSAGE FORMS Injection or infusion of sterile solutions or suspensions.

ADVANTAGES AND DISADVANTAGES The parenteral route is the one of the fastest of all methods for delivering systemic drugs, but it has associated dangers, including traumatic injury from the insertion of the needle or catheter into the body and the potential for introducing toxic agents, microbes, or pyrogens (fever-producing byproducts of microbial metabolism).

MORE ON PARENTERAL ADMINISTRATION

Parenteral forms deserve special attention because of complexity, widespread use, and potential for therapeutic benefit and danger. The term *parenteral* comes from the Greek words *para,* meaning "outside," and *enteron,* meaning "the intestine." The derivation of the word refers to the fact that this route of administration bypasses the alimentary canal. A parenteral preparation is administered directly into the body, generally, but not always, directly into the blood stream. Because of this it is relatively irretrievable. If an adverse reaction occurs, one cannot retrieve or remove the dose from the body.

Characteristics of Parenteral Preparations

Parenteral preparations must be sterile. That is, they must be free of microorganisms and so are prepared using aseptic techniques that ensure sterility. They are either solutions (in which ingredients are dissolved) or, much less commonly, suspensions (in which ingredients are suspended). The body is primarily an aqueous, or water-containing, vehicle, and so most parenteral preparations introduced into the body are made up of ingredients placed in a sterile water medium. In the case of intravenous infusions the vehicle commonly used is dextrose in water, normal saline solution, or dextrose in saline solution. Some parenteral solutions, however, may be oleaginous, or oily. For example, an emulsion containing fat may be administered in some cases to supply extra calories to patients who cannot or will not feed themselves and who need more calories than can be supplied by dextrose in water. Most parenterals are introduced directly into the blood stream and must be free of air bubbles or particulate matter. The introduction of air or particles might cause an embolism, or blockage, in a vessel.

Parenteral preparations must also have chemical properties that will not damage vessels or blood cells nor alter the chemical properties of the blood serum. Generally speaking, parenterals must be iso-osmotic (having the same number of particles in solution per unit volume) and isotonic (having the same osmotic pressure) with blood. The osmolality, or amount of particulate per unit volume of a liquid preparation, is measured in milliosmoles (mOsm). The osmolality of blood serum is approximately 285 mOsm/L. Osmolality and tonicity, while similar, are not exactly the same because blood cells are more or less permeable by various chemical substances. A parenteral solution of greater than normal tonicity is said to be hypertonic. Such a solution has a greater number of particles than the blood cells themselves. A solution of less than normal tonicity is said to be hypotonic. A hypotonic solution has fewer numbers of particles than blood cells. Pharmacists sometimes have to adjust the tonicity of parenteral preparations to ensure that they are not hypertonic or hypotonic. On occasion, it is necessary to administer hypertonic solutions, but this must be done very slowly and cautiously. The degree of acidity or alkalinity of a solution is known as its pH value. If a solution has a pH of less than 7, it is acidic. If it has a pH value of more than 7, it is alkaline. Blood plasma has a pH of 7.4; it is slightly alkaline. Parenteral solutions, if they are not to alter the acidity or alkalinity of the blood, must have a pH value close to neutral.

Methods of Injection

The bolus, or injection, is one of the most common routes of administration. The injection is performed using a syringe. Many injectables come prepackaged in the form of filled, disposable plastic syringes. At other times, the injectable drug must be taken up into the syringe from a single- or multi-dose glass or plastic vial, or from a glass ampule. In some cases, as with lyophilized powder, the solid drug in the vial has to be reconstituted by addition of a liquid (generally sterile water for injection) before use. A vial may be clear, or light amber (to protect the drug from exposure to light).

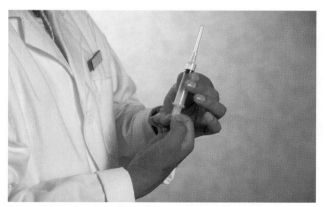
Disposable syringes and needles are used to administer drugs by injection. There are different sizes available depending on the type of medication and injection needed.

Routes of Parenteral Administration

Injections may be made into almost any part of the body. The most common sort of injection is one done by the intravenous (IV) route, directly into a vein. However, other common forms are intradermal (ID) (or intracutaneous) injections made into the skin, subcutaneous (SC, subq., SQ, hypodermic, or hypo) injections made under the skin, and intramuscular (IM) injections made into a muscle.

INTRAVENOUS Intravenous drug administration, by injection or by infusion is an extremely fast-acting route because the drug goes directly into the blood stream. Because of their rapid delivery, intravenous injection and infusion are often used in emergency situations. Commonly, intravenous injections and infusions are given into the superficial veins of the arm on the side opposite the elbow, though other sites are used. Figure 5.1 shows an intravenous injection.

INTRADERMAL Intradermal injections, given into the more capillary-rich layer just below the epidermis (Figure 5.2), are given for local anesthesia and for various diagnostic tests and immunizations. A typical site for such injections is the upper forearm, below the area where intravenous injections are given.

SUBCUTANEOUS Subcutaneous injections, usually of very small amounts (less than 2 mL), are given just beneath the skin (Figure 5.3), usually on the outside of the upper arm, the top of the thigh, or the lower portion of the abdomen. Insulin, the most common of subcutaneous injections, is given using 28 to 30 gauge needles, and the site is varied from injection to injection. A special insulin syringe is used, which has a short needle and measures insulin in units.

INTRAMUSCULAR Intramuscular injections, appropriate in most cases for no more than 3 mL of drug, are slower in delivery but longer in duration than intravenous ones. Care must be taken with deep intramuscular injections to avoid hitting a vein, artery, or nerve. In adults, intramuscular injections are generally given into the upper, outer portion of the gluteus maximus, the large muscle on either side of the buttocks. Another common site, especially for children, is the deltoid muscles of the shoulders. Figure 5.4 shows the needle angle and injection depth for an intramuscular injection.

Not much will be said of parenteral infusions here, as these are treated in detail in Chapter 10. Intravenous infusions, or IVs, deliver large amounts of liquid into the

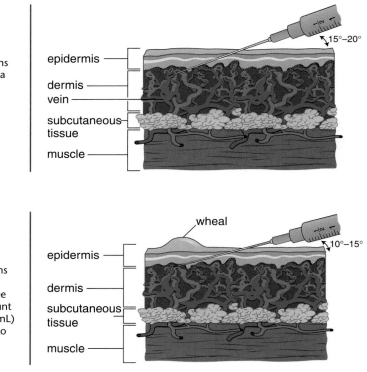

Figure 5.1

Intravenous Injection
Intravenous injections are administered at a fifteen- to twenty-degree angle.

epidermis
dermis
vein
subcutaneous tissue
muscle

15°–20°

Figure 5.2

Intradermal Injection
Intradermal injections pierce the skin at a ten- to fifteen-degree angle. A small amount of medication (0.1 mL) is injected slowly into the dermal layer to form a wheal.

wheal

epidermis
dermis
subcutaneous tissue
muscle

10°–15°

Figure 5.3

Subcutaneous Injection
Subcutaneous injections usually are administered just below the skin at a forty-five-degree angle.

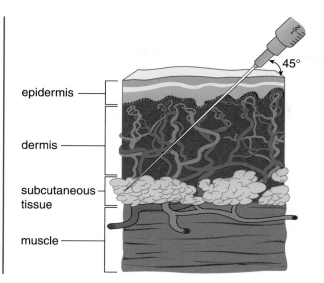

epidermis

dermis

subcutaneous tissue

muscle

45°

Figure 5.4

Intramuscular Injection
Intramuscular injections are administered at a ninety-degree angle.

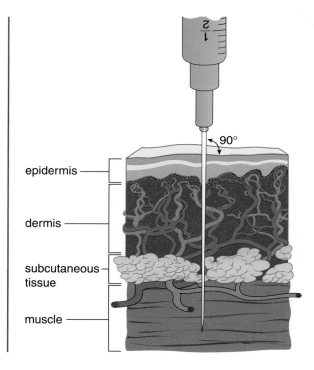

epidermis

dermis

subcutaneous tissue

muscle

90°

bloodstream, over prolonged periods of time. This route of administration is used to deliver blood, water, other fluids, nutrients such as lipids and sugars, electrolytes, and drugs. Infusions are administered using sterile, pyrogen-free IV containers and IV sets. The IV container is a vented or unvented glass bottle or a flexible, vented plastic bottle (see Figure 5.5). The IV set, or IV administration set, is a sterile, pyrogen-free, disposable unit. The set may be sterilized before use by means of radiation or ethylene oxide, or it may come in sterile packaging with a peel-off top cardboard

Figure 5.5

**Different Types of
IV Containers**

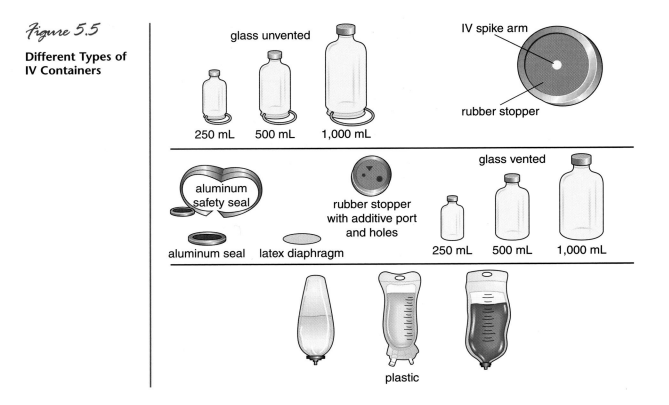

glass unvented

250 mL   500 mL   1,000 mL

IV spike arm

rubber stopper

aluminum
safety seal

rubber stopper
with additive port
and holes

glass vented

aluminum seal   latex diaphragm   250 mL   500 mL   1,000 mL

plastic

and a sealed plastic wrap. Some IV set packaging has a clear wrap for viewing the contents, while other packaging employs a diagram of the enclosed set printed on the outside of the packaging. Sets do not carry expiration dates but do carry the legend "Federal law restricts this device to sale by or on the order of a physician."

Chapter Summary

Many factors influence the decision about the many possible routes of administration chosen to deliver a particular drug or combination of drugs. These factors include patient compliance, ease of administration, site of action (local or systemic), rate of onset of action, duration of action, the quantity to be administered, the susceptibility of the drug to first-pass metabolism by the liver, and the toxicology of the drug. Possible routes of administration are oral and peroral, sublingual, buccal, epicutaneous (including transdermal), ophthalmic (ocular or conjunctival), nasal, otic, rectal, vaginal, urethral, intrarespiratory, and parenteral. Types of parenterals include injections and intravenous infusions.

Parenterals are sterile, pyrogen and particulate free, and are usually aqueous solutions. Parenterals for intravenous injection or infusion generally have osmolality, tonicity, and pH values similar to that of blood. Because parenterals are injected directly into the blood stream, special precautions must be taken in the preparation and administration. Injections are typically given intravenously, intradermally, subcutaneously, or intramuscularly. Infusions are given for a variety of purposes, including delivery of fluids, nutrients, and drugs, are administered by means of IV sets.

Chapter Review

Knowledge Inventory

Choose the best answer from those provided.

1. The willingness of a patient to take a drug in the amounts and on the schedule prescribed is called
   - a. ease of administration.
   - b. compliance.
   - c. route of administration.
   - d. factor of administration.

2. Nausea and vomiting might preclude the use of
   - a. a parenteral route of administration.
   - b. an epicutaneous route of administration.
   - c. a peroral route of administration.
   - d. a urethral route of administration.

3. In the first-pass effect, some drugs taken orally are rapidly metabolized, or broken down, by the
   - a. spleen.
   - b. bowels.
   - c. liver.
   - d. kidneys.

4. The study of adverse effects of drugs or other substances on the body is
   - a. embolism.
   - b. osmolality.
   - c. tonicity.
   - d. toxicology.

5. The most common route of administration of drugs is the
   - a. parenteral route of administration.
   - b. epicutaneous route of administration.
   - c. peroral route of administration.
   - d. intravenous route of administration.

6. A tablet placed between the gums and the inner lining of the cheek is dissolved by the
   - a. conjunctival mucosa.
   - b. sublingual mucosa.
   - c. vaginal mucosa.
   - d. buccal mucosa.

7. A transdermal patch makes use of the
   - a. percutaneous route of administration.
   - b. ophthalmic route of administration.
   - c. otic route of administration.
   - d. conjunctival route of administration.

8. Suppositories are *not* used for
    a. rectal administration.
    b. urethral administration.
    c. buccal administration.
    d. vaginal administration.

9. The word *parenteral* means, literally, "outside the
    a. stomach."
    b. intestine."
    c. mouth."
    d. liver."

10. A solution with a pH of 8 would be
    a. acidic.
    b. alkaline.
    c. hypertonic.
    d. hypotonic.

Pharmacy in Practice

1. Nitroglycerin is an example of a drug that comes in a wide variety of dosage forms appropriate for a wide variety of routes of administration. Do some research on the different routes of administration used for nitroglycerin. Refer to Internet sites to reference works, and to healthcare professionals. Pose the following questions: What are the dosage forms of nitroglycerin? What routes of administration are used? Why do people choose one route of administration over another? For what purposes are the various routes of administration used?

2. The label on a medication contains directions for using the medication, including amounts to be taken, times when these should be taken, and any other information that the prescriber deems necessary. Write a brief report explaining why it is important for a pharmacist to counsel customers or patients with regard to taking medications. How can such counseling improve compliance?

3. In a small group, discuss the advantages and disadvantages of the various routes of administration. Which are the most convenient? Which are the safest? Which are the fastest acting? Which provide for controlled release? Which last a long time? Which pose compliance problems? Present your group's opinions to the class.

4. Create a chart with a schematic diagram of the human body, illustrating the various routes of administration described in this lesson.

5. Do some research into the history of parenterals in Remington's Pharmaceutical Sciences. When were they first used? By whom? What difficulties did they present to the people who first experimented with parenteral administration? How have these difficulties been overcome? Present your findings in a report or class discussion.

Improving Communication Skills

1. A patient has come in to pick up some prescriptions for fertility drugs. Some of the medications are given SC and others IM. The pharmacist has selected the appropriate syringes for them.

   a. Which of the following syringes is for the IM injection, and which is for the SC injection?

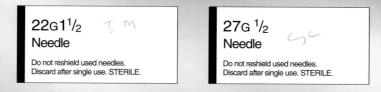

   22G1½ I M
   Needle

   Do not reshield used needles.
   Discard after single use. STERILE.

   27G ½ SC
   Needle

   Do not reshield used needles.
   Discard after single use. STERILE.

   b. Prepare a brief explanation for the patient as to which syringe is used for what, and what the technique and location for each injection is.

2. Antiviral medications are available in a variety of dosage forms and utilize a variety of routes for administration. Often the drug, dosage form, and route of administration are selected due to a specific viral infection in a specific location. Research five antiviral medications that have different dosage forms and routes of administration using a source such as Drug Facts and Comparisons. Make a list of the five drugs you have found and prepare a brief paragraph on the drugs and their indication. Use lay terms to describe the medical terms that you find.

Internet Research

1. Visit a drug information site, such as www.mayoclinic.com or www.Rxlist.com and research the following drugs. For each drug identify the dosage forms and the route by which each dosage form is administered. Each drug is available in at least two dosage forms.

   a. Imitrex
   b. Compazine
   c. Valium
   d. morphine
   e. triamcinolone
   f. Proventil

2. Go to www.baxter.com and research ten specialized delivery systems manufactured by this company and state how each is used.

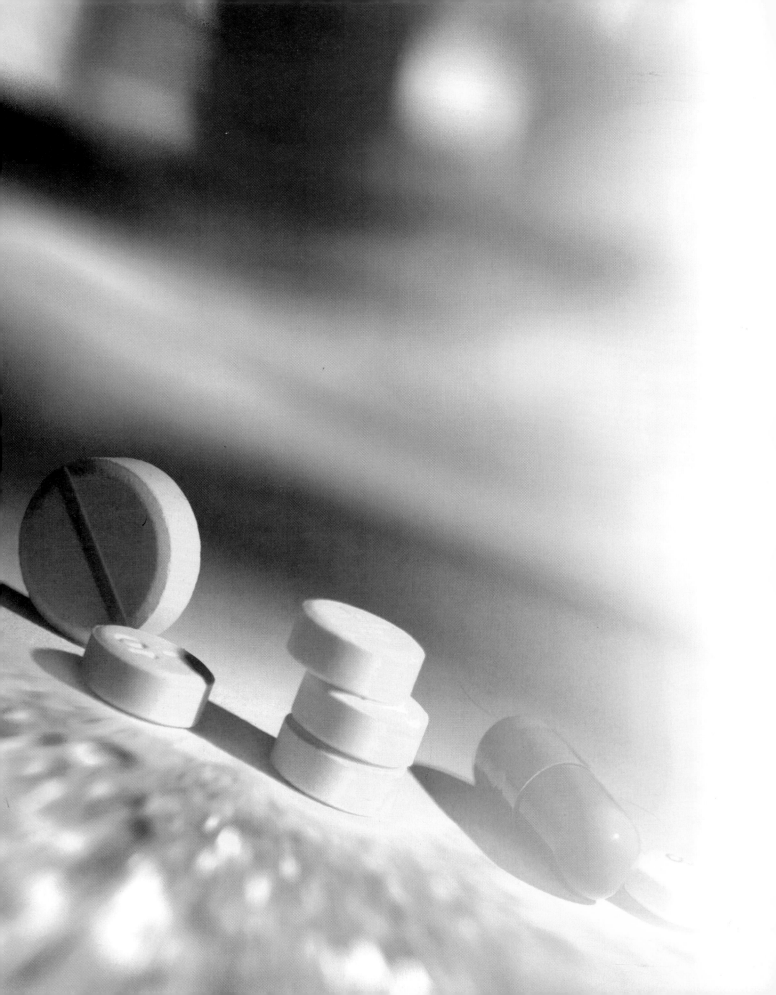

Basic Pharmaceutical Measurements and Calculations

Learning Objectives

◇ Describe four systems of measurement commonly used in pharmacy and be able to convert units from one system to another.

◇ Explain the meanings of the prefixes most commonly used in metric measurement.

◇ Convert from one metric unit to another (e.g., grams to milligrams).

◇ Convert Roman numerals to Arabic numerals.

◇ Distinguish between proper, improper, and compound fractions.

◇ Perform basic operations with fractions, including finding the least common denominator; converting fractions to decimals; and adding, subtracting, multiplying, and dividing fractions.

◇ Perform basic operations with proportions, including identifying equivalent ratios and finding an unknown quantity in a proportion.

◇ Convert percents to and from fractions and ratios and convert percents to decimals.

◇ Perform elementary dosage calculations and conversions.

◇ Calculate the molecular weight of certain substances used in the pharmacy.

◇ Compute the specific gravity of liquids.

◇ Calculate IV rates and administration.

◇ Solve problems involving powder solutions and dilutions.

◇ Use the alligation method.

◇ Calculate markup and markup rate.

◇ Compute discounts.

◇ Apply average wholesale price and capitation fee to profit calculations.

◇ Calculate inventory turnover.

The daily activities of pharmacists and pharmacy technicians require making precise measurements. Because they compound drugs and prepare parenteral infusions, the measurements of amounts or quantities and calculations that involve those quantities must always be precise. A mistake in calculation can have severe consequences. Therefore, it is essential for practicing pharmacists and technicians to grasp the basic measurement systems and mathematical techniques used in the field. This chapter introduces you to the basic systems and methods used in pharmacy.

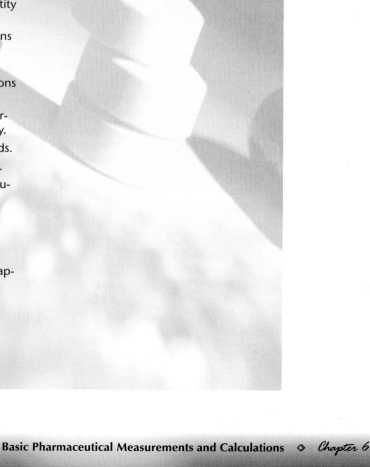

SYSTEMS OF PHARMACEUTICAL MEASUREMENT

Systems of measurement are widely accepted standards used to determine such quantities as area, distance (or length), temperature, time, volume, and weight. Of these, temperature, distance, volume, and weight are the most important for the pharmacy profession. Quantities of temperature and weight are the simplest and most familiar. Distance is a measurement of extension in space in one dimension. Area is a measurement of extension in space in two dimensions. Volume, the least intuitive of these quantities, is a measurement of extension in space in three dimensions.

The Metric System

The metric system is the measurement system most commonly used today for pharmaceutical measurement and calculation. Developed in France in the 1700s, the metric system became the legal standard of measure in the United States in 1893. Since then, it has been the system to which other measurements are compared for legal purposes.

The metric system has several distinct advantages over other measurement systems. First, the metric system is based on decimal notation, in which units are described as multiples of ten (0.001, 0.01, 0.1, 1, 10, 100, 1,000, and so on), and this decimal notation makes calculation simple. Second, the system contains clear correlations among the units of measurement of length, volume, and weight, again simplifying calculation. For example, the standard metric unit for volume, the liter, is almost exactly equivalent to 1,000 cubic centimeters. (A centimeter is a metric unit of length.) Third, with slight variations in notation, the metric system is used worldwide, especially in scientific measurement, and so, like music, is a "universal language."

Like languages, measurement systems tend to evolve by folk processes. Thus a foot was, originally, a length approximately equal to that of the average person's foot. Later, these systems become standardized by governments and professional organizations. The modern metric system makes use of the standardized units of the Système International (SI), adopted by agreement among governments worldwide in 1960. Three basic units in this system are the meter, the liter, and the gram. The meter, the unit for measuring length, has limited use in the pharmacy. The gram, the unit for measuring weight, is used in the pharmacy for measuring the amount of medication in solid form and for indicating the amount of solid medication in a solution. The gram is the weight of one cubic centimeter of water at 4° C. The liter is the unit for measuring the volume of liquid medications and also liquids for solutions. Figure 6.1 shows an application of the metric system in measuring distance, area, and volume. Distance and area are measured in meters, and volume is measured in grams.

Prefixes—syllables placed at the beginnings of words—can be added to these basic units to specify a particular measure. Because SI is a decimal system, the prefixes denote powers of ten, as shown in Table 6.1.

The metric units most commonly used in pharmacy practice, along with their abbreviations, are given in Table 6.2. Note that the same abbreviations are used for both singular and plural (1 g, 3 g).

In prescriptions using the metric system, numbers are expressed as decimals rather than fractions. Weights are generally given in grams, and volumes in milliliters.

For numbers less than 1, a zero is placed before the decimal point to prevent misreading, as in

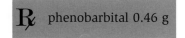

℞   phenobarbital 0.46 g

Figure 6.1

Measurements in the Metric System
(a) Distance or length.
(b) Area. (c) Volume.

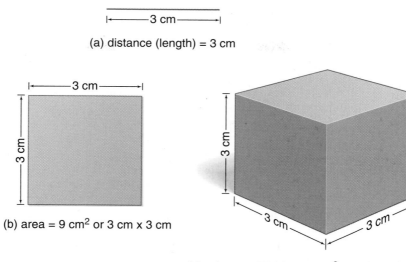

(a) distance (length) = 3 cm

(b) area = 9 cm² or 3 cm x 3 cm

(c) volume = 27 mL or 3 cm³ or 3 cm x 3 cm x 3 cm

Table 6.1   **Système International (SI) Prefixes**

Prefix	Meaning
pico-	one trillionth (basic unit × 10^{-12}, or unit × 0.000,000,000,001)
nano-	one billionth (basic unit × 10^{-9}, or unit × 0.000,000,001)
micro-	one millionth (basic unit × 10^{-6}, or unit × 0.000,001)
milli-	one thousandth (basic unit × 10^{-3}, or unit × 0.001)
centi-	one hundredth (basic unit × 10^{-2}, or unit × 0.01)
deci-	one tenth (basic unit × 10^{-1}, or unit × 0.1)
hecto-	one hundred times (basic unit × 10^{2}, or unit × 100)
kilo-	one thousand times (basic unit × 10^{3}, or unit × 1,000)
mega-	one million times (basic unit × 10^{6}, or unit × 1,000,000)
giga-	one billion times (basic unit × 10^{9}, or unit × 1,000,000,000)
tera-	one trillion times (basic unit × 10^{12}, or unit × 1,000,000,000,000)

Table 6.2   **Common Metric Units**

Weight: Gram

1 gram (g)	= 1,000 milligrams (mg)
1 milligram (mg)	= 1,000 micrograms (mcg or μg), one thousandth of a gram (g)
1 kilogram (kg)	= 1,000 grams (g)

Length: Meter

1 meter (m)	= 100 centimeters (cm)
1 centimeter (cm)	= one hundredth of a meter; 10 millimeters (mm)
1 millimeter (mm)	= one thousandth of a meter; 1,000 micrometers, or microns (mcm or μm)

Volume: Liter

1 liter (L)	= 1,000 milliliters (mL)
1 milliliter (mL)	= one thousandth of a liter, 1,000 microliters (mcL or μL)

Note that an error of a single decimal place is an error by a factor of 10. It is therefore extremely important that decimals be written properly.

To convert from one metric unit to another, simply move the decimal point to the left (to convert to larger units) and to the right (to convert to smaller units). The most common metric calculations in pharmacy involve conversions to and from milliliters and liters, and to and from grams, milligrams, and kilograms. Table 6.3 shows how to do these conversions.

Common Measure

In spite of the fact that the metric system is the legal standard of measure in the United States, many U.S. pharmacies still use the "common" measure system. The United States is practically the only industrialized country that uses this system. Common measure is made up of older systems of measure not widely used in pharmacy today. However, since they do crop up from time to time, it is a good idea to become familiar with those measurement units still used.

Three types of common measure encountered in pharmacy are apothecary measure, avoirdupois measure, and household measure. Tables 6.4, 6.5, and 6.6 provide conversion equivalents for common units in these systems and compare them to the metric system. Note that the only equivalent unit in both the apothecary and avoirdupois systems is the unit of dry measure known as the grain. This is the most commonly encountered nonmetric unit in pharmacy practice. Pharmacists sometimes make use of apothecaries' weights that come in 5-grain, 4-grain, 3-grain, 2-grain, 1-grain, and ½-grain units.

Roman Numerals

A prescription using apothecary measure is commonly written in Roman numerals that follow rather than precede the unit of measurement. Thus "aspirin gr vi" means "six grains of aspirin." Roman numerals are also sometimes used to express other quantities, as in tablets no. C (100 tablets) or tbsp iii (3 tablespoonsful). As we mentioned in Chapter 3, the Roman numerals i, ii, and iii are often written with a line above to prevent errors in interpretation (for example: ī, īi, īii). Table 6.7 summarizes the Roman numeral system and gives equivalents in Arabic numerals.

When juxtaposed, Roman numerals are equal or get smaller reading left to right, the total value equals the sum of their individual values. Thus iii = 3 and xi = 10 + 1 = 11. Otherwise, first subtract the value of each smaller numeral from the value of the larger numeral that it precedes and then add the individual values. Thus iv = 5 − 1 = 4 and xxiv = 10 + 10 + (5 − 1) = 10 + 10 + 4 = 24.

Table 6.3	Common Metric Conversions		
Conversion	**Instruction**		**Example**
kilograms (kg) to grams (g)	multiply by 1,000 (move decimal point three places to the right)		6.25 kg = 6,250 g
grams (g) to milligrams (mg)	multiply by 1,000 (move decimal point three places to the right)		3.56 g = 3,560 mg
milligrams (mg) to grams (g)	multiply by 0.001 (move decimal point three places to the left)		120 mg = 0.120 g
liters (L) to milliliters (mL)	multiply by 1,000 (move decimal point three places to the right)		2.5 L = 2,500 mL
milliliters (mL) to liters (L)	multiply by 0.001 (move decimal point three places to the left)		238 mL = 0.238 L

Table 6.4   **Apothecary System**

Measurement Unit	Equivalent within System	Metric Equivalent
Fluid Measure (volume)		
1 minim (♏)		0.06 mL
1 fluid dram (f℥)	60 minims (♏)	3.6 mL
1 fluid ounce (fl oz)	8 fluid drams (f℥)	approx. 30 mL
1 pt (pt)	16 fluid ounces (fl oz)	480 mL
1 quart (qt)	2 pints (pt) or 32 fluid ounces (fl oz)	960 mL
1 gallon (gal)	4 quarts (qt) or 8 pints (pt)	3,840 mL
Dry Measure (weight)		
1 grain (gr)		65 mg
1 scruple (Э)	20 grains (gr)	1.3 g
1 dram (Ʒ)	3 scruples (Э) or 60 grains (gr)	3.9 g
1 ounce (oz)	8 drams (Ʒ) or 480 grains (gr)	31.1 g
1 pound (#)	12 ounces (oz) or 5,760 grains (gr)	373.2 g
2.2 pounds (#)	26.4 ounces (oz) or 12,672 grains (gr)	1 kg

Table 6.5   **Avoirdupois System**

Measurement Unit	Equivalent within System	Metric Equivalent
1 grain (gr)		65 mg
1 ounce (oz)	437.5 grains (gr)	28.35 g
1 pound (lb)	16 ounces (oz) or 7,000 grains (gr)	454 g

Table 6.6   **Household Measure**

Measurement Unit	Equivalent within System	Metric Equivalent
1 teaspoonful (tsp)		5 mL
1 tablespoonful (tbsp)	3 teaspoonsful (tsp)	15 mL
1 fluid ounce (fl oz)	2 tablespoonsful (tbsp)	30 mL
1 cup	8 fluid ounces (fl oz)	240 mL
1 pint (pt)	2 cups	480 mL
1 quart (qt)	2 pints (pt)	960 mL
1 gallon (gal)	4 quarts (qt)	3.84 L

Table 6.7   **Roman Numerals**

Roman	Arabic	Roman	Arabic
s̄s̄	0.5 or ½	L or l	50
I or i or ī	1	C or c	100
V or v	5	D or d	500
X or x	10	M or m̄	1,000

BASIC MATHEMATICS USED IN PHARMACY PRACTICE

Many tasks in pharmacy—determining dosages, compounding medications, and preparing solutions, for example—use calculations involving the units of measure given in the preceding section. If you are fairly confident about your basic mathematical skills, you may wish to skip this section. However, it never hurts to review fundamental principles before undertaking mathematical work. Pharmacy work often requires performing fundamental operations involving fractions, decimals, ratios, proportions, and percentages.

Fractions

A simple fraction consists of two numbers, a numerator (the number on the top) and a denominator (the number on the bottom).

$$\frac{1}{2} \begin{array}{l} \leftarrow \text{numerator} \\ \leftarrow \text{denominator} \end{array}$$

A fraction is simply a convenient way of representing an operation, the division of the numerator by the denominator. Thus the fraction $\frac{6}{3}$ equals 6 divided by 3, which equals 2. The fraction $\frac{7}{8}$ is 7 divided by 8, which equals 0.875. The number obtained upon dividing the numerator by the denominator is the value of the fraction. Fractions with the same value are said to be equivalent fractions. The following are equivalent fractions.

$$\frac{1}{2} = 1 \div 2 = 0.5 \qquad\qquad \frac{3}{16} = 3 \div 16 = 0.1875$$

$$\frac{2}{4} = 2 \div 4 = 0.5 \qquad\qquad \frac{12}{64} = 12 \div 64 = 0.1875$$

$$\frac{4}{8} = 4 \div 8 = 0.5$$

A fraction with a value of less than 1 (the numerator smaller than the denominator) is called a proper fraction.

$$\frac{1}{4} \qquad \frac{2}{3} \qquad \frac{7}{8} \qquad \frac{9}{10}$$

A fraction with a value greater than 1 (the numerator greater than the denominator) is called an improper fraction.

$$\frac{6}{5} \qquad \frac{7}{5} \qquad \frac{11}{6} \qquad \frac{15}{8}$$

A mixed number, also called a compound fraction, is a whole number and a fraction.

$$5\frac{1}{2} \qquad 13\frac{7}{8} \qquad 99\frac{23}{24} \qquad 111\frac{99}{100}$$

In pharmaceutical work, it is especially important not to misread a compound fraction as a simple one. For example,

$$\text{Do not confuse } 3\frac{3}{8} \text{ with } \frac{33}{8}.$$

ADDING AND SUBTRACTING FRACTIONS To add or subtract fractions, first convert any compound fractions to improper fractions containing no whole numbers. To do this, multiply the whole number part of the compound fraction by the denominator and add the result to the numerator.

$$\text{compound fraction} = \frac{(\text{whole number} \times \text{denominator}) + \text{numerator}}{\text{denominator}}$$

$$3\frac{3}{8} = \frac{(3 \times 8) + 3}{8} = \frac{27}{8} \qquad 4\frac{1}{3} = \frac{(4 \times 3) + 1}{3} = \frac{13}{3}$$

The next step in adding or subtracting fractions is to check if the denominators are equal. If all of the fractions have the same denominator, addition or subtraction can proceed. If not, it is necessary to convert each fraction to an equivalent fraction such that all the fractions have the same denominator, called the least common denominator, or LCD. The least common denominator of a group of fractions is the smallest number that is evenly divisible by all of the denominators. To find the least common denominator, follow the steps shown in the following example.

Example 1 **Find the least common denominator of**

$$\frac{9}{28} \text{ and } \frac{1}{6}$$

Step 1: Find the prime factors (numbers divisible only by 1 and themselves) of each denominator. Make a list of all the different prime factors that you find. Include in the list each different factor as many times as the factor occurs for any one of the denominators of the given fractions.

The prime factors of 28 are 2, 2, and 7 (because $2 \times 2 \times 7 = 28$).
The prime factors of 6 are 2 and 3 (because $2 \times 3 = 6$).

The number 2 occurs twice in one of the denominators, so it must occur twice in the list. The list will also include the unique factors 3 and 7; so the final list is

2, 2, 3, 7

Step 2: Multiply all the prime factors on your list. The result of this multiplication is the least common denominator:

$$2 \times 2 \times 3 \times 7 = 84$$

Step 3: To convert a fraction to an equivalent fraction with the common denominator, first divide the least common denominator by the denominator of the fraction, then multiply both the numerator and denominator by the result (the quotient).

Convert

$$\frac{9}{28} \quad \text{and} \quad \frac{1}{6}$$

to equivalent fractions with a common denominator. The least common denominator of $\frac{9}{28}$ and $\frac{1}{6}$ is 84. In the first fraction, 84 divided by 28 is 3, so multiply both the numerator and the denominator by 3:

$$\frac{9}{28} = \frac{9 \times 3}{28 \times 3} = \frac{27}{84}$$

In the second fraction, 84 divided by 6 is 14, so multiply both the numerator and the denominator by 14:

$$\frac{1}{6} = \frac{1 \times 14}{6 \times 14} = \frac{14}{84}$$

The two equivalent fractions are

$$\frac{27}{84} \quad \text{and} \quad \frac{14}{84}$$

Step 4: Once the fractions are converted to contain equal denominators, adding or subtracting them is straightforward. Simply add or subtract the numerators:

$$\frac{9}{28} + \frac{1}{6} = \frac{27}{84} + \frac{14}{84} = \frac{41}{84}$$

$$\frac{9}{28} - \frac{1}{6} = \frac{27}{84} - \frac{14}{84} = \frac{13}{84}$$

MULTIPLYING AND DIVIDING FRACTIONS To multiply fractions, multiply numerators by numerators and denominators by denominators. Table 6.8 shows some guidelines for multiplying fractions.

$$\frac{1}{8} \times \frac{1}{2} = \frac{1 \times 1}{8 \times 2} = \frac{1}{16}$$

$$\frac{3}{4} \times \frac{12}{17} = \frac{3 \times 12}{4 \times 17} = \frac{36}{68} = \frac{9}{17}$$

$$\frac{1}{8} \times \frac{1}{2} \times \frac{2}{3} = \frac{1 \times 1 \times 2}{8 \times 2 \times 3} = \frac{2}{48} = \frac{1}{24}$$

Table 6.8	Guidelines for Multiplying Fractions

1. Multiplying the numerator by a number increases the value of a fraction.

$$\frac{1}{4} \times \frac{2}{1} = \frac{1 \times 2}{4} = \frac{2}{4} = \frac{1}{2}$$

2. Multiplying the denominator by a number decreases the value of a fraction.

$$\frac{1}{4} \times \frac{1}{2} = \frac{1}{4 \times 2} = \frac{1}{8}$$

3. The value of a fraction is not altered by multiplying or dividing both numerator and denominator by the same number.

$$\frac{1}{4} \times \frac{4}{4} = \frac{1 \times 4}{4 \times 4} = \frac{4}{16} = \frac{1}{4}$$

4. Dividing the denominator by a number is the same as multiplying the numerator by that number.

$$\frac{3}{20/5} = \frac{3}{4} \qquad \frac{3 \times 5}{20} = \frac{15}{20} = \frac{3}{4}$$

5. Dividing the numerator by a number is the same as multiplying the denominator by that number.

$$\frac{6/3}{4} = \frac{2}{4} = \frac{1}{2} \qquad \frac{6}{4 \times 3} = \frac{6}{12} = \frac{1}{2}$$

To divide by a fraction, invert the fraction and multiply. The inverted fraction is known as the reciprocal of the original fraction. Note that if the numerator of the original fraction is 1, the reciprocal will be a whole number.

$$\frac{3}{4} \div \frac{1}{3} = \frac{3}{4} \times \frac{3}{1} = \frac{3 \times 3}{4 \times 1} = \frac{9}{4} = 2\frac{1}{4}$$

$$10 \div \frac{1}{4} = \frac{10}{1} \times \frac{4}{1} = \frac{40}{1} = 40$$

Decimals

A decimal is any number that can be written in decimal notation, using the integers 0, 1, 2, 3, 4, 5, 6, 7, 8, and 9 and a point (.) to divide the ones place from the tenths place.

$$0.131313 \qquad 2.09 \qquad 43.0$$

Notice that in the decimal expansion of a fraction, a zero (0) is placed before the decimal point if the number is less than one. Using the zero helps to prevent errors in reading decimals.

A fraction can be expressed as a decimal by dividing the numerator by the denominator:

$$\frac{1}{2} = 1 \div 2 = 0.5$$

$$\frac{1}{3} = 1 \div 3 = 0.33\overline{33}$$

$$\frac{438}{64} = 438 \div 64 = 6.84375$$

CONVERTING FRACTIONS TO DECIMAL EQUIVALENTS One way to add, subtract, multiply, or divide fractions is to first convert each fraction to a decimal equivalent and then perform the operation.

Example 2 **Multiply the two given fractions:**

$$\frac{24}{3} \times \frac{22}{4}$$

$$\frac{24}{3} = 24 \div 3 = 8$$

$$\frac{22}{4} = 22 \div 4 = 5.5$$

$$\frac{24}{3} \times \frac{22}{4} = 8 \times 5.5 = 44$$

CONVERTING DECIMALS TO FRACTIONS The metric system generally uses numbers in decimal form. Any decimal number can be expressed as a decimal fraction that has a power of 10 as its denominator. (See Table 6.9.)

To express a decimal number as a fraction, remove the decimal point and use the resulting number as the numerator. To obtain the denominator, count the number of places to the right of the decimal point. Use Table 6.9 to find the corresponding power of ten to put in the denominator.

Table 6.9	Decimals and Equivalent Decimal Fractions
$1 = \dfrac{1}{1}$	$0.001 = \dfrac{1}{1,000}$
$0.1 = \dfrac{1}{10}$	$0.0001 = \dfrac{1}{10,000}$
$0.01 = \dfrac{1}{100}$	$0.00001 = \dfrac{1}{100,000}$

$$2.33 = \frac{233}{100}$$

$$0.1234 = \frac{1,234}{10,000}$$

$$0.00367 = \frac{367}{100,000}$$

A decimal fraction can then be reduced to a common fraction:

$$0.84 = \frac{84}{100} = \frac{84}{100} \div \frac{4}{4} = \frac{21}{25}$$

$$0.1234 = \frac{1,234}{10,000} = \frac{1,234}{10,000} \div \frac{2}{2} = \frac{617}{5,000}$$

ADDING AND SUBTRACTING DECIMALS When adding or subtracting decimals, place the numbers in columns so the decimal points are aligned directly under each other. Add or subtract from the far-right column to the left column.

$$
\begin{array}{r}
20.4 \\
+\,21.8 \\
\hline
42.2
\end{array}
\qquad
\begin{array}{r}
11.2 \\
13.6 \\
+\,16.0 \\
\hline
40.8
\end{array}
\qquad
\begin{array}{r}
15.36 \\
-\ \ 3.80 \\
\hline
11.56
\end{array}
$$

MULTIPLYING DECIMALS Multiply the two decimals as whole numbers. Add the total number of decimal places that are in the two numbers being multiplied (count from right to left), count that number of places from right to left in the answer, and insert a decimal point.

$$
\begin{array}{r}
1.23 \\
\times\quad 2.3 \\
\hline
369 \\
+\,2460 \\
\hline
2.829
\end{array}
$$

(A zero is added to align the columns. Note that no value is added to the number.)

DIVIDING DECIMALS To divide decimal numbers, move the decimal point the same number of places in both the denominator and numerator to make them both whole numbers. In the first example, move the decimal point in the divisor (the number doing the dividing) to the right three places to make it a whole number. Move the decimal point in the dividend (the number being divided) the same number of places. In the second example, move the decimal point in the dividend three places to the right to make it a whole number, and move the decimal point in the divisor three places to the right, also.

$$1.45 \div 3.625 = 0.4 \qquad 1.617 \div 2.31 = 0.7$$

$$\frac{1.45}{3.625} = \frac{1450}{3625} = 0.4 \qquad \frac{1.617}{2.31} = \frac{1617}{2310} = 0.7$$

ROUNDING OFF DECIMALS To round off an answer to the nearest tenth, carry the division out two places, to hundredths. If the number in the hundredth place is 5 or greater, add 1 to the tenths. If the number in the hundredth place is less than 5, round the number down by omitting the digit in the hundredth place.

$$5.65 \text{ becomes } 5.7 \qquad 4.24 \text{ becomes } 4.2$$

The same procedure may be used when rounding to the nearest hundredth place or thousandth place.

$$
\begin{aligned}
3.8421 &= 3.84 \quad \text{(hundredth)} \\
41.2674 &= 41.27 \quad \text{(hundredth)} \\
0.3928 &= 0.393 \quad \text{(thousandth)} \\
4.1111 &= 4.111 \quad \text{(thousandth)}
\end{aligned}
$$

When rounding numbers used in pharmacy calculations, it is common to round off to the nearest tenth. However, there are times when a dose is very small and rounding to the narest hundredth or thousandth may be more appropriate.

The exact dose calculated is 0.08752 g.
Rounded to nearest tenth: 0.1 g
Rounded to nearest hundredth: 0.09 g
Rounded to nearest thousandth: 0.088 g

Ratios and Proportions

A ratio is a comparison of two like quantities and can be expressed in fraction or in ratio notation, using a colon. For example, if a beaker contains two parts water and three parts alcohol, then the ratio of water to alcohol in the beaker can be expressed as the fraction ⅔ or as the ratio 2:3. The ratio is read not as a value (2 divided by 3) but as the expression "a ratio of 2 to 3."

One common use of ratios is as follows: the numerator is the number of parts of one substance contained in a known number of parts of another substance, which is the denominator. For example, suppose that 60 mL of sterile solution contains 3 mL of tetrahydrozoline hydrochloride. This can be expressed as the ratio ³⁄₆₀ or ¹⁄₂₀. In other words, the ratio of the active ingredient to the sterile solution is 1 to 20, or 1 part in 20 parts.

Two ratios that have the same value, such as ½ and ²⁄₄, are said to be equivalent ratios. This is similar to the concept of equivalent fractions discussed earlier. When ratios are equivalent, the product of the numerator of the first ratio and the denominator of the second ratio is equal to the product of the numerator of the second ratio and denominator of the first ratio. Therefore if 2:3 = 6:9, then

$$\frac{2}{3} = \frac{6}{9} \qquad \text{and thus} \qquad 2 \times 9 = 3 \times 6 = 18$$

The same thing is true of the reciprocals:

$$\frac{3}{2} = \frac{9}{6} \qquad \text{and thus} \qquad 3 \times 6 = 2 \times 9 = 18$$

Two equivalent ratios are said to be in the same proportion. Equivalent, or proportional, ratios can be expressed in three different ways:

$$\frac{a}{b} = \frac{c}{d} \qquad \left(\text{example: } \frac{1}{2} = \frac{2}{4}\right)$$

$$a\!:\!b = c\!:\!d \qquad (\text{example: } 1\!:\!2 = 2\!:\!4)$$

$$a\!:\!b :: c\!:\!d \qquad (\text{example: } 1\!:\!2 = 2\!:\!4)$$

Pairs of ratios written in this form are called a proportion. The first and fourth, or outside, numbers are called the extremes, and the second and third, or inside, numbers are called the means.

$$3\!:\!4 = 15\!:\!20$$

means

extremes

A very useful fact about proportions was illustrated in the previous examples: the product of the extremes equals the product of the means. If the proportion is expressed as a relationship between fractions, the numerator of the first fraction times the denominator of the second is equal to the denominator of the first fraction times the numerator of the second. This can be stated as a rule:

$$\text{If} \quad \frac{a}{b} = \frac{c}{d}, \quad \text{then} \quad a \times d = b \times c.$$

This equation proves extremely valuable because it can be used to calculate an unknown quantity in a proportion when the other three variables are known. In mathematics, it is common to express unknown quantities using letters from the lower end of the alphabet, especially x, y, and z.

When setting up ratios in the proportion, it is important that the numbers remain in the correct ratio, and that the numbers have the correct units of measurement in both the numerator and denominator. Table 6.10 lists the rules for solving proportions. Table 6.11 lists the steps for solving for an unknown quantity, which we usually label x.

Table 6.10	Rules for Solving Proportions

- Three of the four amounts must be known.
- The numerators must have the same unit of measurement.
- The denominators must have the same unit of measurement.

Table 6.11   **Steps for Solving for** *x*

Step 1. Create the proportion by placing the ratios in fraction form so that the *x* is in the upper-left corner.

Step 2. Be sure to check that the unit of measurement in the numerators is the same and the unit of measurement in the denominators is the same.

Step 3. Solve for *x* by multiplying both sides of the proportion by the denominator of the ratio containing the unknown, and cancel.

Step 4. Check your answer by seeing if the product of the means equals the product of the extremes.

Example 3   Solve for *x*:

$$\frac{x}{35} = \frac{2}{7}$$

By the proportion rule,

$$7x = 70$$

Then, dividing both sides by 7,

$$\frac{7x}{7} = \frac{70}{7}$$

$$x = 10$$

Percents

The word *percent* comes from the Latin words *per centum*, meaning "in one hundred." A percent is a given part or amount in a hundred. Percents can be expressed in many ways:

◆ as an actual percent (example: 3% or 3 percent)
◆ as a fraction with 100 as the denominator (example: $^3/_{100}$)
◆ as a decimal (example: 0.03)
◆ as a ratio (example 3:100)

All of these expressions are equivalent.

CHANGING A RATIO TO A PERCENT To express a ratio as a percent, designate the first number of the ratio as the numerator and the second number as the denominator. Multiply the fraction by 100% (which does not change the value), and simplify as needed.

$$5:1 = \frac{5}{1} \times 100\% = 5 \times 100\% = 500\%$$

$$1:5 = \frac{1}{5} \times 100\% = \frac{100\%}{5} = 20\%$$

$$1:2 = \frac{1}{2} \times 100\% = \frac{100\%}{2} = 50\%$$

CHANGING A PERCENT TO A RATIO To change a percent to a ratio, first change it to a fraction by dividing it by 100 and then reducing it to its lowest terms. Express this as a ratio by making the numerator the first number of the ratio and the denominator the second number.

$$2\% = 2 \div 100 = \frac{2}{100} = \frac{1}{50} = 1{:}50$$

$$10\% = 10 \div 100 = \frac{10}{100} = \frac{1}{10} = 1{:}10$$

$$75\% = 75 \div 100 = \frac{75}{100} = \frac{3}{4} = 3{:}4$$

$$\tfrac{1}{2}\% = \frac{1}{2} \div 100 = \frac{\tfrac{1}{2}}{100} = \frac{1}{2} \times \frac{1}{100} = \frac{1}{200} = 1{:}200$$

CHANGING A PERCENT TO A DECIMAL To convert from a percent to a decimal, divide by 100% or insert a decimal point two places to the left of the last number, inserting zeros if necessary, and drop the percent symbol. To change a decimal to a percent, multiply by 100% or move the decimal point two places to the right and write in the percent symbol. (Just as multiplying or dividing a number by 1 does not change the value of the number, multiplying, or dividing a number by 100% does not change the value of a number.)

Percent to Decimal
4% = 0.04	4 ÷ 100% = 0.04
15% = 0.15	15 ÷ 100% = 0.15
200% = 2.0	200 ÷ 100% = 2.0

Decimal to Percent
0.25 = 25%	0.25 × 100% = 25%
1.35 = 135%	1.35 × 100% = 135%
0.015 = 1.5%	0.015 × 100% = 1.5%

COMMON CALCULATIONS IN THE PHARMACY

Math skills typically used by the pharmacy technician involve converting units and calculating dosages. For nearly all types of mathematics in the pharmacy, decimals and the metric system are preferred over Roman numerals, fractions, and the apothecary or household systems.

Converting Measures between the Metric and Apothecary Systems

Many situations in pharmacy practice call for conversion of quantities within one measurement system or between different measurement systems. When possible, convert to the metric system, since it is the preferred system. To convert between measurements and apothecary units, it is necessary to know the equivalent measures shown in Table 6.12.

Table 6.12 Apothecary and Metric System Equivalents

Apothecary		Metric
16.23 minims	=	1 mL
1 fluid ounce	=	29.57 mL or about 30 mL
1 pint	=	480 mL
1 gallon	=	3,840 mL
1 gram	=	15.432 grains
1 grain	=	65 mg
1 pound (avoirdupois)	=	454 g
1 ounce (apothecary)	=	31.3 g
1 ounce (avoirdupois)	=	28.35 g
1 fluid dram	=	5 mL

When converting from fluid ounces to milliliters in pharmacy calculations, it is common practice to round up, for example, 29.57 mL up to 30 mL. Such calculations are performed on a frequent basis, and rounding makes the conversions easier and more accurate. After some practice, you will be able to perform these calculations in your head. In this chapter use 30 mL when converting from fluid ounces.

A special discrepancy to be aware of is the difference between the true volume of a dram and the commonly used volume of a dram. In Table 6.4 you learned that there are eight drams per fluid ounce. If we use the rounded volume of 30 mL to represent one fluid ounce and divide it by 8, we get that a dram is equal to 3.75 mL. However, in Table 6.12, you see that a dram is 5 mL. For many years, physicians used a dram to represent the common household measure of a teaspoonful. Eventually, 5 mL became the value assigned to both a teaspoonful and a dram. It is common practice to use 5 mL per 1 fluid dram and 6 fluid drams per 30 mL. However at times, we also use 8 fluid drams per 1 fluid ounce. For the purpose of this chapter, use the eight drams/fluid ounce conversion.

Another calculation performed on a frequent basis is a conversion from ounces to grams. The two values for an ounce are 31.1 g and 28.35 g. In both cases it is common practice to round to 30 g. Many physicians are accustomed to writing prescription orders in ounces of medication, in both liquid and solid forms, however the metric system is considered more accurate and is becoming the system of choice in the United States. Also, many pharmacy computer systems are programmed to accept only amounts with metric units.

As stated earlier, it is common practice to round a fluid ounce (29.57 mL) up to 30 mL. When measuring this amount, it is often appropriate to make this estimation as the volume differs by such a small amount. However, the discrepancy becomes far more apparent when measuring multiple fluid ounces that have been rounded up to the 30 mL equivalent. For example if asked to measure a pint (16 fl oz), one would measure roughly 480 mL. This becomes problematic as 29.57 mL multiplied by 16 is equal to only 473.12 mL, not 480 mL. Products in most stock bottles will be labeled 473 mL, yet pharmacies will bill according to the estimation of 480 mL and measure out fluid ounces in 30 mL increments. For the purposes of this chapter, use the rounded 30 mL and 480 mL, and 3,840 mL for a gallon.

Yet another discrepancy you should be aware of is the differing value of a grain. In Table 6.12, the grain is equal to 65 mg, but many other references use 60 mg instead. Most pharmacists use the 65 mg conversion.

Example 4 **Convert 1 gal, 12 fl oz to milliliters.**

$$12 \text{ fl oz} \times \frac{30 \text{ mL}}{\text{fl oz}} = 360 \text{ mL}$$

$$1 \text{ gal} = 3,840 \text{ mL}$$

$$360 \text{ mL} + 3,840 \text{ mL} = 4,200 \text{ mL}$$

Example 5 **A solution is to be used to fill hypodermics containing 60 mL each, and three liters are on hand. How many hypodermics can be filled with the three liters of solution?**

From Table 6.2, one liter is 1,000 mL. The available supply of solution is therefore

$$3 \times 1,000 = 3,000 \text{ mL}$$

Thus

$$3,000 \div 60 = 50$$

Fifty hypodermics can be filled.

Example 6 **You are to dispense 300 mL of a liquid preparation. If the dose is 2 tsp, how many doses will there be in the final preparation?**

From Table 6.6, one teaspoonful is 5 mL. Therefore, one dose is 10 mL. Dividing,

$$\frac{300 \text{ mL}}{10 \text{ mL/dose}} = 30 \text{ doses}$$

Example 7 **A prescription calls for acetaminophen 400 mg. How many grains of acetaminophen should be used in the prescription?**

From Table 6.5, one grain is 65 mg. This can be set up as a proportion. In other words, 1 grain is to 65 milligrams as the unknown number of grains is to 400 milligrams.

$$\frac{x \text{ gr}}{400 \text{ mg}} = \frac{1 \text{ gr}}{65 \text{ mg}}$$

$$65x \text{ gr} = 400 \text{ gr}$$

$$x \text{ gr} = 6.15 \text{ gr}$$

Rounding down, 6 gr should be used in the prescription.

Example 8 A physician wants a patient to be given 0.8 mg of nitroglycerin. On hand are tablets containing nitroglycerin 1/150 gr. How many tablets should the patient be given?

From Table 6.5, one grain is 65 mg. To determine the number of grains in 0.8 mg, set up a proportion:

$$\frac{x \text{ gr}}{0.8 \text{ mg}} = \frac{1 \text{ gr}}{65 \text{ mg}}$$

$$65x \text{ gr} = 0.8 \text{ gr}$$

$$x \text{ gr} = 0.012 \text{ gr}$$

To determine the number of tablets that the patient should receive, set up another proportion:

$$\frac{x \text{ tablets}}{0.012 \text{ gr}} = \frac{1 \text{ tablet}}{1/150 \text{ gr}}$$

$$\frac{x}{150} \text{ tablets} = 0.012 \text{ tablet}$$

$$\cancel{150}\left(\frac{x}{\cancel{150}}\right) \text{ tablets} = 150(0.012) \text{ tablets}$$

$$x \text{ tablets} = 1.8 \text{ tablets}$$

This is almost two tablets, so two tablets will approximate the patient's dose.

Calculation of Dosages

One of the most common calculations in pharmacy practice is that of dosages. The available supply is usually labeled as a ratio of an active ingredient to a solution:

$$\frac{\text{active ingredient (available)}}{\text{solution (available)}}$$

The prescription gives the amount of the active ingredient to be administered. The unknown quantity to be calculated is the amount of solution needed in order to achieve the desired dosage of the active ingredient. This yields another ratio:

$$\frac{\text{active ingredient (to be administered)}}{\text{solution (needed)}}$$

The amount of solution needed can be determined by setting the two ratios equal:

$$\frac{\text{active ingredient (available)}}{\text{solution (available)}} = \frac{\text{active ingredient (to be administered)}}{\text{solution (needed)}}$$

When solving medication-dosing problems, use ratios to describe the amount of drug in a dosage form (tablet, capsule, or volume of solution). It is important to remember that the numerators and denominators of both fractions must be in the same units—for example, mg/mL 5 mg/mL or mg/tablets = mg/tablets.

Example 9 **You have a stock solution that contains 10 mg of active ingredient per 5 mL of solution. The physician orders a dose of 4 mg. How many milliliters of the stock solution will have to be administered?**

Using the information provided, set up a proportion:

$$\frac{x \text{ mL}}{4 \text{ mg}} = \frac{5 \text{ mL}}{10 \text{ mg}}$$

$$10x \text{ mL} = 20 \text{ mL}$$

$$x \text{ mL} = 2 \text{ mL}$$

Thus 2 mL of solution are needed to provide the dose.

Example 10 **An order calls for Demerol 75 mg IM q4h prn pain. (If you find it necessary, review the pharmaceutical abbreviations given in Chapter 3.) The supply available is in Demerol 100 mg/mL syringes. How many milliliters will the nurse give?**

Using the given information, set up a proportion:

$$\frac{x \text{ mg}}{75 \text{ mg}} = \frac{1 \text{ mL}}{100 \text{ mg}}$$

$$100x \text{ mL} = 75 \text{ mL}$$

$$x \text{ mL} = 0.75 \text{ mL}$$

Notice that 0.75 mL is three-quarters of a syringe.

Example 11 **An average adult has a body surface area of 1.72 m² and requires an adult dosage of 12 mg of a given medication. The same medication is to be given to a child in a pediatric dosage. If the child has a body surface area of 0.60 m², and if the proper dosage for pediatric and adult patients is a linear function of the body surface area (in other words, think of the child as a small adult), what is the proper pediatric dosage?**

The assumptions regarding the calculation of pediatric dosages make it possible to use a proportion:

$$\frac{x \text{ mg}}{0.06 \text{ m}^2} = \frac{12 \text{ mg}}{1.72 \text{ m}^2}$$

$$1.72x \text{ mg} = 7.2 \text{ mg}$$

$$x \text{ mg} = 4.2 \text{ mg}$$

Rounding down, since it is for a child, the proper dosage is 4 mg.

Electrolytes

Many fluids used in pharmacy practice contain dissolved mineral salts; such fluids are known as electrolytes. They are so-named because they conduct an electrical charge through the solution when connected to electrodes. Electrolyte solutions and certain drugs, besides being measured in the usual units, are also measured in "millimoles" and "milliequivalents." These types of measures are particularly important in working with IV solutions. In this chapter, you will learn how to perform those calculations and related problems.

UNDERSTANDING MILLIMOLES AND MILLIEQUIVALENTS Most electrolyte solutions are measured by milliequivalents, which are related to molecular weight. Molecular weights are based on the atomic weights of common elements. The atomic weight of an element is the weight of a single atom of that element compared to the weight of one atom of hydrogen, and the valence of an element is a number that represents its capacity to combine to form a molecule of a stable compound. An element can exist in various forms. Valence may vary depending on an elemental form. The molecular weight of a compound is the sum of the atomic weights of all the atoms in one molecule of the compound. Table 6.13 lists the valences and atomic weights of common elements. For pharmaceutical calculations, atomic weights are usually rounded to the nearest tenth, as shown in the fourth column of the table.

One mole (M) of an element is equal to its atomic weight in grams. Thus one mole of sodium (Na) is equal to 22.9898 g, or 23 g. Compounds are also measured in moles. For example, one mole of sodium chloride (NaCl) would equal its grams, which is as follows:

Table 6.13	Valences and Atomic Weights of Common Elements		
Element	**Valence**	**Atomic Weight**	**Rounded-off Value**
Hydrogen (H)	1	1.008	1
Carbon (C)	2, 4	12.011	12
Nitrogen (N)	3, 5	14.007	14
Oxygen (O)	2	15.999	16
Sodium (Na)	1	22.9898	23
Sulphur (S)	2, 4, 6	32.064	32.1
Chlorine (Cl)	1, 3, 5, 7	35.453	35.5
Potassium (K)	1	39.102	39.1
Calcium (Ca)	2	40.08	40.1

atomic weight of sodium (23) + atomic weight of chlorine (35.5) = 58.5 g

One millimole (mM) is the molecular weight expressed in milligrams. Since one gram equals 1,000 milligrams, one mole equals 1,000 millimoles. Thus one millimole of sodium chloride equals 58.5 milligrams.

One equivalent (Eq) is equal to one mole divided by its valence or the number of grams of solute dissolved in one milliliter of solution, as shown in the following formula:

$$equivalent\ weight = \frac{molecular\ weight}{valence}$$

One milliequivalent (mEq) is equal to one millimole divided by its valence. Thus, as before, one equivalent equals 1,000 milliequivalents, or one thousandth of a gram equivalent.

DETERMINING THE MILLIEQUIVALENTS OF COMPOUNDS The first step in determining the number of milliequivalents of a compound is to identify the formula of the compound. The next step is to separate the formula into atoms. The atomic weight of each atom is then multiplied by the number of those atoms, the products are added together, and that sum substituted into the formula for atomic weight.

$$mEq = \frac{molecular\ weight}{valence}$$

Example 12 **The molecular weight of magnesium sulfate ($Mg^{++}SO_4^{--}$) is 120 mg and its valence is 2. How many milligrams does 1 mEq of magnesium sulfate weigh?**

$$1\ mEq = \frac{120\ mg}{2} = 60\ mg$$

In the phosphate ion, both the valence and the oxygen combining quantity may change with the pH of the solution and/or the temperature. Several forms of phosphorus/oxygen combinations may be found in the same solution. These are called phosphates. Because the valence might change, phosphates are measured in millimoles instead of milliequivalents.

Example 13 **Magnesium has an atomic weight of 24. What is the weight of 1 millimole?**

$$1\ mM = 24\ g \div 1,000 = 0.024\ g = 24\ mg$$

CONVERTING BETWEEN MILLIGRAMS AND MILLIEQUIVALENTS To convert back and forth between milligrams and milliequivalents, use the following formula:

$$number\ of\ mEq = \frac{weight\ of\ substance\ in\ mg}{mEq\ weight}$$

Example 14   **Sodium has an atomic weight of 23 and a valence of 1. How many milliequivalents are in 92 mg of sodium?**

By the formula at the end of the previous section,

$$\text{mg of sodium} = \frac{23}{1} = 23 \text{ mg}$$

Then, by the formula just before this example,

$$\text{mEq of 92 mg sodium} = \frac{92 \text{ mg}}{23 \text{ mg}} = 4 \text{ mEq}$$

MEASURING ELECTROLYTES Both milliequivalents and millimoles are used to measure electrolytes in the bloodstream and/or in an IV preparation.

Example 15   **You are requested to add 44 mEq of sodium chloride (NaCl) to an IV bag. Sodium chloride is available as a 4 mEq/mL solution. How many milliliters will you add to the bag?**

$$\frac{x \text{ mL}}{44 \text{ mEq}} = \frac{1 \text{ mL}}{4 \text{ mEq}}$$

$$x \text{ mL} = \frac{(44 \text{ mEq}) \times 1 \text{ mL}}{4 \text{ mEq}}$$

$$x \text{ mL} = 11 \text{ mL}$$

Specific Gravity

Specific gravity can be defined as the ratio of the weight of a substance to the weight of an equal volume of water, the standard, when both have the same temperature. Final weight can be measured in grams, because 1 mL of water weighs 1 g.

> 1 mL volume of water = 1 g weight of water
>
> specific gravity of water = 1.0

The specific gravity represents the weight of 1 mL of the substance. The ratio that we call specific gravity is in essence a comparison of the weight of a liquid to the weight of water when exactly 1 mL of each is measured out. Water is the standard that is used and the specific gravity assigned to it is 1.0. The formula for determining specific gravity is as follows:

> $$\text{specific gravity} = \frac{\text{weight of a substance}}{\text{weight of an equal volume of water}}$$

When the specific gravity is known, certain assumptions can be made regarding the physical properties of a liquid. Solutions that are viscous or have particles floating in them often have a specific gravity higher than 1.0. Solutions that contain volatile chemicals (or something that is prone to quick evaporation), such as alcohol, often have a specific gravity lower than 1.0.

Note that specific gravity has no units.

Example 16 **If the weight of 100 mL of dextrose solution is 117 g, what is the specific gravity of the dextrose solution?**

$$\text{specific gravity} = \frac{117 \text{ g (weight of 100 mL dextrose solution)}}{100 \text{ g (weight of 100 mL of water)}} = 1.17$$

If the specific gravity is known, you can determine the weight of a volume of a liquid.

Example 17 **If a liquid has a specific gravity of 0.85, how much does 125 mL weigh?**

Since the specific gravity of the liquid is 0.85,

$$\text{specific gravity} = 0.85$$

$$= \frac{85 \text{ g (weight of 100 mL of the liquid)}}{100 \text{ g (weight of 100 mL of water)}}$$

Now, setting up a proportion to find the weight of 125 mL,

$$\frac{x \text{ g}}{125 \text{ mL}} = \frac{85 \text{ g}}{100 \text{ mL}}$$

$$x \text{ g} = \frac{(125 \text{ mL}) \times 85 \text{ g}}{100 \text{ mL}}$$

$$x \text{ g} = 106.25 \text{ g}$$

Calculation of IV Rate and Administration

Another common type of calculation in pharmacy practice is the rate of flow for intravenous infusions. Intravenous flow rates are usually described as mL/hr or as drops (gtt) per minute. The pharmacy usually uses the mL/hr method. Nurses generally uses drops/min. The most common intravenous sets dispense at rates of 10 gtt/mL, 15 gtt/mL, and 60 gtt/mL.

Example 18 **A physician orders 4,000 mL of a 5% dextrose and normal saline (D_5NS) IV over a 36 hour period. If the IV set will deliver 15 drops/mL, how many drops must be administered per minute?**

First, determine the number of milliliters the patient is to receive each hour:

$$\frac{4000 \text{ mL}}{36 \text{ hr}} = 111.11 \text{ mL/hr}$$

Round down to 111 mL/hr. Second, use the following formula to determine the number of drops the patient will receive each minute:

$$\frac{(\text{number of mL/hr}) \times (\text{number of drops/mL})}{60 \text{ min/hr}} = x \text{ drops/min}$$

Substituting the given data in the formula,

$$\frac{(111 \text{ mL/hr}) \times (15 \text{ drops/mL})}{60 \text{ min/hr}} = 27.75 \text{ drops/min}$$

Since it is impractical to consider 3/4 of a drop, we round up to 28 drops/min.

Example 19 **If 500 mg of a drug is to be administered from a 50 mL minibag over 30 minutes using a 15 drop set, how many drops/min is that?**

Specified volume of fluid	= 50 mL
Specified fluid delivery time	= 30 min = 0.5 hr
Drops/mL of the administration set	= 15 drops/mL

The rate in mL/hr will need to be calculated before using the formula.

$$\frac{50 \text{ mL}}{0.5 \text{ hr}} = 100 \frac{\text{mL}}{\text{hr}}$$

$$x \text{ drops/min} = \frac{(100 \text{ mL/hr}) \times (15 \text{ drops/mL})}{60 \text{ min/hr}}$$

$$x \text{ drops/min} = 25 \text{ drops/min}$$

Example 20 **You are to prepare 750 mg of medication in 75 mL for infusion over 30 minutes, using a 10-drop set. How many drops/min will that be?**

Specified volume of fluid	= 75 mL
Specified fluid delivery time	= 30 minutes = 0.5 hr
Drops/mL of the administered set	= 10 drops/mL

First calculate the rate in mL/hr:

$$\frac{75 \text{ mL}}{0.5 \text{ hr}} = 150 \frac{\text{mL}}{\text{hr}}$$

Now we can use the formula for drops/minute:

$$x \text{ drops/min} = \frac{(150 \text{ mL/hr}) \times (10 \text{ drops/mL})}{60 \text{ min/hr}}$$

$$x \text{ drops/min} = 25 \text{ drops/min}$$

Example 21   **A one-liter IV is running at 125 mL/hr. How often will a new bag have to be administered?**

The number of hours that the IV will last can be determined by dividing the volume of the IV bag (1 L = 1000 mL) by the flow rate (125 mL/hr):

$$\frac{1000 \text{ mL}}{125 \text{ mL/hr}} = 8 \text{ hr}$$

Preparation of Solutions

When solutions are prepared, even though the active ingredient has units of weight, it also occupies a certain amount of volume, referred to as powder volume. It is defined as the difference between the amount of solution added and the final volume.

PREPARING SOLUTIONS USING POWDERS In preparing solutions, although the active ingredient is discussed in terms of weight, it also occupies a certain amount of space. With dry pharmaceuticals, this space is referred to as powder volume (pv). It is equal to the difference between the final volume (fv) and the volume of the diluting ingredient, or the diluent volume (dv), as expressed in the following equation:

> powder volume = final volume − diluent volume
>
> or
>
> pv = fv − dv

Example 22   **A dry powder antibiotic must be reconstituted for use. The label states that the dry powder occupies 0.5 mL. Using the formula for solving for powder volume, determine the diluent volume (the amount of solvent added). You are given the final volume for three different examples below with the same powder volume:**

Final Volume	Powder Volume
(1) 2 mL	0.5 mL
(2) 5 mL	0.5 mL
(3) 10 mL	0.5 mL

dv = fv − pv
(1) dv = 2 mL − 0.5 mL = 1.5 mL
(2) dv = 5 mL − 0.5 mL = 4.5 mL
(3) dv = 10 mL − 0.5 mL = 9.5 mL

Example 23   **You are to reconstitute 1 g of dry powder. The label states that you are to add 9.3 mL of diluent to make a final solution of 100 mg/mL. What is the powder volume?**

The final solution will have a strength of 100 mg/mL. Then, since you start with 1 g = 1,000 mg of powder, for a final volume x of the solution, it will have strength 1,000 mg/x mL.

$$\frac{x \text{ mL}}{1,000 \text{ mg}} = \frac{1 \text{ mL}}{100 \text{ mg}}$$

$$x \text{ mL} = \frac{(1,000 \text{ mg}) \times 1 \text{ mL}}{100 \text{ mg}}$$

$$x \text{ mL} = 10 \text{ mL}$$

The final volume is 10 mL. You added 9.3 mL of solvent; therefore the difference is

$$\begin{array}{r} 10.0 \text{ mL} \\ - \ 9.3 \text{ mL} \\ \hline 0.7 \text{ mL} \end{array}$$

and the powder volume is 0.7 mL.

WORKING WITH DILUTIONS   Manufacturers usually prepare pharmaceuticals with adult usage as the primary intent. Quite frequently, however, it is necessary to administer these medications to children and infants. Thus the medication must be diluted further so that it can be measured more accurately and easily.

Volumes less than 0.1 mL are usually considered too small to measure accurately. Therefore, there must be further dilution of the preparation. Many pharmacies have a policy as to how much an injection can be diluted. A rule of thumb is for the required dose to have a volume greater than 0.1 mL and less than 1 mL.

Example 24   **Dexamethasone is available as a 4 mg/mL preparation; an infant is to receive 0.35 mg. Prepare a dilution so that the final concentration is 1 mg/mL. How much diluent will you need if the original product is in a 1 mL vial and you use the full vial?**

Step 1:   Determine the volume of the final product. Since the strength of the dexamethasone is 4 mg/mL, a 1 mL vial will contain 4 mg of the active ingredient. Then, for a final volume x of solution, you will have a concentration of $(4/x)$ mg/mL.

| Diluted | Desired |
| solution | concentration |

$$\frac{x \text{ mL}}{4 \text{ mg}} = \frac{1 \text{ mL}}{1 \text{ mg}}$$

$$x \text{ mL} = \frac{(4 \text{ mg}) \times 1 \text{ mL}}{1 \text{ mg}}$$

$$x \text{ mL} = 4 \text{ mL}$$

Step 2: Subtract the volume of the concentrate from the total volume to determine the amount of diluent needed:

$$4 \text{ mL} - 1 \text{ mL} = 3 \text{ mL}$$

Therefore three more milliliters of solution are needed to dilute the original 1 mL of preparation to a strength of 1 mg/mL.

USING ALLIGATION TO PREPARE SOLUTIONS Another method of preparing solutions is by using two solutions of the same active ingredient but of different percent concentrations, and from those, preparing a solution of a prescribed percentage. This method is called the alligation method. This process requires changing the percentages to parts of ratios and then using those ratios and finally proportions to solve for the amounts of the two ingredients. The answer can then be checked by using the following formula:

$$\text{milliliters} \times \text{percent (as a decimal)} = \text{grams}$$

It is important to note that this formula works for any strength solution.

Example 25 **Prepare 250 mL of dextrose 7.5% using dextrose 5% (D_5W) and dextrose 50% ($D_{50}W$). How many milliliters of each will be needed?**

Step 1: Set up a box arrangement and at the upper-left corner, write the percent of the highest concentration (50%) as a whole number. At the lower-left corner, write the percent of the lowest concentration (5%) as a whole number, and in the center, write the desired concentration.

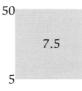

Step 2: Subtract the center number from the upper-left number (note: the smaller from the larger) and put it at the lower right. Now subtract the lower-left number from the center number (again: the smaller from the larger) and put it at the upper right.

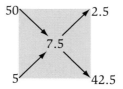

The number 2.5 represents the number of parts of the 50% solution that will be needed to make the final 7.5% solution, while the number 42.5 represents the number of parts of the 5% solution that will be needed. The sum of these two numbers, 2.5 + 42.5 = 45, is the total number of parts of the 7.5% solution. In terms of ratios, the ratio of the 5% solution to the 7.5% solution is 42.5:45, and the ratio of the 50% solution to the 7.5% solution is 2.5:45. Much less of the 50% solution is needed to make the 7.5% solution.

Step 3: Calculate the volume needed of each dextrose solution:

50% Dextrose

$$\frac{x \text{ mL}}{2.5 \text{ parts}} = \frac{250 \text{ mL}}{45 \text{ parts}}$$

$$x \text{ mL} = \frac{(2.5 \text{ parts}) \times 250 \text{ mL}}{45 \text{ parts}}$$

$$x \text{ mL} = 13.89 \text{ mL } D_{50}W$$

5% Dextrose

$$\frac{x \text{ mL}}{42.5 \text{ parts}} = \frac{250 \text{ mL}}{45 \text{ parts}}$$

$$x \text{ mL} = \frac{(42.5)250 \text{ mL}}{45}$$

$$x \text{ mL} = 236.11 \text{ mL } D_5W$$

Step 4: Add the volumes of the two solutions together. The sum should equal the required volume of dextrose 7.5%.

$$
\begin{array}{r}
236.11 \text{ mL} \\
+13.89 \text{ mL} \\
\hline
250.00 \text{ mL}
\end{array}
$$

Step 5: Check your answer by calculating the amount of solute (dextrose) in all three solutions. The number of grams of solute should equal the sum of the grams of solutes from the 50% solution and the 5% solution, using the following formula:

$$\text{mL} \times \% \text{ (as a decimal)} = g$$

$$250 \text{ mL} \times 0.075 = 18.75 \text{ g}$$
$$13.89 \text{ mL} \times 0.5 = 6.945 \text{ g}$$
$$236.11 \text{ mL} \times 0.05 = 11.805 \text{ g}$$

$$
\begin{array}{r}
11.805 \text{ g} \\
+6.945 \text{ g} \\
\hline
18.750 \text{ g}
\end{array}
$$

We will simplify the step method used in Example 25 by combining Steps 1 and 2 into a single step and calculating the ratios right at the square, where it is easy to visualize.

Example 26 You are instructed to make 454 g of 3% cream. You have in stock 10% and 1% cream. How much of each percent will you use?

Step 1:

10 ↘ ↗ 2 parts 10%

3

1 ↗ ↘ +

7 parts 1%
———————
9 parts 3%

Step 2:

10% cream

$$\frac{x \text{ g of } 10\%}{454 \text{ g}} = \frac{2 \text{ parts } 10\%}{9 \text{ parts } 3\%}$$

$$x \text{ g of } 10\% = 101 \text{ g of } 10\% \text{ cream}$$

1% cream

$$\frac{x \text{ g of } 1\%}{454 \text{ g}} = \frac{7 \text{ parts } 1\%}{9 \text{ parts } 3\%}$$

$$x \text{ g of } 1\% = 353 \text{ g of } 1\% \text{ cream}$$

Step 3: Check your work:

$$353 \text{ g} + 101 \text{ g} = 454 \text{ g}$$

BUSINESS MATH USED IN PHARMACY PRACTICE

A pharmacy, whether institutional or community, is controlled by and operates under the same principles as any other business: it deals with expenses and receipts. And like any other business, the pharmacy must make a profit, that is, it must have more receipts than expenses in order to continue to provide customer services. One of the responsibilities of the pharmacy technician is to help ensure that the receipts are greater than the expenses. The technician often takes care of pricing in the pharmacy by marking products up a certain percentage over the cost, or the average wholesale price (AWP), and by marking products down by a percentage discount at other times. Insurance companies most often use either a percentage-based payment for prescription products or a capitation fee. Pharmacy technicians also have the responsibility of monitoring and correcting insurance billing of prescription products. Inventory management is a duty assigned to the seasoned pharmacy technician who understands the movement of drug items on the shelf and how inventory levels are related to the cash flow in the pharmacy.

Markup

Like all businesses, pharmacies purchase their products (drugs) at one price and sell them at a higher price. This difference is called gross profit and it is also referred to as markup. Although pharmacies are subject to governmental laws and regulations regarding the sale of drugs, markup still plays a part in the pricing system.

The markup is computed as

$$\text{selling price} - \text{purchase price} = \text{markup or gross profit}$$

Example 27 **A 30 day supply of an antidiabetic agent sells for $45 and costs the pharmacy $30. What is the markup?**

The markup is computed as follows:

$$\text{selling price} - \text{purchase price} = \text{markup or gross profit}$$
$$\$45 - \$30 = \$15$$

The markup rate is computed as

$$\frac{\text{markup}}{\text{cost}} \times 100\% = \text{markup rate}$$

Discount

Sometimes a manufacturer or a supplier offers an item at a lower price to a pharmacy. This reduced price is a discount. Similarly, a discount, or a deduction from what is normally charged, can be offered by a pharmacy to the consumers as an incentive to purchase an item.

$$\text{purchase price} \times \text{discount rate} = \text{discount}$$

$$\text{purchase price} - \text{discount} = \text{discounted price}$$

Example 28 **Assume five cases of dermatological cream are purchased at $100 per case. If the account is paid in full within 15 days, a 15% discount is offered on the purchase. What is the total discounted purchase price?**

First calculate the full purchase price:

$$\text{quantity of product} \times \text{cost per unit} = \text{total purchase price}$$
$$5 \text{ cases} \times \$100 \text{ per case} = \$500$$

Next calculate the discount for payment within 15 days:

$$\text{total purchase price} \times \text{discount rate} = \text{discount}$$
$$\$500 \times 0.15 = \$75$$

Finally, to obtain the discounted price, subtract the discount from the original price:

$$\text{total purchase price} - \text{discount} = \text{discounted purchase price}$$
$$\$500 \times \$75 = \$425$$

Average Wholesale Price (AWP) Applications

A pharmacy may potentially receive payment from several different sources. Historically, patients have been responsible for paying for their own medications. More recently, health maintenance organizations, and health insurers have become major players in determining the cost of healthcare, including patient medications. The very survival of a pharmacy depends on its ability to contain costs. The average wholesale price (AWP) of a drug is an *average* price that wholesalers charge the pharmacy. Usually, third parties reimburse a pharmacy based upon the AWP. Therefore, there is an incentive for a pharmacy to purchase a drug below its AWP. There are situations when drugs are sold below AWP, such as volume discounts, contract situations, and rebates from manufacturers.

$$\text{prescription reimbursement} = \text{AWP} \pm \text{percentage} + \text{dispensing fee}$$

Example 29 A certain tablet comes in a quantity of 60 and has an AWP of $100.00. The pharmacy has an agreement with the supplier to purchase the drug at the AWP minus 15%. The insurer is willing to pay AWP plus 5% plus a $2.00 dispensing fee. A patient on this insurer's plan purchases 30 tablets for $54.50. How much profit does the pharmacy make on this prescription?

First calculate the amount of the discount:

$$\$100.00 \times 0.15 = \$15.00$$

and then the purchase price of the drug:

$$\$100.00 - \$15.00 = \$85.00$$

Therefore the pharmacy can purchase this drug at $85 per 60 tablets. The insurance company will pay the pharmacy AWP + 5%:

$$\$100.00 + \$100.00 \times 0.05 = \$100.00 + \$5.00$$
$$= \$105.00$$

At that price, the amount the insurance company will pay to fill a prescription for 30 pills is

$$\$105.00 \div 2 + \$2 \text{ (dispensing fee)} = \$52.50 + \$2.00 = \$54.50$$

Compare this to the pharmacy's cost of 30 tablets:

$$\$85.00 \div 2 = \$42.50$$

Therefore the pharmacy's profit on 30 tablets is

$$\$54.50 - \$42.50 = \$12.00$$

Capitation Fee

Some insurers provide a form of reimbursement to the pharmacy in the form of a monthly fee, called a capitation fee, for some patients. The monthly fee is paid to the pharmacy whether or not the patients receive prescriptions during that month. The pharmacy in return must dispense all the patients' prescriptions, even if they cost more than the monthly fee.

Example 30 **The Corner Drug Store receives a monthly capitation fee of $250 for John Jones. During April, Mr. Jones fills three prescriptions totalling $198.75. How much profit does the capitation fee provide?**

In this case the monthly fee exceeds the sum of the prescription costs, yielding a profit for the pharmacy:

$$\$250.00 - \$198.75 = \$51.25$$

Inventory Management

An inventory is a listing of all items that are available for sale in a business. Inventory value is defined as the total value of the drugs and merchandise in stock on a given day. Pharmacies must maintain a record of drugs and other supplies and merchandise purchased and sold to know when to reorder and when to adjust inventory levels of each item. Unlike some businesses, however, a pharmacy may need to keep some very slow-moving drugs in stock as a service to a few customers.

Space must be allocated to maintain inventory. Other considerations include shelving design and refrigeration. Keeping medications on the shelf is a cost to a pharmacy, and a large inventory can hinder cash flow. Inventory management should be designed such that medications arrive shortly before they are dispensed and sold; this minimizes shelf space.

Today most inventory records are computerized. Each time drugs are purchased, the quantity and price are entered into the computer database. As customers buy the drugs, the computer system automatically adjusts the inventory record. Pharmacies usually establish an inventory range for each item, that is, a maximum and a minimum number of units to have on hand. When the inventory drops to the minimum level, the item is purchased to restock the supply. This predetermined order point and the order quantity are based on historical use of each drug.

Example 31 **The maximum inventory level for ampicillin capsules is 1,000 capsules. At the end of the day, the computer prints a list of items to be reordered, which indicates an inventory level of 75 ampicillin capsules. How many capsules should be ordered to restock the inventory to maximum? If the drug wholesaler supplies ampicillin in bottles of 25, 100, 250, and 500 capsules, how many of each bottle size will fill the order (assuming that you begin with one 500-capsule bottle)?**

In order to replenish the ampicillin inventory to maximum levels (1,000), it first must be determined how much the present level differs:

$$1,000 \text{ capsules} - 75 \text{ capsules} = 925 \text{ capsules}$$

Then the idea is to purchase the 925 capsules in bottles of 500, 250, 100, and 25. It is good business practice to do this using the smallest number of bottles, keeping in mind that large-quantity containers are usually a more economical purchase.

$$\underset{\text{1 bottle}}{500 \text{ capsules}} + \underset{\text{1 bottle}}{250 \text{ capsules}} + \underset{\text{1 bottle}}{100 \text{ capsules}} + \underset{\text{3 bottles}}{25 \text{ capsules}} = 925 \text{ capsules}$$

Often today's pharmacies have $75,000 to $200,000 in inventory sitting on the shelves as drug products. If a large chain has ten stores in a particular region, the amount of money in goods sitting on the shelf adds up very quickly. Large companies often set goals for lowering the inventory in order to improve cash flow. One method used to set inventory goals for a pharmacy is called "days' supply," which refers to making the value of the inventory approximately equal to the cost to the pharmacy of the products sold in certain number of days. A common number is in the 25–35 day range. For example, if a pharmacy has a goal of "30 days' supply," it means that the goal is to reduce the value of the inventory to equal the total cost to the pharmacy of the products sold for 30 days.

On the other hand, sometimes a pharmacy does not know the best number of days to use as a goal in calculating costs. What they do know is the current inventory value, and average daily costs are easily calculated (weekly costs ÷ 7). With this information, it can be determined how many days it will take (what is referred to as "days' supply") for the average daily product costs to equal the value of the inventory. Then the pharmacy can revise the goal as necessary.

$$\text{number of days' supply} = \frac{\text{value of inventory}}{\text{average daily cost of products sold}}$$

Example 32 **Tom's Pharmacy has a total inventory value of $103,699. They had sales last week of $37,546, and the cost to the pharmacy of the products sold was $28,837. What should their days' supply be in order to keep their inventory value stable?**

Tom's average daily product costs were

$$\$28,837 \div 7 = \$4,120$$

Now according to the above formula, dividing the value of the inventory by the average daily product costs approximately equals the number of days' supply:

$$\text{number of days' supply} = \frac{\$103,699}{\$4,120} = 25$$

Thus in 25 days, Tom will have sold products approximately equal to the value of his inventory.

Chapter Summary

The daily activities of pharmacists and pharmacy technicians often include measurements and calculations. Pharmacy typically employs the metric system of measurement, which makes use of decimal units, including the basic units of the gram (for weight), the meter (for length and area), and the liter (for volume). Pharmacy also makes use of so-called common measure, including the apothecary, avoirdupois, and household measurement systems.

The most widely used units of measure in pharmacy are the metric units of milligrams, grams, kilograms, milliliters, and liters, as well as the apothecary/avoirdupois unit known as the grain. Pharmacy technicians should be able to convert between these different units and should be familiar with the standard prefixes for abbreviating metric quantities.

To move between units in the metric system, move the decimal to the right to go from larger to smaller units and to the left to go from smaller to larger units. Technicians should also be familiar with the basic rules for adding, subtracting, multiplying, and dividing fractions; with the basic principles for manipulating decimals; including converting to percents, and with procedures for calculating ratios and proportions. Of particular use to the technician is the ability to find an unknown quantity in a proportion when three elements of the proportion are known. The technician should be comfortable converting ratios to and from percents.

These basic mathematical principles and procedures are used in a wide variety of pharmaceutical calculations, such as calculating and converting dosages. At times it may be necessary to use mathematical techniques to calculate the molecular weight of certain substances in the pharmacy, or the specific gravity of various liquids. It is important to know how to compute the size, period, and rates of flow for intravenous solutions. Common in the preparation of pharmaceutical mixtures is the need to solve problems involving powder solutions and also dilutions. One very helpful tool in this case is the alligation method.

The principals of business must be understood in order to run a profitable pharmacy. It will often be the responsibility of the technician to calculate the markup on the products and compute any discounts. In order to deal with insurance companies, there must be an understanding of average wholesale price and capitation fees. And the financial stability of the pharmacy is very dependent on good inventory management, something that involves the technician.

Chapter Review

Knowledge Inventory

Choose the best answer from those provided.

1. The modern metric system makes use of the standardized units of the
   a. avoirdupois system.
   b. Système International (SI).
   c. Système Quebeçois.
   d. apothecaries' system.

2. The metric prefix meaning one millionth is
   a. nano-.
   b. micro-.
   c. milli-.
   d. deci-.

3. A gram is equal to
   a. 1,000 micrograms.
   b. 1,000 milligrams.
   c. 1,000 centigrams.
   d. 1,000 nanograms.

4. The liter is a standard measurement of
   a. distance.
   b. area.
   c. volume.
   d. weight.

5. Given ½, the fraction ²/₁ is its
   a. equivalent fraction.
   b. value.
   c. reciprocal.
   d. least common denominator.

6. A decimal fraction has as its denominator a power of
   a. 2.
   b. 5.
   c. 10.
   d. 25.

7. 58% means 58 out of one
   a. hundred.
   b. thousand.
   c. million.
   d. billion.

8. To find out if two fractions are equivalent,
    a. cross multiply them and check to see if the products of the multiplication are equal.
    b. multiply their denominators and check to see if the product is equal.
    c. multiply their numerators and check to see if the product is equal.
    d. invert them, then cross multiply them and check to see if the products of the multiplication are equal.

9. Intravenous flow rates are usually described as mL/hr or as
    a. mL/min.
    b. gtt/min.
    c. gtt/hr.
    d. mL/sec.

10. The proper pediatric dosage of a medication depends upon the child's
    a. body mass.
    b. weight.
    c. body surface area.
    d. none of the above.

Pharmacy in Practice

1. Convert the following:
    a. 34.6 g = _____ mg
    b. 735 mg = _____ g
    c. 3400 mL = _____ L
    d. 1.2 L = _____ mL
    e. 7.48 kg = _____ g
    f. 4.27 mL = _____ L

2. Convert the following:
    a. 24 oz = _____ pt
    b. 40 gr = _____ Э
    c. 6 oz (avoirdupois) = _____ lb (avoirdupois)
    d. 6.25 tbsp = _____ tsp
    e. 8 qt = _____ gal
    f. viii = _____ (Arabic numeral)
    g. C = _____ (Arabic numeral)

3. Solve the following conversion problems.
    a. You have 2 L of solution in stock. The solution is to be used to fill vials that hold 40 mL each. How many vials can you fill with the 2 L of solution?
    b. The patient has received a bottle containing 400 mL of a liquid medication. The patient is to take 3 tsp of the medication per day. How many days will the bottle last?
    c. A prescription calls for codeine sulfate 40 mg. How many grains of codeine sulfate should be used in the prescription?
    d. A patient takes two $\frac{1}{150}$ gr nitroglycerin tablets per day. How many mg of nitroglycerin does the patient receive each day?

4. Solve the following dosage problems.
   a. In stock, you have a solution that contains 8 mg of active ingredient per 10 mL of solution. A customer has a prescription calling for 4 doses of 6 mg each of the active ingredient. How many mL of the solution should the customer be given?
   b. A medication order calls for phenobarbital 60 mg. The supply available is phenobarbital 100 mg/mL of solution. How many milliliters of the solution will the patient be given?
   c. If the adult dose of a medication is 30 mg and the average adult body surface area is 1.72 m², what would be the appropriate pediatric dosage for a child with a body surface area of 0.50 m²?

5. Solve the following IV rate and administration problems.
   a. A physician orders 3,000 mL of a 10% dextrose and normal saline ($D_{10}NS$) IV over a 48 hour period. If the IV set will deliver 15 drops/mL, how many drops must be administered per minute?
   b. A ½ liter IV is running at a rate of 100 mL/hr. How long will the bag last?

6. Solve the following solution preparation problems.
   a. You have been asked to prepare a solution containing a powder with a volume of 0.7 mL. The total volume of the solution that you are to prepare should be 30 mL. How much diluent will you use in the solution, and what will be the percentage, by volume, of the powder in the solution?
   b. You are instructed to make 240 mL of a 0.45% w/v solution. You have a 100% concentrate in stock. How much of the full-strength solution will you use and how much diluent will be needed?
   c. You must prepare 300 mL of a solution containing 42.5% dextrose. In stock you have solutions containing 5% dextrose (Solution 1) and 50% dextrose (Solution 2). How many milliliters of each stock solution must you use in the solution that you prepare?

7. Solve the following business math problems.
   a. Eye drops with antihistamine are purchased in cases of 36 drop-dispenser bottles. The pharmacy desires a markup of $1.75 per bottle. The purchase price is $111.60 per case. What is the selling price per bottle?
   b. Identify the markup and the selling price of an oral antibiotic suspension that costs the pharmacist $15.60 per bottle if the markup rate is 25%.
   c. An asthma tablet costs the pharmacy $24.80 for a month's supply and the selling price is $30.75. Calculate the markup rate.
   d. John's Drug Shop purchases five cases of dermatological cream at $100/case. The invoice specifies a 15% discount if the account is paid in full within 15 days. What is the discounted price?
   e. There are 24 tubes of cream per case in Exercise d. You are to mark each tube up by 20% based on the discounted cost. What will the selling price be per tube?

f. A prescription is written for a tube of ointment. The AWP is $62.00. Smith's Pharmacy purchases the tube at AWP and Jones' Pharmacy purchases the tube at AWP minus 10%. The insurer will reimburse at AWP plus 2% plus a $1.50 dispensing fee. How much profit does each pharmacy make?

g. Sinus tablets have an AWP of $37.50 per 50 tablets. The Corner Drug Store dispensed prescriptions for a total of 300 sinus tablets during May. They were purchased at AWP minus 15%. The insurer reimburses at AWP plus 1.5% plus a $2.00 dispensing fee. Fifteen prescriptions of 20 tablets each were filled that month. How much profit was made?

h. Mountain Health Maintenance pays a capitation fee of $310.00 per month. Six patients on this plan bring in prescriptions during July. They are as follows with the cost reflected as the pharmacy cost for each.
Patient #1: $15.75, $106.50, $27.80
Patient #2: $210.00
Patient #3: $47.50, $105.25, $160.00, $52.60
Patient #4: $150.00, $210.00, $76.00
Patient #5: $10.50, $28.00, $62.50
Patient #6: $210.00, $210.00, $17.00
   1. What is the total capitation?
   2. What is the pharmacy cost?
   3. Was the profit positive or negative?
   4. What was the profit?

i. In the preceding question, if the drugs dispensed were allowed AWP (assuming all drugs were purchased at AWP) plus 3% and a $2.00 dispensing fee, would more profit have been made? How much total profit would be made? Is it more or less than on capitation? How much more or less?

j. Review the inventory list below and calculate the necessary purchases to reestablish maximum inventory. Write your answers in the "Purchased" column.

	A B	C	D	E	F	G
1	JOHN'S DRUG SHOP					
2	Current Drug	Max.	Dispensed	Min.	Current	Purchased
3	Date	Level	Today	Level	Inventory	
4	Eucerin cream, jars	10	1	3	3	
5	Ampicillin caps	4,500	500	4,000	2,400	
6	Eyedrops, bottles	24	4	4	4	
7	Nystatin oral solution	1,000 mL	100 mL	200 mL	400 mL	
8	Sterile saline	600 mL	315 mL	100 mL	75 mL	
9						
10						
11						
12						
13						

k. Kathy's Pharmacy has an inventory of $184,520. Her cost of sales last week were $28,223, and she made a 26% profit. Her day's supply goal is 34 days.
1. What was the amount sold last week?
2. What is the day's supply?
3. How much is the value above or below inventory in dollars?

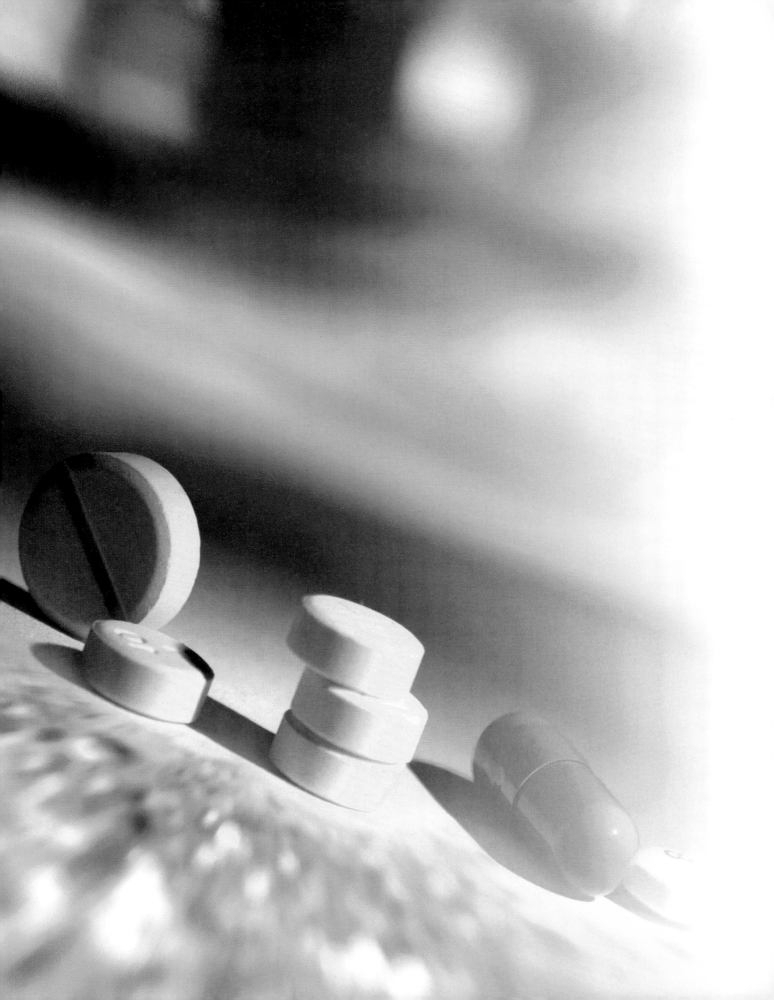

Dispensing, Billing, and Inventory Management

Learning Objectives

◇ Enumerate typical duties of pharmacy technicians with regard to dispensing of over-the-counter and prescription drugs.

◇ Explain the typical procedures for receiving and reviewing prescriptions.

◇ Describe the parts of a prescription and of a typical prescription label.

◇ Describe the parts of a patient profile and detail the steps required to prepare, check, or update a profile.

◇ Explain the parts of a computer system.

◇ Explain the alternatives for third-party administration.

◇ Enumerate some standard approaches to purchasing, receiving, and inventory management.

The primary role of the pharmacy, of course, is to dispense medications safely, accurately, and in accordance with the law. In this chapter you will learn some of what is involved in the dispensing of medications. The chapter also treats the mechanics of billing, purchasing, receiving, and inventory management.

COMMUNITY PHARMACY OPERATIONS

Community pharmacies sell both over-the-counter (OTC) and legend drugs. The former are drugs that can be legally sold without a prescription. The latter are drugs that, under the Durham-Humphrey Amendment of 1951, are required to bear on their labeling the legend, "Caution: Federal law prohibits dispensing without a prescription." Community pharmacies are generally organized into a front area, where OTC drugs, toiletries, cosmetics, greeting cards, and other merchandise are sold and an R̥ area, where prescription merchandise and related items are sold. For obvious reasons, the R̥ area is off limits to customers and may be entered only by authorized employees.

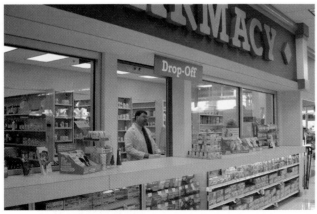

The R̥ area of the pharmacy can only be accessed by authorized employees in order to limit access to legend drugs.

Technician Duties Related to Dispensing Over-the-Counter Drugs

Increasingly, customers are turning to products that they can purchase at will for self-administration. The increase in use of over-the-counter drugs is related to a number of factors, including the increased cost of visits to physicians and the rising cost of prescription medications. In addition, many drugs that once could be purchased only with a prescription are now available over the counter. Although over-the-counter medications may be purchased without a prescription, the active ingredients in these medications are sometimes the same as those found in higher-strength prescription versions. The FDA generally approves an over-the-counter preparation only when the approval process leaves no doubt that the dosage strength is beneficial but unlikely to cause harm when taken as directed. These days, pharmacists devote a greater percentage of their time to recommending over-the-counter products to their customers and to counseling customers about their proper use. Over-the-counter drugs are also becoming an increasingly important part of the technician's responsibilities. Technicians often carry out such functions as stocking over-the-counter drugs, taking inventory of these drugs, removing drugs from stock when their shelf-life has expired, and helping customers to locate drugs on the shelves. However, technicians should avoid counseling customers with regard to use of over-the-counter drugs unless directed to do so by the pharmacist. Questions about the applications, effects, indications, contraindications, and administration of such drugs should be referred to the pharmacist.

Technician Duties Related to Dispensing Prescription Drugs

With regard to legend, or prescription, drugs, the technician may carry out a number of different duties, including greeting customers and receiving written prescriptions from them, answering the telephone and referring call-in prescriptions to the pharmacist, calling up the patient's profile on the computer or retrieving it from files, retrieving products from storage in the ℞ area, assisting the pharmacist with compounding (in some states), packaging of products, preparing labels for prescriptions, entering billing information into the computer, and third-party billing.

Technicians are often responsible for preparing prescription medications, packaging, labeling and preparing a patient bill. These duties are performed and all materials pertaining to a prescription are kept together for the pharmacist to check prior to dispensing to the patient. The process that begins with checking the prescription for completeness and ends with dispensing to the patient will take about 5–10 minutes and 100% accuracy is expected. If prescriptions filled in a given day were 99% correct, that would mean that the average pharmacy filling 200 prescriptions daily would have filled two prescriptions incorrectly. That is not acceptable. The prescription and product selection should be checked several times for accuracy during the fill process, and should be mentally checked again as the stock bottle is returned to the shelf. Table 7.1 explains the path a prescription follows once it crosses the threshold of a pharmacy, and the following sections of this chapter discuss certain steps in greater detail.

RECEIVING AND REVIEWING PRESCRIPTIONS

Prescriptions come into a pharmacy in a variety of ways. Most often, of course, customers carry in written prescriptions or physicians phone them in. A technician may, by law, receive a written prescription from a customer. However, he or she cannot take a prescription by telephone and reduce it to writing. Taking telephone prescriptions, by law, can be done only by a licensed pharmacist, although taking prescription refill information by telephone is, in many instances, considered acceptable.

Table 7.1	The Critical Path of a Prescription

1. The patient drops off the prescription.
2. The pharmacy technician checks the prescription to make sure it is complete and authentic and then verifies that the patient is in the pharmacy database.
3. The pharmacy technician enters the prescription into the computer, bills the insurance company or the patient, and generates the medication label.
4. The pharmacy technician asks the pharmacist to check the drug utilization review (DUR) warning screen when required.
5. **The pharmacy technician selects the appropriate medication and verifies the NDC number on the computer-generated label.**
6. **The pharmacy technician prepares the medication. For example, the prescribed number of tablets are counted.**
7. The pharmacy technician packages the medication.
8. The pharmacy technician labels the prescription container with the computer-generated label.
9. **The pharmacy technician prepares the filled prescription for the pharmacist to check.**
10. **The pharmacist checks the prescription.**
11. The pharmacy technician bags the approved prescription for patient sale and attaches an information sheet about the prescription, including indications, interactions, and possible side effects.
12. **The pharmacy technician returns the bulk product container to the shelf.**
13. **The pharmacy technician delivers the packaged prescription to the cash register area for patient pickup and pharmacist counseling.**

Note: The **bolded** steps should include verification that the proper product has been selected.

When taking a written prescription from a customer, first review it to make sure that it looks legitimate. A physician legally must write out a prescription entirely by hand. However, almost always, the prescription will be on a preprinted prescription form bearing the name, address, and telephone number of the prescribing physician. When receiving a prescription, the pharmacy technician should always check the elements illustrated in Figure 7.1. Table 7.2 details the parts of a prescription. If you have any doubts about the authenticity of a prescription, mention these to the pharmacist. A phone call from the pharmacist to the prescribing physician might be in order. Of course, prescriptions can come into a pharmacy by other means as well. A physician might fax or electronically transmit a prescription. In some drugstore chains, a prescription may be entered into a central database and be accessed at a store other than the one where the prescription was originally received. It is important for pharmacy technicians to be aware of state laws regarding prescription faxing and the transferring of prescriptions electronically or via a database.

Abbreviations used on prescriptions were covered in Chapter 3. You may wish to review that chapter or refer to it as you look at the sample prescriptions in this chapter. The following are some general guidelines with regard to reviewing prescriptions.

The patient's name should be given in full, including at least the full first and last names. Initials alone are not acceptable. If necessary, rewrite the patient's name in full above the name on the prescription and verify the spelling of the patient's name when it is not legible.

The patient's address is needed for patient records. In most states, the address is required for all prescriptions. Federal law requires addresses on prescriptions for controlled substances (substances with a high potential for abuse that are governed by the Controlled Substances Act—see Chapter 4); they must be, for such prescriptions,

Figure 7.1

Parts of a Prescription

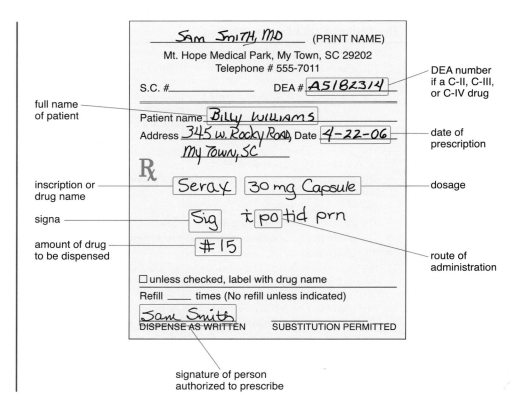

a resident address, not a post office box number even if the patient does not receive mail at this address.

Preprinted prescriptions often contain a space for the patient's birth date. If this space is not filled in, you should ask for the information. The patient's birth date is helpful for third-party billing and for distinguishing among patients with the same name. Knowing the patient's age also helps the pharmacist evaluate the appropriateness of the drug, quantity, and dosage form prescribed.

The date is the date when the physician wrote the prescription. For pharmacy records, the date when the prescription is received should be written on the prescription as well. If no date is written on the prescription, the date the prescription is brought into the pharmacy should be recorded, and noted as such. If the undated prescription is for an antibiotic, the pharmacist may wish to verify that the patient is under the current care of a physician. In addition, state regulations may dictate the length of time a controlled-substance prescription is valid, for example, six months from the date of issue. The date received is especially important for prescriptions for controlled substances, especially Schedule II controlled substances, which are drugs with accepted medical uses that have high potential for abuse. State regulations may control the time period for filling a controlled-substance prescription. In some states, a Schedule II prescription must be filled within seven days of issue and in other states it must be filled within 72 hours. Prescriptions for Schedule II controlled substances may be handwritten or typed. Some states require that the physician fill a prescription by hand and do not allow a nurse or assistant to write the prescription, even if it is signed by the physician. Signatures on all Schedule II prescriptions must be handwritten, not stamped. In an emergency situation, a person with the legal au-

Table 7.2	**Parts of a Prescription**
Prescriber Information	The name, address, telephone number, and other information identifying the prescriber.
Date	The date on which the prescription was written.
Patient Information	The name, address, and other pertinent information about the patient who receives the prescription. If the patient is an infant, a toddler, an elderly person, or someone else with special needs, the prescription may include such information as the age, weight, and body surface area (BSA) of the patient, information needed by the pharmacist in order to calculate appropriate dosages. To assist the pharmacist, if this information is missing the pharmacy technician may query the customer about this information and add it to the prescription.
℞	The symbol ℞, for the Latin word *recipe,* meaning "take."
Inscription	The medication or medications prescribed, including generic or brand names, strengths, and amounts. States and most institutions have regulations and policies allowing pharmacists to substitute cheaper generic equivalents of brand-name medications when appropriate.
Subscription	Instructions to the pharmacist on dispensing the medication, including such information as compounding or packaging instructions, labeling instructions, instructions on allowable refills, and, when a generic equivalent may not be substituted, instructions to that effect (e.g., "No substitutions" or "No substitutions allowed"). The abbreviation PBO means "Prescribe Brand Only." The abbreviation DAW means "Dispense As Written."
Signa	Directions for the patient to follow (commonly called the "sig").
Additional Instructions	Any additional instructions that the prescriber deems necessary.
Signature	The signature of the prescriber.
DEA Number	This number, identifying the prescriber as someone authorized to prescribe controlled substances, is required on all prescriptions for such substances.

thority to issue prescriptions for Schedule II controlled substances may provide oral, rather than written authorization for the prescription. However, the amount prescribed must not exceed the amount necessary for treatment during the emergency period, and the prescriber must provide a written prescription within 72 hours of the oral authorization.

If the prescription is for a controlled substance, the quantity must be limited in some states to 120 units or a 30-day supply or, depending on the state, 34 days or 120 units, whichever is less. A prescription for a Schedule II drug is not refillable. A prescription for a Schedule III or IV drug may be refilled up to five times, but these refills must occur within a six-month period, after which time a new prescription is required. A prescription for a Schedule V controlled substance may be refilled only if authorized by a prescribing physician.

Drugs may be listed on prescriptions using brand names or generic names. A brand, proprietary, or trademark name given to a product by the manufacturer and is the property of that manufacturer. A generic name is a nonproprietary, or nontrademark, name that identifies a drug substance. A given drug (i.e., one with a particular generic name) may be marketed under various brand names. For example, NitroBid and Nitrostat are two brand names under which nitroglycerin is marketed. A generic drug is one that is marketed under the generic name rather than a brand name. Generic drugs are often cheaper than brand name drugs and are often substituted, under regulations now existing in every state, for brand name drugs. Such substitutions can be made, of course, only if the generic drug and the brand name drug are bioequivalent. If the prescription for a brand name drug is filled with a generic equivalent, then the name, strength, and manufacturer of the generic substitution must be written on the label.

The signa, or directions for use, from the prescription must be placed on the label produced for the medication. The label should read exactly as indicated on the prescription. Any signa comments written on the prescription must be included on the label.

If the refill blank on the prescription is left blank, then there can be no refill for the prescription. The words "No Refill" will appear on the prescription label, and an indication of *No Refill* will be entered into the patient's record. If the refill blank on the prescription indicates "as needed" (prn), then this is not construed as indicating an unlimited duration. Most pharmacies and state laws require at least yearly updates on prn prescriptions.

If refills are called for, prescriptions should generally be refilled one or two days before the customer's supply will run out, although this is not a hard-and-fast rule. In some circumstances—as, for example, when a customer is leaving on vacation—an early refill might be appropriate. Insurance companies often will not pay for these early refills, and the patient may need to pay for the prescription up front and send in the receipts for reimbursement.

Regulations in a given state may require two signature lines at the bottom of the prescription, one reading "Dispense As Written," (DAW) and the other reading "Substitution Permitted." If the "Dispense as Written" line is signed, then substitution of a generic equivalent is not permitted. Other states may have only one signature line required, and if a prescriber wishes that only the brand name product be dispensed, "Brand Name Medically Necessary" must be noted on the prescription.

The space for DEA number on the prescription form is for the number issued to the physician authorizing him or her to prescribe controlled substances. Some physicians have this number preprinted on their prescriptions while others write it on the prescription when writing out the order for a narcotic medication. There are some states that require all narcotic prescriptions to be written on authorized "safety paper." Many insurance companies require a pharmacy to have a physician's DEA number on file in order to be reimbursed for prescriptions, even when the drug is for a nonscheduled medication. Pharmacy personnel can check for falsified DEA numbers by following this procedure:

Step 1. Add the first, third, and fifth digits of the DEA number.
Step 2. Add the second, fourth, and sixth digits of the number and multiply the sum by two.
Step 3. Add the two results from Steps 1 and 2. The last digit of this sum should be the same as the last digit of the DEA number.

The patient should be asked whether he or she has any known allergies to drugs or foods. If the answer is negative, the notation NKA, for "No Known Allergies," should be made on the back of the prescription form and on the patient profile. If the answer is positive, the allergy should be listed on the back of the prescription form and on the patient profile. It is good practice to inquire about allergies every time a patient comes to the pharmacy with a prescription for an antibiotic. Antibiotics are the most common medication allergy, and allergies can begin at any age. A patient could have safely taken an antibiotic several times and become allergic to it on a subsequent occasion. Thus it is important to confirm and update the patient's allergies in the profile.

PREPARING, CHECKING, AND UPDATING THE PATIENT PROFILE

A patient profile is a paper form (hard copy) or a computerized record that lists the patient's prescriptions and other relevant information. If the patient is a previous customer, he or she may already have a profile on file that the technician can retrieve. If not, then a new profile will have to be created. Figure 7.2 is an example of a patient profile form. Figure 7.3 shows a computerized profile. The patient profile will generally contain the information listed in Table 7.3.

Figure 7.2

A Patient Profile Form

PATIENT PROFILE

Patient Name

_____ _____ _____
Last   First   Middle Initial

Street or PO Box

_____ _____ _____
City   State   Zip

Phone   **Date of Birth**   **Social Security No.**
( ) __ __   _____   □ Male □ Female   ___ __ ____
                 Month   Day   Year

□ Yes, I would like medication dispensed in a child-resistant container.
□ No, I do not want medication dispensed in a child-resistant container.

Medication Insurance   **Card Holder Name** _____
□ Yes   □ No   □ Card Holder   □ Child   □ Disabled Dependent
                              □ Spouse   □ Dependent Parent   □ Full Time Student

MEDICAL HISTORY

HEALTH   **ALLERGIES AND DRUG REACTIONS**
□ Angina   □ Epilepsy   □ No known drug allergies or
□ Anemia   □ Glaucoma   reactions
□ Arthritis   □ Heart Condition   □ Aspirin
□ Asthma   □ Kidney Disease   □ Cephalosporins
□ Blood Clotting Disorders □ Liver Disease   □ Codeine
□ High Blood Pressure □ Lung Disease   □ Erythromycin
□ Breast Feeding   □ Parkinson's Disease   □ Penicillin
□ Cancer   □ Pregnancy   □ Sulfa Drugs
□ Diabetes   □ Ulcers   □ Tetracyclines
Other Conditions _____   □ Xanthines
_____   Other Allergies/Reactions _____
_____   _____

Prescription Medication Being Taken   **OTC Medication Currently Being Taken**
_____   _____
_____   _____
_____   _____

Would You Like Generic Medication Where Possible? □ Yes □ No

Comments
_____

Health information changes periodically. Please notify the pharmacy of any new medications, allergies, drug reactions, or health conditions.
_____ Signature _____ Date □ I do not wish to provide this information.

167-B

Figure 7.3

A Computerized Patient Profile

```
04-21-20XX                    PATIENT MEDICATION PROFILE        DR: JONES

NAME: SMITH, GEORGE                    ROOM: 276            SEX: M    HT:  73 IN
DIAGNOSIS: PNEUMONIA                                        AGE:  46  WT: 195 LB
ALLERGIES: NKA
COMMENTS:

    ********************************* ACTIVE MEDICATIONS ********************
    *********** MEDICATIONS PRECEDED BY '*' WILL BE STOPPED TODAY UNLESS REORDER

    MEDICATION        STRENGTH    FORMULARY        RT    DOSAGE   FREQUENCY      START  R
    ==============    =========   ==============   ==    ======   ============   =====  =
    APRESOLINE        75MG        HYDRALAZINE      PO    TAB      TID            04/21
    ASA EC                        ACETYL SALICYL   PO    TAB      QD             04/21
    LANOXIN           .125MG      DIGOXIN          PO    TAB      QD             04/21
    MAALOX            30ML                         PO    LIQ      Q4H            04/21
    TYLENOL           650MG       ACETAMINOPHEN    PO    CAPLET   Q4H PRN        04/21
    ZANTAC            150MG       RANITIDINE       PO    TAB      BID            04/21
    -----------------------------------------------------------------------------


    **************** INACTIVE MEDICATIONS (STOPPED WITHIN LAST THREE DAYS) ****

    -----------------------------------------------------------------------------
```

Policies and Procedures for Patient Profiles

Different pharmacies follow different policies and procedures, generally explained in a policies and procedures manual. This manual reflects not only the requirements of the relevant state laws and regulations but also the guidelines for safe and effective operation established by the pharmacy itself. Part of the technician's job, as described in the policies and procedures manual, might be to enter data from a new prescription into the patient profile. Completing a patient profile might require asking questions related to each of the items indicated in Table 7.2. If a patient profile information sheet is not complete, the technician may need to interview the patient to obtain necessary information. Any time you notice a patient having difficulty with filling out the form, offer assistance in filling it out.

Updating the Patient Profile

When the prescription is filled, the patient profile must be updated to reflect that prescription. A technician who has received sufficient training may be given the task of recording the new prescription in the profile to provide such information as the prescription number; the name of the drug prescribed; the dosage form; the quantity; the number of refills authorized, if any; and the charge for the prescription.

Occasionally, a patient will need to update information regarding insurance or changing medical conditions. The technician too may perform this, however, confirming this new information with the on-duty pharmacist is essential so that the pharmacist may conduct a drug utilization review (DUR) regarding a change of medical condition.

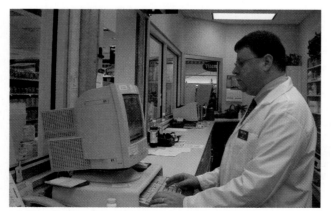

It is important to keep records such as the patient profile up-to-date.

MANAGING COMPUTER SYSTEMS

Contemporary pharmacies, both community and institutional, often use computer sys-

Table 7.3   Parts of the Patient Profile

Identifying Information	Includes the patient's full name with the middle initial; address; telephone number; social security number; birth date; and gender.
Insurance/Billing Information	Records information necessary for billing. If the patient has prescription insurance, this should be indicated, along with information such as the name of the insurer, the group number, the patient's ID or card number, the effective date and expiration date of the insurance, the cardholder's name, the patient's relationship to the cardholder, and the persons covered by the insurance, and other relevant information.
Medical History	Contains information on existing conditions (such as epilepsy or glaucoma) and on known allergies and adverse drug reactions the patient has experienced. An allergy is a hypersensitivity to a specific substance that is manifested in a physiological disorder. Common allergic reactions include sweating, rashes, swelling, and difficulty in breathing. In extreme cases, allergic reactions can lead to shock, coma, or death. An adverse drug reaction is any negative consequence to any individual from taking a particular drug. The pharmacist reviews the medical history information on the profile to make sure that the prescription is safe to fill for a given patient.
Medication/Prescription History	Describes any prescription and OTC medications currently being taken and provides a list of previous prescriptions filled for this patient, including information on refills. The pharmacist reviews this information to make sure that the prescription will not cause adverse drug interactions (negative consequences) due to the combined effects of drugs and/or drugs and foods.
Prescription Preferences	Indicates patient preferences with regard to his or her prescriptions, such as child-resistant or non–child-resistant containers or generic substitutions.
Refusal of Information	Statement of refusal by the patient to provide any or all of the above information. This statement is for the protection of the pharmacy.

tems to carry out a wide variety of functions, such as checking and updating patient profile information, checking for possible allergies and drug interactions, printing labels, calculating charges, and completing automated third-party billing. The process of billing insurance companies "online" has greatly lessened the quantity of paperwork in the average retail pharmacy. This online billing process is called adjudication. From their beginnings as simple order-input devices, pharmacy computer systems have evolved into complex systems offering a wide range of functions. Today, some systems are capable of tracking expenses, doing pharmacokinetic calculations, tracking inventory, generating controlled substances reports, retrieving literature, and controlling automatic or robotic dispensing and compounding devices. Systems vary from pharmacy to pharmacy. A computer system within an institution is often networked with other departments, such as nursing, laboratory, and administration, thus providing the opportunity for transmitting and sharing of information, including patient data, medication orders, pharmacy literature, and adverse reaction reports.

Because of the widespread use of computers in pharmacy, the aspiring technician should become familiar with computer systems and how they work. Becoming competent at basic keyboarding is also essential. This section provides some elementary information about computer systems, but a thorough introduction to computers is beyond the scope of this book.

The Parts of a Computer System

A computer is an electronic device for inputting, storing, processing, and/or outputting information. A digital computer represents information internally using binary numbers, which are constructed of strings of ones and zeros. Many types of digital computers exist today. In order of size and power, some types of computers available today include supercomputers, mainframe computers, minicomputers, workstations, personal computers, network computers, laptop computers, and handheld or palmtop computers. Some of the more important parts of a typical computer system include the following (see Figure 7.4):

◇ one or more input devices, such as a keyboard, a mouse, or a touch screen, for getting information into the computer
◇ a central processing unit (CPU) for processing (manipulating) data that is input prior to output or storage
◇ one or more storage devices, such as a floppy disk drive, hard drive, tape drive, or removable disk drive (such as a Zip, Jaz, Syquest, Bernoulli, or optical drive), for storing information that has been input into the computer
◇ random-access memory (RAM), which is the temporary, nonpermanent memory of the computer in which information is held while it is being input and processed
◇ read-only memory (ROM), which is permanent memory containing essential operating instructions for the computer
◇ a monitor, or display, providing a visual representation of data that has been input and/or processed
◇ a printer, for creating hard copy, or paper output, such as patient profiles, medication labels, and receipts
◇ a scanner, for inputting a photo version of the prescription into the computer system, utilized in some pharmacies to save the step of pulling out a hard copy of the prescription if there is a question about its original intent.
◇ a modem, a device for connecting a computer to a remote network via telephone lines
◇ an operating system, a software program that performs essential functions such as maintaining a list of file names, issuing processing instructions, and controlling output
◇ applications, software programs that perform particular functions, such as word processing

An application that allows one to enter, retrieve, and query records is known as a database management system, or DBMS. Database management systems are the kind of application most commonly used in pharmacy. Often the DBMS used in a particular community or institutional pharmacy was specifically written and/or al-

Figure 7.4

A Desktop Computer System

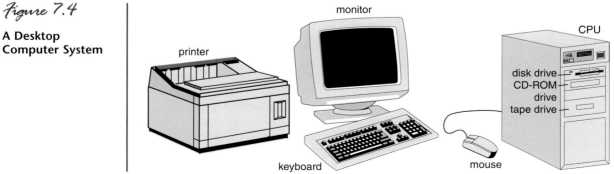

tered to meet the needs of the pharmacy. Such a program, known as a vertically integrated application, meets a wide variety of needs within an organization from customer record keeping to inventory control and billing. Often, the pharmacy DBMS is menu-driven, allowing the operator to choose functions from a menu of options on the screen by typing a single number, letter, or function key on the keyboard.

How Pharmacy Computer Systems Work

In many pharmacies the operator works at a dumb terminal, a computer device that contains a keyboard and a monitor but does not contain its own storage and processing capabilities. A terminal is connected to a remote computer—often a mini-computer or a mainframe—that stores and processes data.

Pharmacy computer systems differ dramatically from one another. In large retail chains, it is not uncommon for computers to be connected to a single large mainframe system at the company headquarters or home office. In such systems, customer records are stored remotely and backed up at the home office computer site and are accessed via telecommunications, connecting to the remote computer via telephone lines, DSL, cable, or wireless connections. Wireless communications involve the transmission of data or voice signals through the air and involve transmitters, receivers, and often, satellites.

Pharmacy computer systems often allow the operator to call up patient profiles onscreen and to enter new prescription information. A hard-copy patient profile might then be generated for backup filing. In addition, the system may automatically print labels containing information keyed into the profile for a given prescription. Many systems in use today contain automatic capabilities to compare the patient profile with new prescription information entered and warn of possible adverse drug interactions or potential problems with allergic reactions to a given prescription (Figure 7.5). Such systems typically prevent the filling of an order until a pharmacist intervenes. In no situation should a pharmacy technician override such a warning on his or her own initiative. In all cases, the pharmacist should review the warning and make the decision as to whether the prescription should be filled. Drugs are generally identified on computer screens by product name, manufacturer, strength, and unique National Drug Code (NDC) number.

Computers are fallible machines. They often break down and are susceptible to such problems as power failures and surges. Therefore, it is important that copies, or backups, of all data be made at regular intervals. Often, pharmacy computer systems make use of tape backup devices. A tape backup device stores backup data on reels or cassettes of magnetic tape.

Figure 7.5

Computerized Drug Interaction Warning
Many pharmacy computer systems contain features that will warn, automatically, of possible allergic reactions or adverse food or drug interactions based on information in the patient profile and on a database of known contraindications for given medications.

```
                    DRUG INTERACTIONS
PHARMACY
PATIENT: George Smith
PHYSICIAN: Jones
ALLERGIES: NKA

SIGNIFICANCE RATING 1 Drug interactions have been identified (1 interaction)

    1. ASA interacts with coumadin


REFERENCE: 'Drug Interaction Facts' by Facts and Comparsions
```

SELECTING AND PREPARING MEDICATIONS

After the information for a new prescription or refill has been entered into the patient profile, the customer is given a time at which the prescription will be ready for pickup, and the prescription is ready to be filled. A given prescription may require either dispensing of drugs that come prepackaged in given dosage forms (e.g., tablets, prefilled capsules, transdermal patches, etc.) or compounding prior to dispensing. Once the printed prescription bill, or label, is available, the proper product should be selected from the stock area, and often the NDC number will be available for comparison to insure that the correct product has been located.

Preparing Oral Dosage Forms

Oral drug products are available in many different dosage forms, and each dosage form has its own dispensing requirements. Syrups and suspensions are used frequently for pediatric medications. Liquid products commonly are poured directly into the dispensing bottle or are dispensed in their original packaging. The most commonly used dosage form is the oral tablet or capsule. Often, tablets and capsules must be counted out and placed in the appropriately sized vial. The vials are sized according to the approximate number of drams they can contain.

Figure 7.6 shows the equipment and procedure for counting tablets and capsules. A special counting tray is used. It has a trough on one side to hold counted tablets or capsules and a spout on the opposite side to pour unused medication back into the stock bottle. The technician should not touch the medication with his or her fingers as oils from the skin as well as germs could contaminate the medication. Therefore, the tablets and capsules should always be counted with a clean spatula and picked up with forceps if they are dropped on the counter. The spatula, tray, and forceps should be cleaned often throughout the workday with 70 % isopropyl alcohol. They should also be cleaned after counting a sulfa or penicillin product or any product that leaves visible powder on the surfaces.

Extemporaneous Compounding

In some cases, filling the prescription requires extemporaneous compounding, the actual preparation of the medication by pharmacy personnel. Compounding might

Figure 7.6

Counting Tablets
(a) Tablets should be counted by fives and moved to the trough with a spatula. (b) The unneeded tablets are returned to the stock container by pouring them from the spout. (c) The counted tablets are then poured into the appropriately sized medication vial.

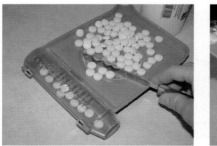
(a)

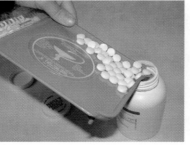
(b)

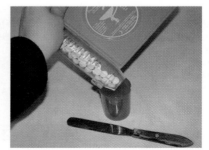
(c)

involve, for example, mixing a powdered active ingredient with a diluent powder and filling a given number of capsules with the combined materials, which is known as an admixture. The pharmacy technician may be required to retrieve from storage in the pharmacy area the necessary constituents of a compound (liquids, powders, capsules, containers, etc.), to prepare necessary equipment for the compounding process, to count or weigh materials, to compound the prescription, and to return products and clean up the compounding area and equipment after the procedure. In any case, compounding duties undertaken by the technician must be directly supervised and checked by the pharmacist. Extemporaneous compounding is treated in Chapter 8.

Dispensing of Prepackaged Drugs

Filling a prescription often involves simply retrieving from stock a drug with the right name, manufacturer, and strength. Sometimes, drugs come in prepackaged, unit dose form. (A unit dose is a single dose of a drug.) This is true, for example, of transdermal patches, of tablets, and of prefilled capsules. Filling the prescription thus amounts to little more than locating the correct drug, in the correct strength, in storage; counting out the number of doses called for by the prescription; and, if necessary, placing these in a container with a label. Sometimes filling a prescription involves retrieving a multiple-dose container of a premixed drug and then measuring out the prescribed quantity and placing it into a container with a label. This would be true, for example, of some powders and liquids. Again, the pharmacist must verify that the proper drug, in the proper dosage form, in the proper amount, in the proper container, and with the proper label has been chosen and prepared.

Choosing Containers

A wide variety of amber vial sizes are available and are named according to approximate "dram" size, even though the dram is a measure that is no longer used. Selecting the proper vial size is a skill that will be learned quickly. Most containers in the pharmacy are colored to prevent UV light exposure and subsequent degradation of the medication. Other containers common to the retail pharmacy include amber liquid containers and solid white ointment jars. Cardboard boxes may be available as well for products such as suppositories or tubes of cream. Many products such as metered dose inhalers and oral contraceptives will not need a container, and the prescription label will be attached directly to the product. Some pharmacists prefer to apply prescription labels for topical products to the tube or jar itself, while others prefer to have the label placed on the box in which the product is packaged.

Pediatric medications should always be dispensed in child-resistant containers, which are designed to be difficult for children to open. The Poison Prevention Packaging Act of 1970 requires, with some exceptions such as nitroglycerin for angina, that prescription drugs be packaged in child-resistant containers but states that a non-child-resistant container may be used if the physician prescribing the drug or the patient receiving it makes a request for such a container. The regulations of a given state may require the patient to make a special request for dispensing a prescription in a non-child-resistant container. Some pharmacies allow patients to complete a blanket request form for non-child-resistant containers. Others require patients to sign such a request for each prescription. Often pharmacies make use of a stamp on the back of the prescription for this purpose.

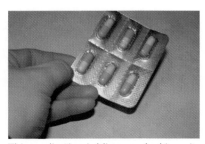

This medication is blister packed in unit dose form so that an individual dose may be prepared for the patient.

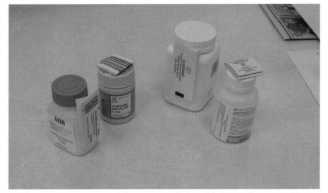

Package inserts are attached to stock bottles, and they provide detailed information about the drug. This information is regulated and is used to create patient information sheets.

PREPARING LABELS

From a technical, legal point of view, a label consists of all information provided with a drug by a manufacturer or pharmacist, including the label on the container and the package insert, which contains information on the product's pharmacological properties and uses contraindications, and side effects.

Manufactures provide information on the package inserts included with prescription drug products. Legally, these package inserts are extensions of the labeling on the drug product, and laws and regulations involving misbranding or mislabeling apply to them. These inserts are required by FDA regulation to contain the information listed in Table 7.4, in the order shown.

The *Physician's Desk Reference*, published by Medical Economics of Oradell, New Jersey, is primarily a compilation of package inserts. It provides, in an easy accessed form, a great deal of information about prescription drugs.

Before or after the preparation of the order, according to the policy of the individual pharmacy, a container label must be generated. This label may either be affixed directly to the container by the person generating the label, or it may be kept separate for review by the pharmacist before being affixed. Figure 7.7 compares a prescription and a container label.

Many pharmacies generate labels by computer. In other cases, labels are typed. Less commonly, preprinted labels are used, requiring that information for a specific prescription be added, checked, or circled. Preprinted labels are generally discouraged because of the potential for labeling error. It is too easy to check the wrong box on a preprinted label.

The information required on a label depends upon the laws and regulations of a given state. As was indicated above, manufacturers' labels for prescription medica-

Table 7.4	Organization of Package Insert Information
	description
	clinical pharmacology
	indications and usage
	contraindications
	warnings
	precautions
	adverse reactions
	drug abuse and dependence
	overdosage
	dosage and administration
	how supplied
	date of the most recent revision of the labeling

Figure 7.7

Prescription and Label Comparison
(a) The original prescription contains the information that should be included on the label. (b) The medication container label translates the instructions for the patient.

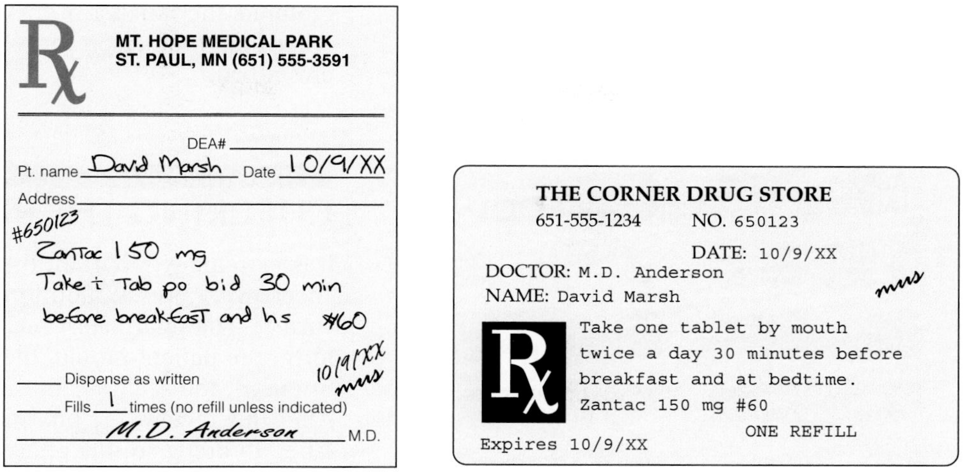

℞ MT. HOPE MEDICAL PARK
ST. PAUL, MN (651) 555-3591

DEA# ______
Pt. name David Marsh Date 10/9/XX
Address ______
#650123
Zantac 150 mg
Take i Tab po bid 30 min
before breakfast and hs #60
10/9/XX mws
____ Dispense as written
____ Fills 1 times (no refill unless indicated)
M.D. Anderson M.D.

THE CORNER DRUG STORE
651-555-1234 NO. 650123
DATE: 10/9/XX
DOCTOR: M.D. Anderson
NAME: David Marsh
mws
℞ Take one tablet by mouth
twice a day 30 minutes before
breakfast and at bedtime.
Zantac 150 mg #60
ONE REFILL
Expires 10/9/XX

(a) (b)

tions must carry the legend, "Caution: Federal law prohibits dispensing without a prescription." Typical information required on a container label prepared by a pharmacy includes the information in Table 7.5.

Auxiliary labels, attached at the pharmacist's discretion, provide additional usage or precautionary information for the patient. For Schedule II, III, and IV controlled substances, the auxiliary label "TRANSFER WARNING" is required.

Labels for Schedule II controlled substances must contain the fill date. Labels for Schedule III, IV, or V drugs must show the date of initial filling. Labels for all prescriptions for controlled substances should include the pharmacy name and address, the serial number of the prescription, the name of the patient, the name of the prescriber, and directions for use and cautionary statements. Labels for Schedule II, III, and IV drugs should contain the cautionary statement, "Caution: Federal law

Table 7.5	Label Information
	date when the prescription was filled
	serial number of the prescription
	name and address of the pharmacy
	name of the patient
	name of the prescribing physician
	all directions for use given on the prescription
	any necessary auxiliary labels, containing patient precautions
	generic or brand name of the medication
	strength of the medication
	name of the drug manufacturer
	quantity of the drug
	expiration date of the drug, or date after which the drug should not be used because of possible loss of potency or efficacy
	initials of the licensed pharmacist
	number of refills allowed or the phrase "No Refills"

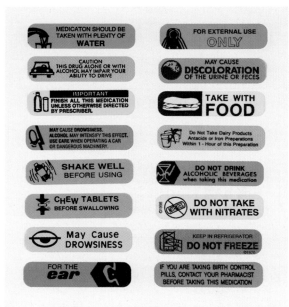

Prescription medications sometimes include labels that provide instructions for how to properly self-administer or store the medication. These labels use color and logos to communicate their message.

prohibits the transfer of this drug to any person other than the person for whom it was prescribed."

CHECKING THE PRESCRIPTION

It is extremely important that the pharmacist check every prescription to make sure that it is correct. The pharmacist reviews the prescription form, the patient profile, the drug and drug quantity used, the accuracy of the label, and the price. After this review, the pharmacist initials the label. In doing so, the pharmacist assumes responsibility for the correctness of the prescription. However, the pharmacist does not necessarily assume, by this action, sole responsibility. Technicians have in the past been held legally responsible for dispensing and labeling mistakes, especially in situations in which the dispensing error was due to negligence on the part of the technician (such as improperly overriding a computerized adverse interaction warning).

BILLING AND THIRD-PARTY ADMINISTRATION

When a new prescription is received, it is important for the pharmacy technician to obtain from the customer all necessary insurance information, including any co-pay amount. Once the prescription has been filled and the label prepared, the billing can be done. Billing policies and procedures differ from pharmacy to pharmacy and from customer to customer. In some cases, the customer pays for the prescription at the time he or she receives it. The customer may or may not then be reimbursed by an insurer for the cost. In other cases, billing involves third-party administration (TPA), or billing by the pharmacist to the third party, the customer's insurer. After the price of the prescription is calculated, based on existing pricing schedules, the prescription is ready for review by the pharmacist.

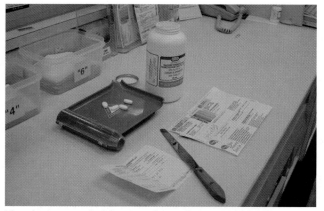

The pharmacy technician must have all prepared prescriptions checked by the supervising pharmacist.

Many pharmacy customers have prescription drug insurance, and billing must be done to a third party. If the customer has such insurance, then he or she may carry a prescription card containing information such as the following: the name of the insured person, the insurance carrier, a group number, a cardholder identification number, information on dependents covered, an expiration date, and the amount of the co-payment. The technician must request this information and either enter it into the computer system or, if the pharmacy uses a manual system for third-party billing, onto a form, generally a universal claim form (UCF). Billing of the third party may be handled in a variety of ways. The bill may be transferred to the third party electronically, via modem, or placed on a computer diskette that is then mailed to the insurer. In other cases, the computer may generate a bill that is mailed to the third party, or a manually prepared bill, usually one on a UCF, may be sent to the insurer.

When the prescription is billed to the insurance company or Prescription Benefits Manager (PBM), the pharmacy will be notified within a few minutes what amount they should charge the patient and what amount the pharmacy will be reimbursed. A PBM is a company that administers prescription drug benefits for covered individuals from many different insurance companies that have contracted the PBM to provide this service. This process, called online adjudication, takes only a few minutes during the prescription fill process and saves the pharmacy a great deal of paperwork when performed properly. In some cases the insurance company advises the pharmacy that a deductible needs to be met before benefits will be paid. The deductible is an amount that must be paid by the insured, usually at the beginning of the year, before the insurance company will consider paying its portion of the prescription. The insurance company may also inform the pharmacy of the appropriate co-pay or co-insurance that the patient is responsible for paying. A co-pay is a flat amount that the patient pays for each prescription. In some cases a patient may have a dual co-pay, or a co-pay for brand names and a lower one for generics (e.g., $10.00 for brand names and $5.00 for generics.) Co-insurance is the term for a percentage-based plan whereby the patient must pay a certain percentage of the prescription price, and again dual co-insurance where one percentage is in effect for brand name medications and usually a lower percentage for generic medications (e.g., 30% for brand names, and 10% for generics.)

Often insurance companies have a formulary of preferred medication for which they will pay maximum benefits and a list of drugs that are either not fully covered or not covered at all. This too will be a part of the online adjudication process. Patients are often provided with these lists and encouraged to give the list to their physician so that appropriate medications may be selected from the list. When the physician decides the patient must have a medication that is not on the insurance company's formulary, it may be necessary to obtain an override number of some sort from the insurance company in order for the prescription to be properly covered. In some cases these prescriptions can not be adjudicated online, and must be hand billed on a UCF to the appropriate insurance company. There are cases where the medication selected by the physician and needed by the patient is not covered by the insurance under any circumstance. If such a question arises, it is often helpful to have on file a photocopy of the patient's insurance card, and appropriate phone numbers for the insurance company.

PURCHASING, RECEIVING, AND INVENTORY CONTROL

The purposes of purchasing and inventory control are to obtain pharmaceutical materials in a timely manner and to establish and maintain appropriate levels of materials in stock. Purchasing, receiving, and inventory processes should be as uncomplicated as possible so as not to disrupt or to interfere with the other activities of the pharmacy.

Pharmaceutical products can be selected by a variety of methods. In an institutional setting, for example, the pharmacy and therapeutics committee (P & T) determines which agents are to be maintained in stock. This committee prepares a list of agents accepted for use in the institution. Such a list is called a formulary. For each product, a formulary lists the product name, dosage form, concentration, and package size.

Purchasing

Purchasing, the ordering of products for use or sale by the pharmacy or institution, is usually carried out in either of two ways. In independent purchasing, the pharmacist or technician works alone or with a purchasing agent and deals directly with pharmaceutical companies regarding matters such as price. In group purchasing, a number of institutions or pharmacies work together to negotiate discounts for high-volume purchases and other benefits. Some independent purchasing exists in almost all pharmacy settings because some products are not available through group purchasing and some settings have unique needs for specialty products.

Several purchasing methods or systems are used in pharmacies. Direct purchasing requires completion of a purchase order, generally a preprinted form with a unique number, on which the product name(s), amount(s), and price(s) are entered. If the pharmacy uses a purchasing agent, then a purchase requisition is sent to that agent. The order is then transmitted directly to the manufacturer. An advantage of direct purchasing is the lack of add-on fees. A disadvantage is the commitment of time and staff on the part of the pharmacy. Wholesaler purchasing enables the pharmacy to use a single source to purchase numerous products from numerous manufacturers. Advantages to wholesaler purchasing include reduced turnaround time for orders, lower inventory and lower associated costs, and reduced commitment of time and staff. Disadvantages include higher purchase cost, supply difficulties, loss of the control provided by in-house purchase orders, and unavailability of some medicinals. Prime vendor purchasing involves an agreement made by an institution or pharmacy for a specified percentage or dollar volume of purchases. Such a system offers the advantages of competitive service fees, electronic order entry, and emergency delivery services. Just-in-time (JIT) purchasing involves frequent purchasing in quantities that just meet supply needs until the next ordering time. JIT reduces the quantity of each product on the shelves and thus reduces the amount of money tied up in inventory. However, such a system can be used only when supplies are readily available and needs can be accurately predicted.

Receiving

Delivery of an order of products initiates a series of procedures known as receiving. It is important for institutions and pharmacies to have a system of checks and balances for purchasing and receiving. In other words, full control should not reside with a single person, and the person ordering should not be the same as the person receiving. The pharmaceutical products received must be carefully checked against the purchase order or requisition. The shipment should be compared for name of product, quantity, product strength, and product package size. Products damaged in shipment or improperly shipped must be reported immediately. Stringent laws regulate the return of pharmaceuticals to manufacturers. In the case of a damaged or incorrect shipment, the manufacturer should be notified immediately and authorization should be secured for the return of the defective shipment.

Pharmaceuticals in a shipment should be checked for expiration dates. Each pharmacy has a policy for acceptable product expiration dates. A typical requirement might be that products have expiration dates of at least six months from the date of receipt. After products are received and checked, they are then placed in a proper storage location. The expiration dates of stored products are periodically checked, and expired products are removed. An accepted method for stocking pharmaceuticals is to position the units of product with the shortest expiration dates where they will be the first units selected for use.

Pharmacy technicians handle and prepare medications more often than pharmacists do and are therefore in a better position to identify potential sources of error related to packaging and storage. A common error is the selection of the wrong pharmaceutical because two products look alike or have names that sound alike. (Look back to Table 3.5 for some examples of near homonyms and homographs among drug names.) A good work habit is to read each label three times and to avoid basing product identification on size, color, package shape, or label design. The technician should make three checks: (1) when the product is initially being pulled from the inventory shelf, (2) at the time of preparation, and (3) when the product is returned to the shelf.

Occasionally, a pharmaceutical product will be unavailable or temporarily unavailable from a supplier. It then becomes necessary to borrow or purchase a small quantity from another institution or pharmacy. A detailed procedure for control of and accountability with regard to loaned or borrowed products is necessary.

Two types of pharmaceuticals require special consideration: controlled substances and investigational drugs. The Controlled Substances Act defines ordering and inventory requirements. Purchase of Schedule II controlled substances must be authorized by a pharmacist and executed on a DEA form. A physical inventory of Schedule II substances is required every two years. Investigational drugs—ones that are being used in clinical trials and have not yet been approved by the FDA for use in the general population—require special ordering and handling procedures.

Inventory Control

As we explained in Chapter 6, the entire stock of products on hand at a given time in an institution or business is known as inventory. Several important issues with regard to inventory include how much inventory should be maintained, when inventory levels should be adjusted, and where inventory should be stored. Factors that bear upon decisions regarding these issues include floor space allocation, design and arrangement of shelves, and demands upon available refrigerator or freezer space.

Keeping excess inventory in stock has a number of associated costs, including the capital that is tied up in the inventory, waste due to product expiration, and increased likelihood of theft or contamination. In an ideal system, pharmaceuticals would arrive shortly before they were needed. Today, a variety of methods may be used for inventory management. In some systems, the dispenser of a product determines when a product needs to be reordered and enters it into an order book. Other systems make use of inventory cards or papers on which an ongoing history of use and purchase is kept. Some systems make use of predetermined minimum and maximum product levels based upon historical use. In still other systems, purchasing is based upon calculation of the most economical order quantity or

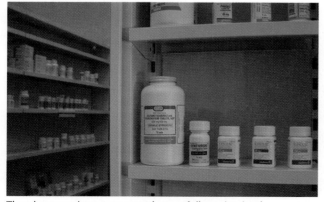
The pharmacy inventory must be carefully maintained.

value. Computerized inventory control systems can automatically generate purchase orders under predetermined conditions. One goal of computerized inventory control is to reduce the time and staff required for inventory management. Ideally, such a system would require only periodic review and adjustment.

A physical inventory, or counting of items in stock, is taken when no perpetual inventory system is in place. Most pharmacies take the inventory once or twice a year. An inventory value is used to determine average inventory and turnover rate. The average inventory allows a pharmacy to determine the number of times that pharmaceuticals are repurchased in a specific period of time, usually annually.

$$\text{average inventory} = \frac{\text{beginning inventory} + \text{ending inventory}}{2}$$

Turnover rate is the number of times the entire stock is used and replaced each year.

$$\text{turnover rate} = \frac{\text{annual dollar purchases}}{\text{average inventory}}$$

Chapter Summary

Pharmacy technicians assume a number of responsibilities related to both over-the-counter and legend drugs. The precise responsibilities a technician may assume depend on the laws and regulations of the state in which he or she is working. Usually, a technician can take written prescriptions from walk-in customers but cannot take new prescriptions by telephone and reduce them to writing. The parts of a prescription include prescriber information, the date, patient information, the symbol ℞, the inscription (the medication or medications prescribed and their amounts), the subscription (instructions to the pharmacist), the signa (directions to the patient), additional instructions, and the signature. After the prescription is checked, it is entered into the patient profile. If no patient profile already exists, a new one, with all necessary information, is created. Patient profiles may be in hard-copy or computerized form and include identifying information, insurance/billing information, medical history, medication/prescription history, and prescription preferences for each patient. Some pharmacy computer systems contain automatic warnings about possible allergic or other adverse reactions.

After the patient profile is created or updated, the prescription may be filled. Filling the prescription may involve any of a number of tasks, including retrieving drugs, supplies, containers, or equipment; setting up equipment; weighing and measuring; compounding; filling containers; and preparing labels. Container labels must contain a unique prescription number, the name of the patient, the date of the prescription, directions for use, the name and strength of the medication, the manufacturer of the medication, the quantity of the drug, the expiration date, the initials of the pharmacist, the number of refills, and auxiliary labels. After the label is prepared, a price for the prescription is calculated from existing tables, or schedules, in the pharmacy. Then the pharmacist checks the prescription form, the patient profile, the drug and drug quantity used, the accuracy of the label, and the price. Billing often must be done to a third party, the customer's insurer. The process of conducting such billing is called third-party administration. In addition to carrying out dispensing and billing functions, technicians are often involved in purchasing, receiving, and inventory functions.

Chapter Review

Knowledge Inventory

Choose the best answer from those provided.

1. Technicians' duties with regard to over-the-counter drugs typically include
   a. stocking them.
   b. taking inventory of them.
   c. removing expired drugs from the shelves.
   d. All of the above

2. In a prescription, the signa is the
   a. signature of the prescribing physician.
   b. initials of the pharmacist.
   c. directions for the patient to follow.
   d. instructions to the pharmacist on dispensing the medication.

3. The symbol ℞ stands for the Latin word *recipe* and means
   a. give.
   b. take.
   c. prepare.
   d. mix.

4. A signature on a prescription for a Schedule II controlled substance
   a. may be stamped.
   b. must be handwritten.
   c. must include the DEA number.
   d. may be that of the prescriber or his or her agent.

5. In most states, a generic drug may be substituted for a brand name or proprietary drug provided that the
   a. generic drug is cheaper.
   b. generic drug has undergone clinical trials
   c. generic drug is bioequivalent to the brand name or proprietary drug.
   d. generic drug is nontoxic.

6. Pharmacy personnel can check to see if a DEA number has been falsified by
   a. looking up the number in the *Orange Book*.
   b. performing a mathematical calculation.
   c. checking the number in *Facts and Comparisons*.
   d. using a code to translate the number into an alphabetical form—the name of the prescriber.

7. An important purpose of the medication/prescription history on the patient profile is to
   a. identify potential adverse drug interactions.
   b. verify the authenticity of the current prescription.
   c. provide information on existing conditions, known allergies, and history of adverse drug interactions.
   d. provide the information used in the pharmacy's record of the controlled substances that it has dispensed.

8. A computer application program that allows one to enter, retrieve, and query records is known as a(n)
   a. vertically integrated application.
   b. operating system.
   c. menu-driven application.
   d. database management system.

9. Child-resistant containers are required by the
   a. Controlled Substances Act.
   b. Federal Anti-Tampering Act.
   c. Durham-Humphrey Amendment to the Food, Drug, and Cosmetic Act.
   d. Poison Prevention Packaging Act.

10. In a manual third-party administration system, billing is typically done by means of a
    a. computer-generated form.
    b. purchase order.
    c. purchase requisition.
    d. universal claim form.

Pharmacy in Practice

1. For each of the prescriptions below, answer the following questions:
    a. Is any essential item missing from the prescription? If so, what is this item?
    b. What medication is prescribed, in what strength, and in what amount?
    c. What special instructions, if any, are provided in the subscription?
    d. What directions are given for the patient to follow?

MT. HOPE MEDICAL PARK
MY TOWN, USA   555-3591

\# *127352*   DEA \#_____

PT. NAME *Fred Figule*   DATE_____

ADDRESS _____

Rₓ   Hydrocortisone 20mg tabs
Take AM   5 tabs day 1
                3   "   2
                2   "   3
                1 tab   "   4 and 5

REFILLS ___ TIMES   (NO REFILL UNLESS INDICATED)
_____ M.D. _____ M.D.
DISPENSE AS WRITTEN   SUBSTITUTE PERMITTED

MT. HOPE MEDICAL PARK
MY TOWN, USA   555-3591

\# *42573*   DEA \#_____

PT. NAME *H. R. Robbins*   DATE *11-24-XX*

ADDRESS _____

Rₓ   Tylenol/codeine No 4
Take 1 prn pain q 4-6h

REFILLS ___ TIMES   (NO REFILL UNLESS INDICATED)
_____ M.D. _____ M.D.
DISPENSE AS WRITTEN   SUBSTITUTE PERMITTED

MT. HOPE MEDICAL PARK
MY TOWN, USA   555-3591

\#_____   DEA \#_____

PT. NAME *Abby Gee*   DATE *9-10-XX*

ADDRESS _____

Rₓ   Prilosec 20mg
Take 1cap before eating qd
                                    \#30

REFILLS ___ TIMES   (NO REFILL UNLESS INDICATED)
_____ M.D. _____ M.D.
DISPENSE AS WRITTEN   SUBSTITUTE PERMITTED

2. Prepare a label for each prescription given on the previous page.

a.

Paragon Pharmacy	AP 1111111
670 Main Street	220-555-3245
Anytown, USA	

Patient: _____   Prescriber: _____

Drug: _____

Date: _____   Refills: _____

b.

Paragon Pharmacy	AP 1111111
670 Main Street	220-555-3245
Anytown, USA	

Patient: _____   Prescriber: _____

Drug: _____

Date: _____   Refills: _____

c.

Paragon Pharmacy	AP 1111111
670 Main Street	220-555-3245
Anytown, USA	

Patient: _____   Prescriber: _____

Drug: _____

Date: _____   Refills: _____

3. Review the patient profile that follows. Then answer the following questions:
   a. What essential information is missing from this profile? What questions should you ask of the customer to complete the profile?
   b. What allergies and drug reactions does the patient have?
   c. What known medical conditions does the patient have?
   d. What prescription and OTC medications is the patient currently taking?
   e. Should the customer's prescription be filled in a child-resistant container?
   f. Does the customer have prescription insurance? If so, in whose name is this insurance held?

PATIENT PROFILE

Patient Name

Frames _____ _Ted_ _____ _R._
  Last   First   Middle Initial

****

111 Black Road
  Street or PO Box

Gaston _____ _SC_ _____ _29052_
  City   State   Zip

****

Phone _(803) 555 7989_   **Date of Birth** _07_ _28_ _38_   ☒ Male ☐ Female   **Social Security No.** _249 00 0012_
                                Month Day Year

☒ Yes, I would like medication dispensed in a child-resistant container.
☐ No, I do not want medication dispensed in a child-resistant container.

Medication Insurance   **Card Holder Name** _Ted Frames_
☒ Yes ☐ No   ☒ Card Holder   ☐ Child   ☐ Disabled Dependent
                  ☐ Spouse   ☐ Dependent Parent ☐ Full Time Student

MEDICAL HISTORY

HEALTH
☐ Angina	☐ Epilepsy
☐ Anemia	☐ Glaucoma
☒ Arthritis	☒ Heart Condition
☐ Asthma	☐ Kidney Disease
☐ Blood Clotting Disorders	☐ Liver Disease
☐ High Blood Pressure	☐ Lung Disease
☐ Breast Feeding	☐ Parkinson's Disease
☐ Cancer	☐ Pregnancy
☐ Diabetes	☐ Ulcers

Other Conditions _____
_____

ALLERGIES AND DRUG REACTIONS
☐ No known drug allergies or reactions
☒ Aspirin
☐ Cephalosporins
☐ Codeine
☐ Erythromycin
☐ Penicillin
☒ Sulfa Drugs
☐ Tetracyclines
☐ Xanthines
Other Allergies/Reactions _____
_____

Prescription Medication Being Taken
Feldene 20mg
Iseptin 80mg

OTC Medication Currently Being Taken
Nasalcrom

Would You Like Generic Medication Where Possible? ☒ Yes ☐ No

Comments

Health information changes periodically. Please notify the pharmacy of any new medications, allergies, drug reactions, or health conditions.
Ted Frames _____ Signature _9-9-XX_ Date ☒ I do not wish to provide this information.

167-B

4. Create a diagram of a typical computer system. Label the following parts: the keyboard, the mouse, the central processing unit, the floppy disk drive, the monitor, the printer, and the modem.

5. Determine which of the following is a valid DEA number:

1234563

2749122

Improving Communication Skills

1. Sometimes customers have difficulty identifying the pharmacist and do not understand that different roles of the pharmacist and the pharmacy technician. This can be frustrating for a customer seeking assistance. What types of things could you do as a pharmacy technician to help the customers?

2. A pharmacy technician working in a retail environment should be familiar with various terms related to health insurance. Patients often have a difficult time understanding how their insurance works, and the technician can often act as an intermediary and advocate for the patient with regards to prescription drug benefits. Research the following insurance terms and define them in words that would be easily understood by a customer of the pharmacy.
   a. major medical insurance
   b. Medicare, Parts A and B
   c. Medicaid
   d. deductible
   e. co-pay
   f. co-insurance
   g. formulary
   h. PBM
   i. usual and customary

Internet Research

1. Visit the Web site of a local pharmacy chain drugstore.
   a. What types of services does the site provide?
   b. Does the site offer online counseling services?
   c. Does the site offer information regarding specific medications?

2. Visit the AmerisourceBergan Web site at www.amerisourcebergen.net. Take the iECHO tour.
   a. What type of company is this?
   b. What online services are available?

Extemporaneous Compounding

Learning Objectives

◇ Define the term extemporaneous compounding and describe common situations in which compounding is required.

◇ Enumerate and describe the equipment used for the weighing, measuring, and compounding of pharmaceuticals.

◇ Use the proper technique for weighing pharmaceutical ingredients.

◇ Use the proper technique for measuring liquid volumes.

◇ Explain the common methods used for comminution and blending of pharmaceutical ingredients.

◇ Explain the use of the geometric dilution method.

◇ Explain the processes by which solutions, suspensions, ointments, creams, powders, suppositories, and capsules are prepared.

Until the emergence of modern, large-scale pharmaceutical manufacturing in the nineteenth century, all medications were prepared (compounded) by individuals from raw pharmaceutical ingredients. Compounding remains an important part of pharmacy practice, and in many states, pharmacy technicians assist in or carry out compounding tasks. Proper compounding requires an intimate knowledge of pharmaceutical equipment and of the techniques for using that equipment properly to weigh, measure, reduce, and combine ingredients.

THE NEED FOR EXTEMPORANEOUS COMPOUNDING

Extemporaneous compounding is the production of medication on demand in an appropriate quantity and dosage form from pharmaceutical ingredients. In the past, compounding accounted for much of a pharmacist's job. With the emergence of widespread industrial pharmaceutical manufacturing, the need for extemporaneous compounding has decreased, but not to the vanishing point. In fact, on many occasions the pharmacist and his or her technician are called upon to practice this ancient art.

The law addresses compounding and quality issues by defining and requiring Good Manufacturing Practices (GMP). GMP are skills that are learned in pharmacy schools, and on the job. It is the pharmacist's duty to ensure all compounded products prepared are made using GMP. The law also addresses the issue of pharmacies making certain compounds ahead of time, or in anticipation of prescriptions. In most cases, compounds are not made until the prescription is received by the pharmacy. However some pharmacies specialize their business by making special orders for a community, and often make the prescription product in bulk in advance.

Some examples of situations that require extemporaneous compounding include the following:

◇ The prescription calls for unit doses smaller than those that are commercially available, as is sometimes the case with pediatric medications. For example, a prescription might call for 15 mg per unit dose of a medication available only in tablets containing 30 mg of the active ingredient. The pharmacist might thus have to pulverize, or triturate, the tablets, mix the resultant powder with a suitable diluent, and then use the diluted powder to fill 15 mg capsules.

⬦ A medication normally available in a solid dosage form might have to be prepared in another dosage form, such as a liquid or a suppository, for administration to a patient who can not or will not swallow the solid form.

⬦ A medication with an unpleasant taste might have to be prepared in a tasty, masking syrup base to ensure compliance by a pediatric patient.

⬦ A medication may be available only in commercial forms containing preservatives, colorings, or other materials to which a patient is allergic, and so an alternative without the unwanted ingredients might need to be prepared.

⬦ The strength or dosage form called for in the prescription may not be in stock or readily available.

⬦ A dosage form other than those commercially available may be desired in order to customize the rate of delivery, rate of onset, site of action, or other pharmacokinetic properties of the drug.

⬦ A non-commercially available medication must be prepared for a veterinary application.

This chapter deals with the extemporaneous compounding of nonsterile products, ones compounded without using special aseptic techniques.

EQUIPMENT FOR WEIGHING, MEASURING, AND COMPOUNDING

To carry out a compounding operation, a pharmacist or pharmacy technician makes use of a number of conventional instruments and supplies.

Balances

A Class III prescription balance, formerly known as a Class A prescription balance, is required equipment in every pharmacy. The Class III prescription balance is a two-pan balance that can be used for weighing small amounts of material (120 g or less) and that has a sensitivity requirement (SR) of 6 mg. This means that a 6 mg weight will move the indicator on the balance one degree.

A counter balance, which also has two pans, is used for weighing larger amounts of material, up to about 5 kg. It has a sensitivity requirement of 100 mg. Because of its lesser sensitivity, a counter balance is not used in prescription compounding but rather for tasks such as measuring bulk products, for instance Epsom salts.

Balance measurements are made using sets of standardized pharmaceutical weights. Typical weight sets contain both metric weights and apothecaries' weights (for infor-

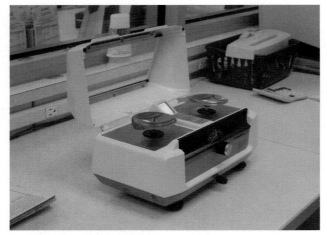

The Class III prescription balance accurately weighs small amounts of material.

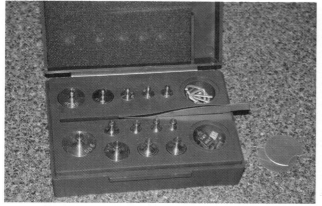

This is a set of pharmacy weights. Metric weights are in the front row and apothecary weights are in the back row.

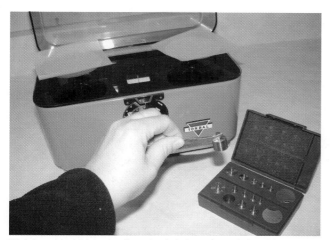

Weights should be transferred using forceps and should not be touched with bare skin. Moisture or oils will affect their accuracy.

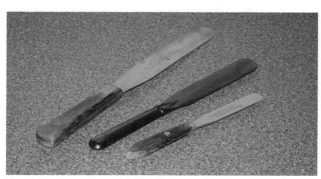

Spatulas are a common tool in the pharmacy.

mation about the metric and apothecary measurement systems, see Chapter 6). Weights are generally made of polished brass and may be coated with a noncorrosive material such as nickel or chromium. Typical metric sets may contain gram weights of 1, 2, 5, 10, 20, 50, and 100 g, which are conically shaped, with a handle and flattened top. Fractional gram weights (10, 20, 50, 100, 200, and 500 mg, for example) are also available. These are made of aluminum and are usually flat, with one raised edge to facilitate picking up the weight using forceps. Avoirdupois weights (again, see Chapter 6) of $\frac{1}{32}$, $\frac{1}{16}$, $\frac{1}{8}$, $\frac{1}{4}$, $\frac{1}{2}$, 1, 2, 4, and 8 oz may also be used. Weights come in a container in which they should be stored when not in use. Care should be taken not to touch or drop a weight or otherwise expose it to damage or contamination.

Forceps and Spatulas

Forceps are instruments for grasping small objects. They are provided with weight sets to use for picking up weights and transferring them to and from balances in order to avoid transferring moisture or oil to the weights, thereby changing their weight. Weights should not be transferred using the hands and fingers. Product and the weights should always be placed on weighing papers. Weighing papers are placed on balances to avoid contact between pharmaceutical ingredients and the balance tray. Typically, glassine paper is used. Glassine paper is a thin paper coated with nonabsorbent paraffin wax.

Spatulas are stainless steel, plastic, or hard rubber instruments used for transferring solid pharmaceutical ingredients to weighing pans and for various compounding tasks such as preparing ointments and creams or loosening material from the surfaces of a mortar and pestle. Hard rubber spatulas are used when corrosive materials such as iodine and mercuric salts are handled.

Compounding Slab

A compounding slab, also known as an ointment slab, is a plate made of ground glass that has a flat, hard, nonabsorbent surface

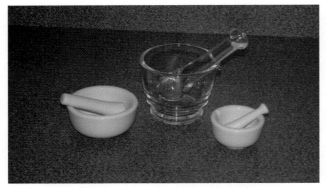

The mortar and pestle are used to mix or grind substances.

ideal for mixing compounds. In lieu of a compounding or ointment slab, compounding may be performed on special nonabsorbent parchment paper that is then disposed of after the compounding operation is finished.

Mortar and Pestle

A mortar and pestle are used for grinding and mixing pharmaceutical ingredients. These devices come in glass, porcelain, and Wedgwood varieties. Paradoxically, the coarser the surface of the mortar and pestle, the finer the trituration, or grinding, that can be done. As a result, a coarse-grained porcelain or Wedgwood mortar and pestle set is used for trituration of crystals, granules, and powders, whereas a glass mortar and pestle, with its smooth surface, is preferred for mixing of liquids and semisolid dosage forms. A glass mortar and pestle also has the advantages of being nonporous and nonstaining.

Graduates and Pipettes

Graduates are glass or polypropylene flasks used for measuring liquids. They come in two varieties. Conical graduates have wide tops and wide bases and taper from the top to the bottom. Cylindrical graduates, which are more accurate, have the shape of a uniform column. Both kinds of graduates are available in a wide variety of sizes, ranging from 5 mL to more than 1,000 mL. Cylindrical graduates are generally calibrated in metric units (cubic centimeters), whereas conical graduates may be calibrated in both metric and apothecary units or using either one of these two systems.

A pipette is a long, thin, calibrated hollow tube used for measurement of volumes of liquid less than 1.5 mL. A pipette filler is a device used instead of the mouth for drawing a dangerous solution, such as an acid, into the pipette.

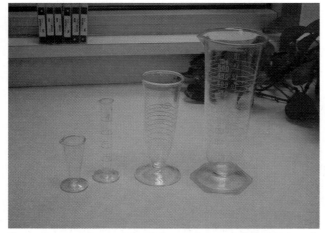

Graduates come in a variety of sizes and shapes. Cylindrical graduates are more accurate than conical graduates. The second graduate is cylindrical.

Master Formula Sheet

Of course, in addition to the equipment described above, the compounding of a medication requires the necessary ingredients. Figure 8.1 shows an example of a master formula sheet, also known as a pharmacy compounding log. The master formula sheet, prepared by the pharmacist, will indicate the amount of each ingredient needed, list the procedures to follow, and provide the labeling instructions. The example in Figure 8.1 lists the directions and ingredients for compounding a preparation called "Magic Mouthwash." Some pharmacies keep this information on large index cards, similar to recipe cards.

Figure 8.1

Master Formula Sheet
This formula sheet is for Magic Mouthwash, a commonly made formula.

MASTER FORMULA SHEET

PRODUCT _____ MTC LOT NUMBER _____

LABEL: Date MFG:
MAGIC MOUTHWASH

Take 1 teaspoonful 3 times daily. Swish and swallow.

STRENGTH: _____

QUANTITY MFG: _____

	MANUFACTURER'S LOT NUMBER	INGREDIENTS	AMOUNT NEEDED	WEIGHED OR MEASURED BY	CHECKED BY
1		Decadron or hydrocortisone	4.5 mg 120 mg		
2		nystatin (Mycostatin)	2,000,000 units		
3		tetracycline	1g		
4		diphenhydramine (Benadryl	qs to 120 mL		
5					
6					
7					
8					

DIRECTIONS FOR MANUFACTURING

1. Draw up, by syringe, 4.5 mg Decadron or 120 mg of hydrocortisone or equivalent steroid.
2. Crush nystatin tablets and mix with 5 mL sterile water or measure 2,000,000 units of liquid.
3. Measure 1 g of liquid tetracycline or dissolve tablets or capsules in 5 mL sterile water.
4. Add each ingredient to liquid container and qs with diphenhydramine to 120 mL.
5. Attach label.

Manufactured by _____
Approved by _____
Date _____

Auxiliary Labeling: SHAKE WELL

TECHNIQUE FOR WEIGHING PHARMACEUTICAL INGREDIENTS

Weighing of the product is one of the most essential parts of the compounding process. One must practice over the period of several weeks, or even months to feel comfortable with weighing products on a prescription balance. The balance is accurate to within a very small quantity, and variations in technique could easily result in a slight but serious error. Weighing the exact amount prescribed is essential in

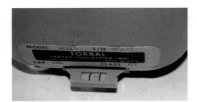

The balance is leveled front to back when the bubble is centered.

compounds for several reasons: the product can not be "checked" for content once mixed, the quantities weighed out are often very small, and a slight overage could mean a serious overdose for the patient.

Table 8.1 outlines the procedure for weighing pharmaceutical ingredients. A pharmacist or second experienced technician may need to check your weighing technique and results for awhile after you begin training.

The balance should be placed on a secure, level surface, at waist height, where it cannot be easily jarred. It should be in the locked or "arrested" position when not in use and when moved. The area where the balance is placed should be well lighted and free from drafts, dust, corrosive vapors, or high humidity that might affect the ingredients or the measurements. Avoid spilling materials onto the balance. If any materials are spilled on the balance, wipe them off immediately. Do not place materials onto the balance while it is released (unlocked), as doing so may force the pan down suddenly and cause damage to the instrument.

The balance must be perfectly level, both side to side and front to back. Leveling is often the most time consuming process for beginners. The front-to-back leveling is done by adjusting the pegs on the front of the scale so that the leveling bubble is centered. The side-to-side leveling is adjusted in a similar way. The released, empty scales will register as equal when the scale is balanced. The levelness should be checked often throughout the day when the balance is heavily used. Remember that the scale must be in a arrested (locked) position whenever the balance is moved or the pegs are adjusted.

Table 8.1	Weighing Pharmaceutical Ingredients

1. Unlock the balance and confirm that it is leveled, front-to-back and side-to-side, using the leveling screws at its base. Once this is done, the balance is ready to use. Lock the balance once again, before transferring weight to it.

2. Place weighing papers on the two pans of the balance. These papers should be of roughly the same size and weight. The edges of the paper on the left-hand pan of may be folded upward, to hold the substance to be weighed. Do not place any materials on the weighing pans without using weighing papers.

3. Unlock the balance to confirm that the balance is still leveled, and then lock it again.

4. Add the desired weight to the right-hand pan, using forceps to transfer the weight from the weight container.

5. Place an approximate amount of the material to be weighed to the left-hand pan, using a spatula to transfer it.

6. Slowly release the beam using the unlocking device at the front of the balance, and check the balance.

7. If the amount of the substance being weighed is too great or too small, lock the balance again and use a spatula to add or remove material. See Figure 8.2 (a).

8. Slowly release the beam using the unlocking device and check for equilibrium.

9. Once a nearly precise amount of material has been transferred to the pan, a very small adjustment upward can be made by placing a small amount of material on the spatula, holding the spatula over the left pan, and lightly tapping the spatula with the forefinger to knock a bit of the substance onto the pan. This is done with the balance unlocked and the balance beam free to move.

10. Lock the balance, close the lid, and then unlock the balance to make a final measurement. (At this point, have the pharmacist check the measurement.) See Figure 8.2 (b).

11. Lock the balance before removing the measured substance. Use transfer forceps to remove the weights and return them to their storage case.

Figure 8.2

A Prescription Balance
(a) Transferring a substance to the scale.
(b) The final measurement is taken with the lid closed.

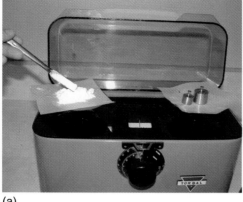
(a)

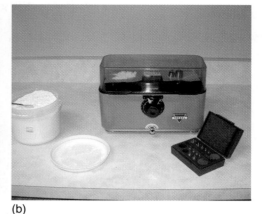
(b)

TECHNIQUE FOR MEASURING LIQUID VOLUMES

Liquid volumes are often much easier to measure than solid volumes that must be weighed, and a wide variety of containers are available to assist in volumetric measurement. A general rule of thumb is to always select the device that will give you the most accurate volume. It is good practice to select a container that will be at least half full when you are measuring.

Bear in mind that most commonly the upper surface of the liquid will be a meniscus, or moon-shaped body, that is slightly concave, or bowed inward toward the center (see Figure 8.2). In other words, the level of the liquid will be slightly higher at the edges. Therefore, do not measure the level by looking down on the graduate. Instead, measure by placing the eyes at the level of the liquid. Read the level of the liquid at the *bottom* of the meniscus.

Table 8.2 outlines the procedure for measuring liquid volumes.

Table 8.2	Measuring Liquid Volumes

1. Choose a graduate with a capacity that equals or very slightly exceeds the total volume of the liquid to be measured. Doing so, for reasons too complex for explanation here, reduces the percentage of error in the measurement. In no case should the volume to be measured be less than 20 percent of the total capacity of the graduate. For example, 10 mL of liquid should not be measured in a graduate exceeding 50 mL in capacity. Again, the closer the total capacity of the graduate to the volume to be measured, the more accurate the measurement will be.

2. Bear in mind that the more narrow the column of liquid in the graduate, the less substantial any reading error will be. Thus, for very small volume measurement a pipette is preferable to a cylindrical graduate, and for larger measurements a cylindrical graduate is preferable to a conical graduate.

3. Pour the liquid to be measured slowly into the graduate, watching the level of the liquid in the graduate as you do so. If the liquid is viscous, or thick, attempt to pour it toward the center of the graduate to avoid having some of the liquid cling to the sides.

4. Wait for liquid clinging to the sides of the graduate to settle before taking a measurement.

5. Measure the level of the liquid at eye level and read the liquid at the bottom of the meniscus, Figure 8.3.

6. When pouring the liquid out of the graduate, allow ample time for all of the liquid to drain. Bear in mind that depending on the viscosity of the liquid, more or less will cling to the sides of the graduate. For a particularly viscous liquid, some compensation or adjustment for this clinging may have to be made.

Figure 8.3

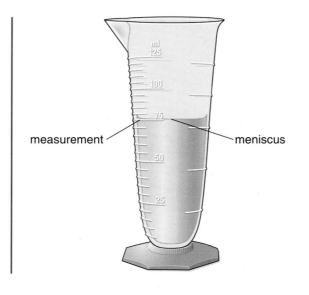

Meniscus
Liquid in a narrow column usually forms a concave meniscus. Measurements should be taken at the bottom of the concavity when read at eye level.

measurement ⎯ meniscus

COMMINUTION AND BLENDING OF DRUGS

Comminution is the act of reducing a substance to small, fine particles. Blending is the act of combining two substances. Techniques for comminution and blending include trituration, levigation, pulverization by intervention, spatulation, sifting, and tumbling. Trituration is the process of rubbing, grinding, or pulverizing a substance to create fine particles, generally by means of a mortar and pestle. A rapid motion with minimal pressure provides the best results. Other forms of comminution include levigation and pulverization by intervention. Levigation is typically used when reducing the particle size of a solid during the preparation of an ointment. A paste is formed of a solid material and a tiny amount of a liquid levigating agent, such as castor oil or mineral oil, that is miscible, or mixable, with the solid but in which the solid is not soluble. The paste is then triturated to reduce the particle size and added to the ointment base. The levigating agent becomes part of the final product.

Pulverization by intervention is the process of reducing the size of particles in a solid with the aid of an additional material in which the substance is soluble—a volatile solvent such as camphor and alcohol or iodine and ether. The solvent is added. The mixture is triturated. The solvent is then permitted to evaporate and so does not become part of the final product. Spatulation is the process of combining substances by means of a spatula, generally on an ointment tile. Sifting, like the sifting of flour in baking, can be used to blend or combine powders. Powders can also be combined by tumbling—placing the powders into a bag or container and shaking it.

Geometric Dilution Method

Often a mortar and pestle are used to combine more than one drug. To combine drugs in a mortar and pestle, you can use the geometric dilution method. Place the most potent ingredient, which will most likely be the ingredient that occurs in the smallest amount, into the mortar first. Then add an equal amount of the next most potent ingredient and mix well. Continue in this manner, adding, each time, an amount equal to the amount in the mortar, until successively larger amounts of all the ingredients are added. Then add any excess amount of any ingredient and mix well.

Some Examples of Compounding

Thorough instruction in the complex art of extemporaneous compounding is beyond the scope of this book. Refer to the standard reference work on the subject such as *Remington: The Science and Practice of Pharmacy* by Gennaro and to the World Wide Web sites of the International Academy of Compounding Pharmacists and Secundum Artem: Current and Practical Compounding Information for the Pharmacist. In practice, a pharmacy technician will, if the laws of the state allow, assist in compounding only after instruction by a pharmacist in specific techniques for specific preparations, and compounding will be done in accordance with instructions in a master formula sheet. Of course, any compounding tasks undertaken by the technician must, in any case, be supervised and checked by the pharmacist. That said, the following are some examples of compounding tasks.

Web Link

International Academy of Compounding Pharmacists www.iacprx.com See the Secundum Artem article in the publications section at www.paddocklabs.com

PREPARATION OF SOLUTIONS A solution is a liquid dosage form in which active ingredients are dissolved in a liquid vehicle. The vehicle that makes up the greater part of a solution is known as a solvent. An ingredient dissolved in a solution is known as a solute. Solutions may be aqueous, alcoholic, or hydroalcoholic. Solutions are prepared by dissolving the solute in the liquid solvent or by combining or diluting existing solutions. Careful measurement is, of course, important for solutions, as it is for all extemporaneous compounding. Colorings or flavoring agents may be added to solutions.

When mixing solids and liquids, it is important to remember that reducing the particle size of the solid through trituration or gently heating the liquid (if the liquid is stable, or nonvolatile) will generally make the solid dissolve faster, more uniformly, and with less precipitation or clinging together of the solute into particles of unacceptably large size. When mixing two liquids, a possible precipitation of solutes within the liquids can sometimes be avoided by making each portion as dilute as possible before mixing the liquids together.

Before preparing a solution for compounding, the technician should gather the master formula sheet, ingredients, equipment, glassware, and packaging material. It is also important that the person compounding the prescription have adequate time to prepare the product. Compounding should never be rushed. Figure 8.4 (a) shows an example of a master formula sheet for a prescription for a dog. In order to prepare this medication, the technician would follow the steps in Table 8.1 for weighing the product (potassium bromide), Figure 8.4 (b). Then, the product is placed in a mortar to be triturated and combined with the flavoring, Figure 8.4 (c). Figure 8.4 (d) shows the mixed ingredients, but at this stage, more trituration is needed in order to get the particles to an even texture. The mixed and triturated ingredients are put into an amber bottle using a glass funnel. In Figure 8.4 (e), 240 mL of distilled water is added using a mounted reconstitube. Then, the bottle is shaken well and labeled, and the preparation is checked by the pharmacist before the bottle is bagged for customer pick up, Figure 8.4 (f).

PREPARATION OF SUSPENSIONS In a suspension, as opposed to a solution, the active ingredient is not dissolved in the liquid vehicle but rather is dispersed throughout it. An obvious problem with suspensions is the tendency of the active ingredient to settle. To avoid settling of the insoluble drug, a suspending agent is sometimes added. Such suspending agents include tragacanth, acacia, carboxymethylcellulose (CMC), bentonite, and Cab-O-Sil. The point at which the suspending agent is added in the mixing procedure can be crucial. Therefore, the technician must always remember to add the ingredients in the proper order, according to the master formula sheet.

04-Feb-04	Ron Holly				3659.69	62
RX NO.	6600008				AQ COST	13.05
PATIENT	LLOYD, SPARKY K-9		01/01/1992 12Yrs		$ PROFIT	2.04
	3000 MAPLE RD, FORT WAYNE, IN				Tax	
	(219) 555-1234				Discount	
	09/03/99 ALLERGY NOT KNOWN—NO MED INFO				New total	15.09!

```
DOCTOR                    ┌────── [ Notes ] ──────┐
                          │ Prescription:          │              15.09
Product                   │     Patient:           │
Disp                      │ Prescriber:            │
                          │     Product: 48GM KBR QS TO 240ML W/ H20 + │
Disp Qty                  │     Product: 1 TEASPOONFUL BEEF FLAVOR POWDER │
G 134                     │ Std PC KT:             │  KT
Give 1                    └────────────────────────┘  KT

# Days  60                                       Total O/R
  Refills      Auth      Remain        Total #   Copay O/R
  DAW   0              First  02/04/04    Comply  P Code O/R KT
Drug Exp 02/04/05      Last   02/04/04[ 1 ]  Status
Rx Exp  02/03/05      Labels 01 166 002       #RX/OR Y
Written 02/04/04 Auth by                      TECH
Exit Enter: Select
```

(a)

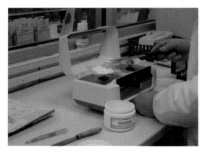

(b)

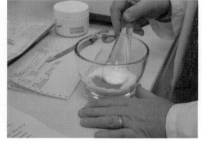

(c)

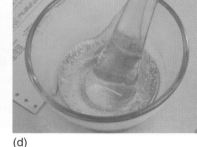

(d)

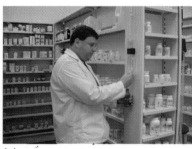

(e)

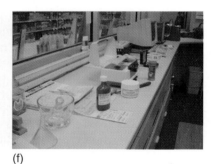

(f)

Figure 8.4

Preparing a Solution for Sparky the Dog
(a) Master formula sheet.
(b) Weighing the potassium bromide.
(c) Potassium bromide and beef flavoring. (d) Not yet fully triturated.
(e) Adding distilled water. (f) Prepared prescription waiting for pharmacist approval.

Regardless of their apparent stability, all suspensions should be dispensed with an auxiliary label reading "Shake Well."

PREPARATION OF OINTMENTS AND CREAMS Ointments, or unguents, and creams are semisolid dosage forms meant for topical application. Many commercially unavailable pediatric suspensions can be extemporaneously prepared in the pharmacy from adult tablets or capsules. In addition, dermatological therapies may call for combining existing ointments or creams. Most ointments and creams are prepared via mechanical incorporation of materials, levigation, or mixing in a mortar and pestle. Levigation involves forming a paste containing a small amount of liquid, generally using a spatula and an ointment slab, prior to addition to the base of the ointment or cream. In some cases, the dry ingredients of an ointment or cream may have to be triturated, or reduced to a fine powder, in a mortar and pestle before being added to the ointment or cream base. When placing a powder into an ointment, it is impor-

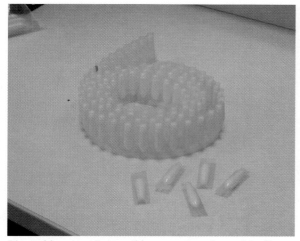

Disposable suppository molds are commonly used to dispense and shape suppositories.

tant to add the powder in small amounts, constantly working the mixture with the spatula or pestle to reduce particle size and to obtain a smooth, nongritty product. When an ointment slab and spatula are used, the edge of the spatula should press against the slab to provide a shearing force, which allows for a smoother product.

PREPARATION OF POWDERS Spatulation, or blending with a spatula, is used for small amounts of powder having a uniform and desired particle size and density. Trituration is used when a potent drug is mixed with a diluent. At first equal amounts of the potent drug and the diluent are triturated with a mortar and pestle. When these are thoroughly mixed, more of the diluent is added, equal to the amount already in the mortar. This process is continued until all of the diluent is incorporated. Tumbling is used to combine powders that have little or no toxic potential. The powders to be combined are placed in a bag or in a wide-mouthed container and shaken well.

PREPARATION OF SUPPOSITORIES Suppositories are solid dosage forms that are inserted into bodily orifices, generally the rectum or the vagina or, less commonly, the urethra. They are composed of one or more active ingredients placed into a base, such as cocoa butter, hydrogenated vegetable oils, or glycerinated gelatin, that melts or dissolves when exposed to body heat and fluids. The preparation of suppositories involves melting the base material, adding the active ingredient(s), pouring the resultant liquid into a mold, and then chilling the mold immediately to solidify the suppository before the suspended ingredients have time to settle.

PREPARATION AND FILLING OF CAPSULES A capsule is a solid dosage form consisting of a gelatin shell that encloses the medicinal preparation, which may be a powder, granules, a liquid, or some combination thereof. Extemporaneous compounding of ingredients for capsules is often done to provide unusual dosage forms, such as dosage forms containing less of an active ingredient than is readily available in commercial tablets or capsules.

Figure 8.5

Types of Hard Shell Capsules
(a) Regular (b) Snap Fit

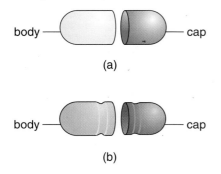

body — cap

(a)

body — cap

(b)

Hard gelatin shells consist of two parts: the body, which is the longer and narrower part, and the cap, which is shorter and fits over the body. In some cases, capsules have a snap-fit design, with grooves on the cap and the body that fit into one another to ensure proper closure (see Figure 8.5).

When hand-filling a capsule with powder, a pharmacist or technician generally uses the punch method. First, the number of capsules to be filled is counted out. Then, the powder is placed on a clean surface of paper, porcelain, or glass and formed into a cake with a spatula. The cake should be approximately ¼ to ⅓ the height of the capsule body. The body of the capsule is then punched into the cake repeatedly until the capsule is full (see Figure 8.6). The cap is then placed snugly over the body. Granules are generally poured into the capsule body from a piece of paper. Sometimes, hand-operated capsule filling machines are used.

Figure 8.6

The Punch Method for Extemporaneous Filling of Capsules
(a) The body of the capsule is filled by "punching" into a cake of the powder. (b) Then, the filled capsule is weighed to verify the dosage.

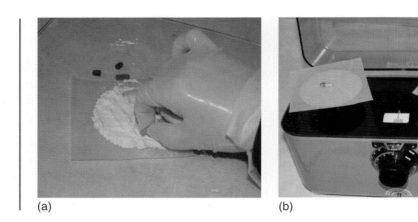

(a)

(b)

Labeling, Record Keeping, and Cleanup

After the compounding operation, the product must be labeled with a prescription label containing all information required by the governing laws and regulations of the state in which the compounding is done. For more information on proper labeling, see Chapter 7. The ingredients of the compound and the amounts of these ingredients should be clearly stated on the label, and in lieu of an expiration date from a manufacturer, the date of the compounding should also appear on the label. A careful record of the compounding operation, including ingredients and amounts of ingredients used, the preparer of the compound, and the name of the supervising pharmacist should be kept. Master formula sheets, such as the one shown in Figure 8.1, provide a means for keeping such a record.

Once the compounding operation is finished, equipment and the work area should be thoroughly cleaned, and ingredients should be returned to their proper places in storage. The prescription balance, when not in use, should be covered, and weights must be placed back in their original container.

Chapter Summary

Extemporaneous compounding, once the major source of medicines, is still used today to prepare medications in strengths, combinations, or dosage forms not commercially available. Instruments for extemporaneous compounding include the Class III prescription balance, weights, forceps, spatulas, weighing papers, the compounding or ointment slab, parchment paper, the mortar and pestle, graduates, and pipettes. Mortars and pestles come in glass, Wedgwood, and porcelain varieties. Graduates come in conical and cylindrical shapes, the latter being the more accurate.

When weighing pharmaceutical ingredients, one must take precautions to ensure that no damage is done to the delicate prescription balance, which is kept locked except when a measurement is taken. With the balance locked, the desired weight is placed onto the right pan of the balance. Then, amounts of the substance to be weighed are placed onto the left pan, and the balance is unlocked to check for equilibrium. The balance is then relocked, and substance is added or removed. Repeat this process until the balance has a reading of zero, indicating an equilibrium between the weight and the drug substance. When measuring liquid volumes, choose a graduate as close as possible in capacity to the volume of liquid to be measured and measure at eye level from the bottom of the meniscus, the concavity at the top of the column of liquid. When combining dry ingredients, one generally uses the geometric dilution method.

Extemporaneous compounding is an art to be learned under the tutelage of an experienced pharmacist and to be practiced according to formulas given on master formula sheets. Procedures vary for preparing the many kinds of extemporaneous compounds, such as solutions, suspensions, ointments, creams, powders, suppositories, and capsules.

Chapter Review

Knowledge Inventory

Choose the best answer from those provided.

1. A large amount of material, such as 2 kg of Epsom salts, would be weighed using a
   a. Class III prescription balance.
   b. Class A prescription balance.
   c. counter balance.
   d. Any of the above

2. Two pharmaceutical ingredients are combined, one a solid and the other a soluble, volatile liquid. The mixture is pulverized to reduce the particle size of the solid, and the liquid is allowed to evaporate in a process known as
   a. levigation.
   b. trituration.
   c. spatulation.
   d. pulverization by intervention.

3. An alternative to the ointment slab is
   a. weighing paper.
   b. parchment paper.
   c. a graduate.
   d. a pipette.

4. A prescription balance is unlocked, temporarily, when the technician
   a. adds weighing papers to the trays.
   b. adds pharmaceutical ingredients to the trays.
   c. moves the balance from one place to another.
   d. checks a measurement.

5. When measuring the amount of liquid in a graduate, one should place the eyes at the level of the liquid and measure the level of the meniscus from the
   a. top.
   b. bottom.
   c. back.
   d. front.

6. When using the geometric dilution method, the most potent ingredient, usually the one that occurs in the smallest amount, is placed into the mortar
   a. half at the beginning and half at the end.
   b. in stages throughout the compounding process.
   c. last.
   d. first.

7. An ingredient dissolved in a solution is known as a
    a. suspension.
    b. precipitate.
    c. solute.
    d. solvent.

8. A suppository mold is chilled immediately after filling to
    a. solidify the compound before its volatile components evaporate.
    b. reduce the possibility of spoilage.
    c. prevent contamination of the compound.
    d. solidify the compound before suspended ingredients have time to settle.

9. The punch method is used for filling
    a. hypodermics.
    b. capsules.
    c. graduates.
    d. unit dose containers.

10. An appropriate auxiliary label for a suspension is
    a. "Take with food."
    b. "For topical use only; Do not swallow."
    c. "Shake well before using."
    d. "May cause drowsiness."

Pharmacy in Practice

1. Practice using a Class III prescription balance and a mortar and pestle to prepare the following amounts of ingredients:
    a. 2.75 g of ground cinnamon
    b. 8.5 g of sugar
    c. 75 g of ground nutmeg
    d. 1.5 g of allspice
    e. 2.5 g of triturated anise seed or clove
Combine the ingredients and use the punch method to fill capsules with this "pumpkin pie spice" compound.

2. Explain why it is important to use proper technique, and weigh ingredients with accuracy while preparing special compounds in the pharmacy.

3. Select the most appropriate size graduate to measure the following volumes: You have the following available in the pharmacy: 1 fl oz (30 mL), 2 fl oz (60 mL), 4 fl oz (120 mL), 8 fl oz (240 mL), 500 mL, and 1,000 mL.
    a. 45 mL
    b. 75 mL
    c. 125 mL
    d. 450 mL
    e. 550 mL
    f. 890 mL

Improving Communication Skills

1. The art of compounding utilizes a whole different language, and you have been asked to describe the following terms to a pharmacy student who is visiting your pharmacy. Use simple terms.
   a. levigate
   b. punch method
   c. triturate
   d. spatulation
   e. diluent
   f. tumbling
   g. solute
   h. solvent
   i. geometric dilution
   j. comminution

2. A patient has arrived at the retail pharmacy where you work and has a prescription for a compound that your store makes often. You are very busy right now, and will not be able to get to this compound for at least an hour. The patient is frustrated from waiting so long at the doctor's office, and is now frustrated that you will not prepare her prescription immediately. What will you tell this patient? Explain why special compounded prescriptions take longer than other prescriptions. Write out your responses.

Internet Research

1. Visit the Web site for Secundum Artem: Current and Practical Compounding Information for the Pharmacist at www.paddocklabs.com. Choose the secundum articles and select three of the listed topics. Read the articles posted on this site and use the information to write, in your own words, directions for the products selected.
   compounding ointments
   topical antibiotics
   oral suspensions
   suppositories
   emulsions
   capsules

2. Visit the USP Web site at www.usp.org, and describe the resources available to assist in compounding prescriptions. Which ones would you choose to rely on?

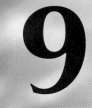

Human Relations and Communications

Chapter 9

Learning Objectives

◇ Explain the role of the pharmacy technician as a member of the customer care team in a retail pharmacy.

◇ State the primary rule of retail merchandising and explain its corollaries.

◇ Provide guidelines for proper use of the telephone in a retail pharmacy.

◇ Explain the appropriate responses to rude behavior on the part of others in a workplace situation.

◇ Define discrimination and harassment and explain the proper procedures for dealing with these.

In addition to being an important part of the healthcare system, the community or retail pharmacy is also a place of business, and the technician must take on customer service responsibilities similar to those appropriate in any retail setting. This chapter begins by noting a recent shift in the orientation of retail merchandisers away from the mass merchandising model and back to the customer service model. It then explains some important aspects of providing first-rate customer service.

PERSONAL SERVICE IN THE CONTEMPORARY COMMUNITY PHARMACY

As you read in Chapter 1, since the Millis Report in 1975, the pharmacy profession has undergone an extensive self-analysis and reevaluation of its duties and goals. The upshot of this reexamination of the profession has been an increased emphasis on clinical pharmacy, the provision by the pharmacist of information and counseling regarding medications. It is now almost universally recognized that the pharmacist is far more than a dispenser of drugs. The pharmacist has the following equally important duties.

◇ to make certain that a given medication will not be harmful to a patient given that patient's medical and prescription history

◇ to identify any known allergies, drug interactions, or other contraindications for a given prescription

◇ to ensure that a patient understands what medication he or she is taking, why he or she is taking it, how it should be taken, and when it should be taken

Just as the pharmacist increasingly plays a clinical role, so the pharmacy technician increasingly is expected to be much more than simply an operator of cash registers, a stock person, and an all-around pharmacy "gofer." Instead, today the technician is viewed as an important part of the customer service team within the pharmacy. In the 1960s and 1970s, at the height of the mass merchandising era, customers grew used to large, impersonal supermarkets, department stores, and pharmacy superstores, with their numbered rows of merchandise and automated, bar-coded checkout stations. In the 1980s, retail merchandisers began to realize that the mass merchandising model adopted in the 1960s was terribly flawed. Customers missed the days of personal service—attention to individual customer needs—associated with the small, independent, neighborhood retail operations of the past. For this reason, many of the large department store chains reorganized their operations to create separate small operational entities, known as boutiques, within their larger stores. They also began extensive training programs to improve the quality of customer service. In pharmacy, as well, a new and welcome emphasis on personal service has returned.

One mass marketing research firm conducted an experiment involving bank tellers. In the experiment, one group of tellers was instructed to lightly touch customers on the hand or wrist at some point during each teller transaction. A second control group was instructed to carry out transactions as usual, without this "personal touch." Exit surveys of customer satisfaction were then conducted, with dramatic results. Though largely unaware that they had been touched during their teller transactions, those customers who had been touched reported a 40 percent higher satisfaction rate with the overall quality of service of their banks. The lesson to be learned from this research is not that one should make a habit of touching customers. Indeed, touching should probably be avoided, in most cases. However, it is clear that a little personal attention goes a long way. A courteous tone of voice, a smile, eye contact, a listening ear, and a bit of assistance finding merchandise or holding a door can go a long way toward making customers think of the pharmacy in which you work as a pleasant place in which to shop.

Attitude and Appearance

Attitude is the overall emotional stance a worker adopts toward his or her job duties, customers, employer, and co-workers. Appearance is the overall look an employee has on the job, including dress and grooming. Pharmacy technicians often conduct their jobs unobtrusively—behind the scenes, as it were—stocking items in the pharmacy area, retrieving stock for compounding operations, maintaining records, filling bottles, cleaning up, and so on. Even if the immediate task is not customer-oriented, the technician should remember the primary rule of retail merchandising, which is this:

> *At all times, you are representing your company to the patient or customer. Remember that in a pharmacy, you are in a legal sense, an agent of your employer, and entering into a contract to provide care to the patient. Your employer must "answer" for all of your actions.*

This rule has a number of corollaries, and these are presented in the following sections.

APPEAR PROFESSIONAL Customers hope for the highest degree of cleanliness and professionalism from their pharmacy. After all, they are entrusting their health or the health of their loved ones to the operation for which you work. A pharmacy employee with unkempt hair or a uniform smock thrown over a pair of jeans makes a bad impression. The customer may not directly register these facts and yet goes away with a vague impression that the pharmacy is not a professional operation. You should wear a smock or lab coat and name tag at all times. This sets the desired pro-

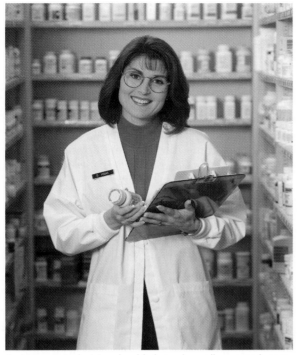

A pharmacy technician should always be well-groomed, neat, and professional-looking while working in the pharmacy.

fessional atmosphere and immediately identifies you as an employee of the pharmacy. However, the technician must follow the dress code of the pharmacy. The dress code may be crisp and professional or more relaxed and casual.

RESPOND TO CUSTOMERS Modern community pharmacies are often large, complex places. When customers enter, the first thing they often do is stand in the middle of the floor, looking around, a bit confused, for the part of the store where the product they seek is to be found. A good pharmacy employee thus continually scans the area around him or her, looking for customers who are lost, confused, or need help.

Consider the following example: Imagine that you are in a diner and want some ketchup for your french fries. Three or four times, a waiter passes your table, but each time, the waiter is concentrating on the immediate concern of taking a meal or a check to another table. In such a situation, you rapidly become frustrated and, perhaps, angry. The same principle—keep your eye on the customer—applies to any retail operation.

KNOW YOUR PHARMACY Few things are as frustrating to a customer as asking for help and getting an insufficient or inaccurate response. Often a customer is uncertain about what he or she is looking for or whom to ask for help. Once you spot that uncertain look, ask courteously, "May I help you?" Then, after the customer's response, you may have to ask some clarifying questions. If, for example, the customer is looking for aspirin, he or she may need to know not only where over-the-counter analgesic products are stocked in the store but also may need some help locating a specific analgesic such as a liquid form for children or an enteric-coated form for persons whose stomachs cannot tolerate conventional analgesic dosage forms. If possible, escort the customer to the place where the merchandise is located and help him or her to find it.

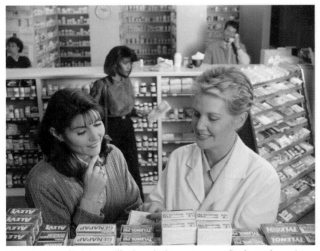

Pharmacy technician will often help customers find products in the retail pharmacy.

RESPECT THE CUSTOMER'S PRIVACY Pharmacies sell many products related to private bodily functions and conditions—condoms and other contraceptives, feminine hygiene and menstrual products, suppositories, hemorrhoid remedies, enemas, adult diapers, catheters, bed pans, scabicides, and so on. Often customers find asking about such products embarrassing and have to get up the nerve to request assistance. If you find discussing such matters embarrassing, get over it. As a pharmacy employee, you are part of the healthcare profession, and you must adopt a helpful, nononsense, professional attitude toward the

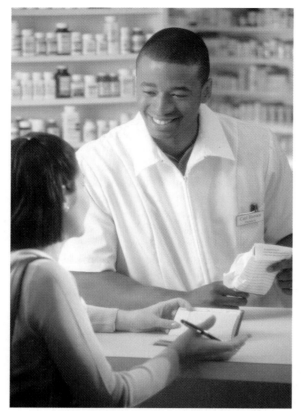

The pharmacy technician should make every effort to make the customer comfortable. This includes maintaining customer privacy by appropriately bagging medications and other purchases.

body and its functions. Responding to an inquiry about such a product with promptness, courtesy, respect, and a certain degree of nonchalance often relieves your customer's embarrassment and demonstrates your professionalism. Speak in a clear voice, but not so loudly that other customers or employees will be privy to your private interchange with the customer.

Privacy of the patient's medical record and information regarding medical conditions and prescriptions is also a legal issue. A patient has the right to expect such information will be kept confidential. When a patient is picking up a prescription, it is good to confirm his identity, and what he is picking up, but you should keep your tone of voice low so as not to broadcast to all nearby customers what the patient is picking up. Many pharmacies now have a private counseling area for prescription pick up, where the patient can have a high degree of privacy.

Privacy should be maintained as you update customer information. If, for example, you are stationed at a pharmacy window and need information for the customer's patient profile, let the customer know why you need the information. Tell the customer, for example, "I need some information for your prescription profile so that we can serve you better. May I ask you a few questions? Thank you. What is your full name and address?" You may also need to verify insurance information, and most customers are accustomed to presenting their card or proof of insurance regularly at the physician's office, and will not be upset once the procedure is explained.

SMILE AND MAKE EYE CONTACT The goodwill you communicate will come back to you. Making a personal connection to the customer is very important. Patients are far more likely to return to a pharmacy where they have received personal attention than to one where they have not. Eye contact is especially important to older patients and

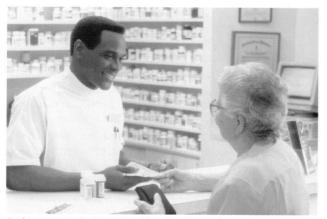

A pharmacy technician should maintain good eye contact and pleasant attitude while talking with patient.

patients who may be hard of hearing. A person who is hard of hearing learns to informally "read lips" to supplement the voice that they hear. If you speak with your head turned away, the person may hear you but not be able to fully interpret what you have said. Remembering to make eye contact will ensure you are looking directly at the person. Also, older generations of Americans often associate eye contact with honesty, sincerity, and respect.

USE COMMON COURTESIES In every interaction with a customer, use courteous words and phrases. Begin and end interactions, even the briefest ones, with ceremonial courtesies such as "Good afternoon" and "Have a nice day." "Please" and "Thank you" should become a part of your regular vocabulary. In between, practice courteous speech, as demonstrated in these examples:

Poor: What do you want?
Better: May I help you?
Poor: It's over there.
Better: That's in aisle three. Follow me, and I'll show you.
Poor: It's $8.39.
Better: That will be $8.39 please.
Poor: Next?
Better: May I help whoever is next?

BE SENSITIVE TO CULTURAL AND LANGUAGE DIFFERENCES Often pharmacies are located in areas catering to a diverse customer base. If you cannot understand a customer because of a language difference, do not speak louder or in an exaggeratedly slow and punctuated manner. Simply enunciate your words and avoid using slang terms or abbreviations, as the person may not be familiar with them. If necessary, apologize courteously for your language deficiency and find another store employee who can communicate in the customer's native tongue. If a translator is not available, the pharmacist may have available some simple counseling sheets that utilize drawings, diagrams, and clocks made especially for this purpose.

Cultural differences should also be taken into account. If the pharmacy where you are employed has a large group of patients from a particular culture, you should make an effort to become familiar with that culture's diet, health habits or beliefs, and courtesies. Knowing more about the culture will help you to provide higher quality service and will show the customer that you care about them.

FOLLOW THE POLICIES AND PROCEDURES Many pharmacies, especially within large retail chains, have policies and procedures manuals covering a wide range of activities. Make sure you are thoroughly familiar with these guidelines and abide by them in your routine interactions. Individual pharmacists also have preferences about how prescriptions are prepared and dispensed under their guidance, and although not written, these guidelines will be learned and followed as you are trained in a particular pharmacy.

DO NOT DISPENSE MEDICAL OR PHARMACEUTICAL ADVICE Remember that you are not trained or licensed to advise customers with regard to medications and their use. Use common sense to determine whether a given query from a customer exceeds the bounds of common knowledge. As a rule of thumb you should refer to a pharmacist any questions involving the proper administration, uses, or effects of a medication, whether prescription or over-the-counter, or any questions regarding a professional "opinion or judgment."

Do not be afraid of admitting your lack of expertise. Customers will appreciate that you are concerned enough to make sure they receive accurate information. When a question deals with the effects or administration of a medication, ask the customer to wait for a moment while you get someone who can

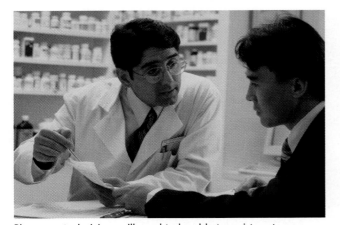

Pharmacy technicians will need to be able to assist customers from other cultural groups.

provide a professional answer to the question. In some instances technicians may provide medication-related information when providing refills and when directed to do so by a pharmacist.

Of course, a technician should use common sense with regard to providing customers with information. In the case of over-the-counter medications, sometimes customers simply need basic information that is readily available on the OTC packaging. For example, a customer might ask what an analgesic is, when an enteric-coated analgesic is appropriate, which alternative brands are available, and other such routine questions. Such questions can be safely answered without referring the customer to the pharmacist.

Customers will also arrive at the pharmacy, and speak or inquire about physicians, specialists, and other healthcare professionals. General information may be given, but opinions as to how good or bad a particular physician or healthcare provider is should not be given out by anyone in the pharmacy. You should at all times avoid making disparaging comments about other healthcare providers. If such comments are made, and the person's professional reputation is questioned, the person may sue you for slander.

Telephone Courtesies

Customers and healthcare professionals often contact pharmacies by telephone. The following are some guidelines for using the telephone properly.

- ◇ Always begin and end the conversation with a conventional courtesy, such as "Good morning" and "Thank you for calling." Stay alert to what the caller is saying and use a natural, conversational voice. You should be friendly, but not too familiar with the caller. When speaking to patients who are hard of hearing, speak clearly, pronounce each word distinctly, and be prepared to repeat yourself.
- ◇ When you answer the phone, identify yourself and the pharmacy, as follows: "Good morning. This is Arden Community Pharmacy. My name is Andrea. How may I help you?"
- ◇ If the caller is calling in a prescription, you may need to turn over the phone to a licensed pharmacist. In most states technicians are not allowed by law to take prescriptions over the telephone. However, you should learn the regulations for the state in which you are employed.
- ◇ If the caller has questions about the administration or effects of a medication or about a medical condition, adverse reaction, or adverse interaction, refer the call to a licensed pharmacist.
- ◇ Make sure that any information you provide is accurate. Giving incorrect directions to a customer in need of a prescription can be a life-threatening mistake.
- ◇ Depending on the regulations in your state and the procedures of your pharmacy, you may be authorized to handle prescription transfers or to provide information related to prescription refills.
- Follow the procedures outlined by your supervising pharmacist.

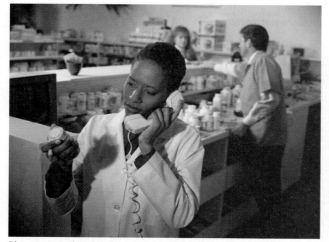

Pharmacy technicians need to be able to communicate effectively over the phone, to both customers and healthcare professionals.

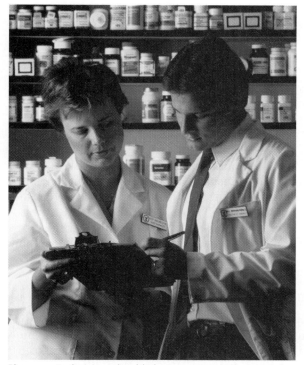
Pharmacy technicians should always approach the supervisory pharmacist with respect.

◇ If a customer is calling about a medical emergency or a prescription error, refer the call to your supervising pharmacist.

Interprofessional Relations

In the course of their duties, pharmacy technicians encounter, personally or on the telephone, many other professionals and paraprofessionals, including pharmacists, doctors, nurses, administrators, store managers, sales representatives, insurance personnel, and other technicians. Healthcare is a demanding industry, often requiring long hours and involving stressful, emergency situations. As a result, practitioners in the industry often suffer from fatigue and stress. Sometimes, this stress shows itself in unintentionally rude behavior. As a matter of course, busy healthcare professionals sometimes, unfortunately, speak to subordinates as though they were not whole, complete human beings but rather part of the machine that must be kept turning to get the job done. Remember that the degree to which you maintain your courtesy and respect, even in the face of rudeness, is a measure of your professionalism. Return rudeness with kindness, and you will often find that, immediately or over time, the quality of your interactions improves. If you answer the telephone and someone barks a command at you, demonstrate your professionalism by attending to the content of the message and not to its tone. Always refer to physicians using the title "Doctor." Refer to a supervising pharmacist, as well, as "Doctor," as a sign of respect for his or her professional attainment in having achieved the Doctor of Pharmacy degree. Refer to other supervisors using appropriate courtesy titles such as "Sir" or "Madam" or "Ma'am." When the technician refers to the pharmacist as "Doctor," this raises customers' level of respect not only for the pharmacist but also for the technician, who is the doctor's assistant. A degree of formality is always in order until you are requested to use more informal modes of address.

OTHER ASPECTS OF PROFESSIONALISM

Other aspects of professionalism include appropriate behavior, verbal and nonverbal communication, and conflict resolution.

Professional Behavior

In any situation there is an expected behavior and this is true in healthcare as well. Healthcare professionals of all levels are expected to abide by both written laws and ethical guidelines. Another set of unwritten rules to be followed is often referred to as etiquette. Etiquette is difficult to describe, and is often recognized most easily when it is not being followed. For example, being disrespectful to a physician would be an obvious violation of etiquette.

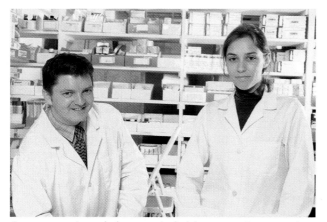
A more experienced pharmacy technician may act as a mentor for a new technician.

Respect should be shown to all who work in a healthcare facility, as each has an important job to do that contributes to the healthcare provided to the patient. However additional respect should be shown to those with a high level of medical training and those responsible for managing the facility where you are employed. Also avoid being overly familiar with all co-workers.

Personal phone calls and visits should be made only during breaks. Telling jokes and making disparaging comments about others is not acceptable. When in doubt as to what the expected behavior is in a situation, it is best to be quiet, watch, learn from someone else in the pharmacy who is a suitable model, and perform your assigned task.

Verbal and Nonverbal Communication

Communicating effectively takes practice. Once you have the knowledge and vocabulary needed to function effectively in the pharmacy, you will acquire verbal communication skills with time. Model yourself after someone whom you admire, but keep in mind that some of your co-workers have a different role, and thus different communication needs and styles. Verbal communication skills take practice, and pronouncing medical terms and drug names is one hurdle that you can overcome with study. Listening and asking a co-worker to pronounce words for you are the best ways to learn. Repeat difficult words to yourself several times. You may also find it helpful to keep a pocket-size reference on drug names handy and make notes in it regarding pronunciation and usage.

Nonverbal communication is easy to understand and one needs only to pay attention to the other party to interpret what is being conveyed. From the time we are small children we learn how to interpret nonverbal communication. Facial expression, eye contact, body position, and tone of voice are all methods of communicating without using words. Mannerisms and gestures often indicate agreement or disagreement. Mood of the other party can often be determined through nonverbal communication. Although each individual is unique and may exhibit unusual habits with certain moods, there are many generalizations that can be made regarding nonverbal communication. Simple observation and listening can be a very effective way to supplement the verbal portion of what you are hearing.

The flip side of verbal communication is, of course, listening. Listening to the words and the voice that you are hearing is important. You should maintain eye contact with the person speaking, and send the speaker nonverbal communication signals to indicate that you are genuinely interested in what he is saying. Learn to tolerate your own silence. When it is necessary to ask questions, ask to clarify issues and repeat portions of the conversation to confirm that you have heard what was said. Always use a nonjudgmental expression and tone of voice. Never let the other person think that your time is more valuable than his or that he is imposing.

Harassment and Disputes

As with any job, you should bear in mind that discrimination (preferential treatment or mistreatment) and harassment (mistreatment, sexual or otherwise) are not only unethical but against the law. If you find yourself the object of discrimination or harassment, first try to resolve the issue with the person or persons involved. Do your best to maintain your composure and to express your discomfort calmly and rationally. If discrimination or harassment persists, you may need to discuss the matter with a supervisor and make inquiries regarding the discrimination and harassment laws and procedures in your state.

The law requires all businesses, pharmacies included, to post information related to workplace discrimination and harassment. Bear in mind that in the past, sexual harassment was defined as unwanted physical contact or as the act of making sexual conduct a condition for advancement, preferential treatment, or other work-related outcomes. Recently, however, the Supreme Court redefined sexual harassment more generally as the creation of an unpleasant or uncomfortable work environment through sexual action, innuendo, or related means. Know, therefore, that you do not have to put up with off-color jokes if you do not wish to hear them, and be aware that you must not contribute in any way to creating an environment that is uncomfortable for your co-workers. One person's innocent remark, made in a spirit of fun, can be another person's grounds for a legal action.

Generally speaking, romantic or sexual involvements with co-workers, and especially with co-workers in supervisory or subordinate positions, is inadvisable.

Disputes involving duties, hours, pay, and other matters are common occurrences in occupations of all kinds. If possible, try to resolve work-related disputes through rational, calm discussion with the parties involved. Most large pharmacies, including chain stores and institutional pharmacies, will have personnel policy manuals detailing procedures for resolving disputes.

Chapter Summary

In recent years, many community pharmacies have made a concerted attempt to return to the spirit, if not the physical reality, of the small, customer-oriented neighborhood pharmacy of the past. An important part of this trend is an increased emphasis on personal service—attention to the needs of individual customers. A customer orientation on the part of the technician is in order at all times. Customer orientation involves dressing and grooming oneself neatly, maintaining a constant lookout for customers in need of assistance, knowing the layout of the store and the locations of its merchandise, respecting the customer's sense of privacy and decorum, smiling and using courteous language, providing explanations as necessary to customers, being sensitive to language differences, following established policies and procedures, and referring requests for medical or pharmaceutical advice to competent professionals. Common courtesy should be used in all telephone communications and conversations regarding prescriptions, medical or pharmaceutical emergencies, medication administration and effects, and adverse reactions. A request for information about adverse interactions should be referred to a supervising pharmacist. At all times, it is important to maintain courteous, respectful relationships with other professionals and paraprofessionals. A pharmacy is a professional workplace. Therefore, a no-tolerance policy with regard to discrimination and harassment is in order.

Chapter Review

Knowledge Inventory

Choose the best answer from those provided.

1. The provision by the pharmacist of information and counseling regarding medications is the primary concern of
   a. a contemporary pharmacy.
   b. pharmacology.
   c. pharmacognosy.
   d. a clinical pharmacy.

2. In the 1980s, retail merchandisers began to rethink their previous
   a. personal service merchandising model.
   b. mass merchandising model.
   c. customer service model.
   d. retail service model.

3. The emotional stance that a worker adopts toward his or her job duties is called
   a. tone.
   b. mood.
   c. attitude.
   d. appearance.

4. Which of the following is the primary rule of retail merchandising?
   a. Always dress and groom yourself neatly.
   b. Respect the customer's privacy and sense of decorum.
   c. Explain necessary interactions to the customer.
   d. At all times, you are representing your company to the customer.

5. Decorum means
   a. proper or polite behavior, or behavior that is in good taste
   b. dissatisfaction with services provided
   c. lack of understanding of the options available
   d. ability to negotiate for goods and services

6. A pharmacy technician should never
   a. waste time walking a customer across the store to show him or her the location of an item on the shelves.
   b. dispense advice regarding the use of a medication.
   c. attempt to speak to a customer in the customer's native language.
   d. take a written prescription from a customer.

7. When asking a customer for information for the patient profile, the pharmacy technician should explain
   a. how and when the prescription should be administered.
   b. why the pharmacy needs this information.
   c. the parts of the label of the prescription.
   d. the differences between the payment policies of various third-party insurance providers.

8. Preferential treatment or mistreatment based upon race, gender, age, or other criteria is known as
   a. harassment.
   b. discrimination.
   c. innuendo.
   d. decorum.

9. When answering a drugstore telephone, a person should identify himself or herself and the name of the
   a. supervising pharmacist.
   b. pharmacy.
   c. customer.
   d. prescribing physician

10. When customers enter a pharmacy, the first thing they typically do is
    a. look around to orient themselves.
    b. head for the cashier.
    c. head for the Rx area.
    d. seek out a store employee to ask for information.

Pharmacy in Practice

1. Working in a small group, recall your own experiences visiting drugstores or pharmacies. Make a list of problems you have encountered in pharmacies (e.g., slow service, lack of a comfortable place in which to wait while a prescription is being filled, difficulty in finding an item). As a group, brainstorm some ways to solve such problems and to improve customer service.

2. Imagine you are a drugstore manager who operates a 24-hour pharmacy in a big-city, urban neighborhood with the following demographics:
   10% Vietnamese-speaking customers
   26% Spanish-speaking customers
   16% Korean-speaking customers
   32% English-speaking customers
   16% customers who speak other languages (Thai, Laotian, Hmong, Russian, Latvian, Polish, etc.)

   With other students, brainstorm a list of steps you might need to take to meet the needs of the customers whom you serve.

3. With other students in a small group, brainstorm a list of positive experiences you have had in retail merchandising establishments of all kinds. Using this list, draw up a list of recommendations for making a customer's experience in a retail establishment a positive one.

Improving Communication Skills

1. Identify four students to play the following roles involving typical pharmacy scenarios: a customer calling to find out when a prescription will be ready, a physician calling in a prescription, a pharmacy technician, and a supervising pharmacist. Act out for other students in the class some typical telephone calls to the pharmacy; including a customer asking medical advice, a customer asking for signs of overdose, and a customer with a complaint. After each call, have other students in the class critique what was said and done by the technician taking the telephone call.

2. Conduct a role-play activity with other students in which a person who is obviously embarrassed asks a store employee for an over-the-counter product related to bodily functions. After each scenario is played out, critique the technician's response. Discuss the kinds of problems that can arise in such situations and how they might be avoided.

3. Tone of voice can communicate many different types of feelings. Consider how you would say the following sentences out loud to communicate the feeling in parentheses.

   a. I love my job.   (Nobody else may love it, but I do.)
   b. I love my job.   (I more than like my job—I love it.)
   c. I love my job.   (I may not like anything else, but I love my job.)
   d. I love my job.   (I don't like my boss, but I like my job.)
   e. I love my job.   (You have got to be kidding!)

   Try repeating the sentence using your own feelings and see if your classmates can interpret your true feelings about your job. Ask yourself if you know how you sound.

Internet Research

1. Visit the Keirsey Web site at www.keirsey.com and take the self evaluation test.
   a. What type person are you?
   b. Were the descriptions of your personality type accurate?
   c. How will knowing your own type and the type of your co-workers assist your communication skills?
   d. Which personality types do you communicate with easily, and which are more difficult for you?

2. Visit one of the many pharmacy magazine Web sites, such as Pharmacy Times or US Pharmacist, and locate the patient education materials.
   a. How is this educational material different from what you may find in one of your textbooks or reference books?
   b. How will material such as this improve communication between the patient and the pharmacy employees?
   c. Does providing this type of written patient education material meet the requirement of the counseling law?

Hospital and Institutional Pharmacy Practice

Learning Objectives

◇ Understand the origins and purpose of the hospital formulary.

◇ Describe the types of materials stored in a drug information center.

◇ List common universal precautions to avoid contamination.

◇ Explain the germ theory of disease— the role of pathogenic organisms in causing disease.

◇ Distinguish among viruses, bacteria, fungi, and protozoa.

◇ Describe proper aseptic technique, including the use of laminar, horizontal, and vertical airflow hoods.

◇ Describe the equipment and procedures used in preparing parenterals.

◇ Describe unit dose and floor stock distribution systems.

◇ Explain the proper procedure for repackaging of medications.

◇ Understand the techniques for handling and disposing of hazardous agents.

Many of the functions carried out by community or retail pharmacies are also carried out in hospital or institutional settings. However, such settings do have some unique functions and procedures. Of particular importance to pharmacy operations in hospital and institutional settings are use of aseptic technique, preparation of parenterals, proper handling of hazardous agents, and understanding systems such as unit dose, floor stock, and repackaging.

THE FUNCTIONS OF THE HOSPITAL OR INSTITUTIONAL PHARMACY

As you learned in Chapter 1, pharmacists and pharmacy technicians work in a wide variety of settings beyond the community pharmacy. One of these sites is the hospital or institutional pharmacy. Of course, some similarities exist between the functions of a hospital pharmacy and those of a community pharmacy. Some functions carried out by both kinds of pharmacy include:

◇ maintaining drug treatment records
◇ ordering and stocking medications and medical supplies
◇ repackaging medications
◇ dispensing medications

- providing information about the proper use of medications
- collecting and evaluating information about adverse drug reactions and interactions
- preparing medications in various dosage forms for dispensing

Some functions either unique to or most commonly performed in a hospital or institutional setting are as follows:

- Preparing and maintaining a formulary, or list of drugs used by the hospital or institution, and conducting drug usage evaluations.
- Following proper procedures, known as universal precautions, as a guard against infection by disease-causing microorganisms, or pathogens, in blood or bodily fluids.
- Preparing the products using aseptic techniques. The sterile parenteral solutions may be bolus or intravenous solutions (IVs). These preparations are for various purposes, such as delivery of medications or nutrition. Pharmacists and technicians in other work settings, such as home healthcare, also prepare such solutions.
- Following proper procedures to ensure that hazardous agents, such as drugs and other chemicals and waste, are handled and disposed of properly.
- Filling medication orders (as opposed to prescriptions) and routinely preparing 24-hour supplies of patient medications in unit dose form, a form appropriate for a single administration to a patient.
- Stocking nursing stations with medications and supplies.
- Delivering medications to patients' rooms.
- Maintaining an institutional drug information center and providing drug information to the other healthcare professionals in the institution.
- Educating and counseling inpatients and outpatients about their drug therapies.
- Participating in clinical drug investigations and research.
- Providing in-service drug-related education.
- Reviewing or auditing prescription services that the pharmacy offers for evaluation of service accuracy and quality.
- Providing expert consultations in such areas as pediatric pharmacology and pharmacokinetics (the study of the absorption, distribution, and elimination of drugs by the body).

THE FORMULARY AND INFORMATION CENTER

Since ancient times, one of the functions of the healer has been to compile a list of medications (such as plants and mineral substances) that are efficacious, or useful, for treating particular conditions. Such a list is known as a formulary. One of the earliest known formularies was listed in the *Papyrus Ebers,* a scroll from ancient Egypt. Today, in a hospital or other institution, the formulary is the official list of medications approved for use in that institution. The formulary is generally established and periodically reviewed by the hospital's Pharmacy and Therapeutics Committee and represents a consensus within the institution as to the medications appropriate for treatment of its patients. Considerations in preparing and maintaining a formulary include the latest technical information regarding the risks and benefits of a drug; information about the costs, risks, and benefits of new drugs; ongoing drug usage evaluations providing information about drug usage patterns and costs within the institution; and ongoing new drug research within the institution.

In order to fulfill its clinical functions, a hospital or institutional pharmacy may maintain a drug information center, which is basically a library containing reference works, including books, periodicals, microfilm, CD-ROMs, and databases providing information about drugs and their uses. Types of references that might be kept in the drug information center are described in Appendix D of this text.

UNIVERSAL PRECAUTIONS

Healthcare workers run the risk of contamination by pathogens, or disease-causing organisms, carried in blood and other bodily fluids such as saliva, semen, gastrointestinal fluid, lymphatic fluid, sebum, mucus, and excrement. Examples of diseases that can be spread by means of bodily fluids include acquired immunodeficiency syndrome (AIDS) and hepatitis B. Procedures followed in hospitals, doctors' offices, long-term care facilities, and other healthcare settings to prevent infection due to exposure to blood or other bodily fluids are known as universal precautions. The following are some common general guidelines:

- ◇ Universal precautions apply to all persons within the institution.
- ◇ Universal precautions apply to all contact or potential contact with blood, other bodily fluids, or body substances.
- ◇ Disposable latex gloves must be worn when contact with blood or other bodily fluids is anticipated or possible.
- ◇ Hands must be washed thoroughly after removing the latex gloves.
- ◇ Blood-soaked or contaminated materials, such as gloves, towels, or bandages, must be disposed of in a wastebasket lined with a plastic bag.
- ◇ Properly trained custodial personnel must be called if cleanup or removal of contaminated waste is necessary.
- ◇ Contaminated materials such as needles, syringes, swabs, and catheters must be placed into red plastic containers labeled for disposal of biohazardous materials. Proper institutional procedures generally involve incineration.
- ◇ A first-aid kit must be kept on hand in any area in which contact with blood or other bodily fluids is possible. The kit should contain, at minimum, the following items:
  - adhesive bandages for covering small wounds
  - alcohol
  - antiseptic/disinfectant
  - bottle of bleach, which will be diluted at time of use to create a solution containing one part bleach to ten parts water, for use in cleaning up blood spills
  - box of disposable latex gloves
  - disposable towels
  - medical tape
  - plastic bag or container for contaminated waste disposal
  - sterile gauze for covering large wounds

Web Link

Review the NIH Universal Precautions at www.niehs.nih. gov/odhsb/biosafe/ univers.htm

Pharmacy personnel generally do not have the kind of patient contact as described above. Universal precautions are applied more by those healthcare workers with direct patient contact or by those who handle patient body fluids and tissues such as physicians, nurses, laboratory staff, respiratory care technicians, and x-ray technicians. Instead, pharmacy personnel are very concerned about exposure to toxic drugs. Handling of toxic materials will be described later in this chapter.

DISEASE, STERILIZATION, AND ASEPTIC TECHNIQUE

Hospitals and other institutions make use of sterile preparations. To understand what, exactly, a sterile preparation is, one needs to know something of microbiology and the germ theory of disease. The comprehension of the potential dangers of contaminants will make the processes of sterilization and aseptic technique more easily understood.

The Development of the Germ Theory of Disease

In ancient days, people had no understanding of the causes of illness and disease, and so they attributed them to evil or malign spiritual influences. Knowledge of the actual causes of disease progressed slowly, over the centuries. In the seventeenth century, the Dutch merchant Anton van Leeuwenhoek made the first crude microscope. In 1673, he wrote the first of a series of letters to the Royal Society of London describing the "animalcules" that he observed through his microscope, which we would today call microorganisms. While van Leeuwenhoek observed microbes, the Englishman Robert Hooke used a microscope to observe thin slices of cork, which is composed of the walls of dead plant cells. Hooke called the pores between the walls "little cells." His discovery of this structure marked the beginning of a cell theory.

Until the second half of the nineteenth century, it was generally believed that some forms of life could arise spontaneously from matter. This process was known as spontaneous generation. People thought that toads, snakes, and mice could be born from moist soil, that flies could emerge from manure, and that maggots could arise from decaying flesh. In 1668, the Italian physician Francesco Redi demonstrated that maggots could not arise spontaneously from decaying meat by conducting a simple experiment in which jars containing meat were left open, sealed, or covered with a fine net. Redi showed that maggots appeared only when the jars were left open, allowing flies to enter to lay eggs.

In 1798, Edward Jenner discovered the principle of immunization against disease. He noticed that milkmaids who had caught cowpox from cows were then immune to contracting smallpox from humans. By infecting healthy persons with cowpox, Jenner successfully inoculated them against smallpox. However, since microorganisms had not yet been identified as disease-causing agents, the reasons behind the success of Jenner's immunizations were not understood.

In 1861, Louis Pasteur demonstrated that microorganisms are present in the air and that they can contaminate seemingly sterile solutions, but that the air itself does not give rise, spontaneously, to microbial life. Pasteur filled several short-necked flasks with beef broth and boiled ham. Some flasks were left open and allowed to cool. In a few days, these flasks were contaminated with microbes. The other flasks, sealed after boiling, remained free of microorganisms. In Pasteur's time, wine making was a hit and miss affair. One year, the wine would be sweet. The next year, it would be sour. No uniform method had been discovered to ensure the same quality year after year. While experimenting along the lines employed in his broth experiment, Pasteur discovered that if grape juice were heated to a certain temperature, cooled, and then treated with a certain yeast, the wine would be consistent year after year. This procedure established the basis for pasteurization and for the development of aseptic technique.

The realization that yeasts play a crucial role in fermentation led people to link the activity of microorganisms with physical and chemical changes in organic materials. This discovery alerted scientists to the possibility that microorganisms might affect plants and animals. The idea that microorganisms cause diseases came to be known as the germ theory of disease. Pasteur, the originator of the theory, designed

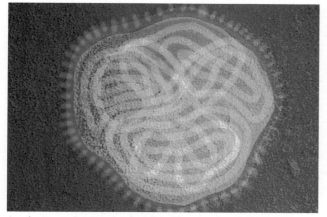

An electron micrograph of a virus. The virus is much smaller than a bacterium and can only be viewed with an electron microscope. It does not have all the components of a cell and requires other living cells to replicate itself. This virus that infects bacteria is called a bacteriophage.

experiments to prove it. In one experiment, he successfully immunized chickens against chicken cholera.

Joseph Lister, an English surgeon, built upon Pasteur's work and applied it to human medicine. Lister knew that carbolic acid (phenol) kills the bacterium, one type of microorganism, so he began soaking surgical dressings in a mild carbolic acid solution. This practice reduced surgical infections and was widely and quickly adopted. In 1876, Robert Koch defined a series of steps, known as Koch's postulates, that could be taken to prove that a certain disease was caused by a specific microorganism. Koch discovered rod-shaped bacteria in cattle that had died from anthrax. He cultured the bacteria in artificial media, then used them to infect healthy animals. When these animals became sick and died, Koch isolated the bacteria in their blood, compared them with the bacteria originally isolated, and found them to be the same.

Microorganisms and Disease

Since the days of Pasteur, Lister, and Koch, thousands of pathogenic, or disease-causing, microorganisms have been identified. Not all microorganisms cause disease. Some, in fact, perform essential functions, such as creating byproducts that are used as medicines, fermenting wine, fixing nitrogen in the soil, or helping the body to break down various food substances. However, some organisms of each of the following types are pathogenic.

VIRUSES Viruses are very small microorganisms, each of which consists of little more than a bit of genetic material enclosed by a casing of protein. Viruses need a living host in which to reproduce, and they cause a wide variety of diseases, including colds, mumps, measles, chicken pox, influenza, and AIDS.

BACTERIA Bacteria are small, single-celled microorganisms that exist in three main forms: spherical (cocci), rod-shaped (bacilli), and spiral (spirilla). See Figure 10.1. Bacteria cause a wide variety of illnesses, such as salmonella poisoning, strep throat, whooping cough, undulant fever, botulism, diphtheria, syphilis, rheumatic fever, meningitis, scarlet fever, pinkeye, boils, bubonic plague, pneumonia, typhoid, leprosy, pimples, and anthrax infection.

FUNGI Fungi, microscopic plants, occur as molds, mildews, mushrooms, rusts, and smuts, are parasites on living organisms or feed upon dead organic material and reproduce by means of spores. Spores and some fungi are microscopic and travel through

Figure 10.1

Characteristic Bacterial Shapes
(a) Round cocci.
(b) Rod-like bacilli.
(c) Spiral-shaped spirochetes.

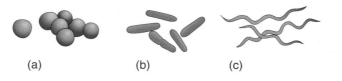

(a)   (b)   (c)

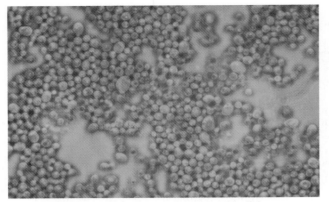
A photomicrograph of a fungus. Fungi are multicellular organisms, unlike bacteria or viruses.

the air. Some are implicated in disease conditions such as athlete's foot and ringworm.

PROTOZOA Protozoa are microscopic animals made up of a single cell or of a group of more or less identical cells; they live in water or as parasites inside other creatures. Examples of protozoa include paramecia and amoebae. Amoebic dysentery, malaria, and sleeping sickness are examples of illnesses caused by protozoa.

Asepsis and Sterilization

Asepsis is the absence of disease-causing microorganisms. The condition of asepsis is brought about by sterilization, any process that destroys the microorganisms in a substance. The scientific control of harmful microorganisms began only about one hundred years ago. Prior to that time, epidemics or pandemics caused by microorganisms (e.g., smallpox or cholera) killed millions of people. For example, the native population of the Americas was decimated by European diseases such as smallpox and syphilis. Prior to the modern era, in some hospitals, 25 percent of delivering mothers died of infections carried by the hands and instruments of attending nurses and physicians. During the American Civil War, surgeons sometimes cleaned their scalpels on their boot soles between incisions.

HEAT STERILIZATION When we sterilize an object, we do not bother to identify the species of microbes on it. Instead, we use an approach that is strong enough to kill the most resistant microbial life forms present. The most common method for killing microbes is heat sterilization. Heat is available, effective, economical, and easily controlled. One way to kill microorganisms is by boiling. Boiling kills vegetative forms, many viruses, and fungi in about ten minutes. Much more time is required to kill some organisms, such as spores and the hepatitis viruses. Most commonly this type of sterilization utilizes an autoclave, a device that generates heat and pressure to sterilize. When moist heat of 121°C or 270°F under pressure of 15 pounds per square inch (psi) is applied to instruments, solutions, powders, etc., most known organisms—including spores and viruses—will be killed in about 15 minutes.

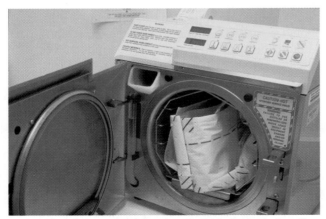
An autoclave is a commonly used and reliable method of sterilizing instruments and equipment. The three vital elements in the autoclave's sterilization cycle are time, temperature, and pressure.

DRY HEAT STERILIZATION Dry heat, such as direct flaming, also destroys all microorganisms. Dry heat is impractical for many substances but is practical as a means for disposal of contaminated objects, which are often incinerated. For proper sterilization using hot, dry air, a temperature of 170°C must be maintained for nearly two hours. Note that a higher temperature is necessary for dry heat, since a heated liquid more readily transfers heat to a cool object.

MECHANICAL STERILIZATION Mechanical sterilization is achieved by means of filtration, which is the passage of a liquid or gas through a screenlike material with pores small enough to block microorganisms. This method of sterilization is used for heat-sensitive materials such as culture media (used for growing colonies of bacteria or other microorganisms), enzymes, vaccines, and antibiotic solutions. Filter pore sizes are 0.22 μ for bacteria and 0.01 μ for viruses and some large proteins.

GAS STERILIZATION Gas sterilization makes use of the gas *ethylene oxide* and is used for objects that are liable, or subject to, destruction by heat. Gas sterilization requires special equipment and aeration of materials after application of the gas. This gas is highly flammable and is used only in large institutions and manufacturing facilities that have adequate equipment to handle the gas. Many prepackaged IV products, and bandages are manufactured and sterilized using this type of sterilization. Ethylene oxide will leave a slight nonharmful residue that can be detected as an odor, such as the odor present on simple adhesive bandages.

CHEMICAL STERILIZATION Chemical sterilization is the destruction of microorganisms on inanimate objects by chemical means. Few chemicals produce complete sterility, but many reduce microbial numbers to safe levels. A chemical applied to an object or topically to the body for sterilization purposes is known as a disinfectant. Alcohol, bleach, iodine, and Mercurochrome are often used as disinfectants.

Contamination

The most important thing to remember about aseptics is that harmful microorganisms, especially bacteria, are everywhere in large numbers. For example, the Harvard biologist E. O. Wilson estimates that as many as 30 billion bacteria are to be found in a single cubic gram of soil. It is extremely easy to introduce bacteria or other contaminants onto a sterile object or device or into a sterile solution. Contamination in a pharmacy occurs by three primary means: touch, air, and water.

TOUCH Millions of bacteria live on our skin, in our hair, and under our nails. Proper scrubbing to reduce the numbers of bacteria on the hands prior to handling sterile materials is very important. Touching is the most common method of contamination, and it is the easiest to prevent.

AIR Microorganisms are commonly found in the air, in dust particles, and in moisture droplets. It is important to prepare sterile materials in a special area in which the numbers of possible contaminants are maintained at a low level.

WATER Tap water is not free of microorganisms. Moisture droplets in the air, especially after a sneeze, often contain harmful microbes. It is important not to contaminate sterile materials by exposure to droplets of tap water or other sources of contaminated moisture.

Aseptic Technique and Equipment

Aseptic technique is the manipulation of sterile products and sterile devices in such a way as to avoid introducing pathogens, or disease-causing microorganisms. Sterile products include fluids stored in vials, ampules, prefilled syringes, and other containers. Sterile devices include syringes, needles, and IV sets. Aseptic technique is used for the preparation of parenteral admixtures, combinations of fluids and/or medications or nutrients, that are administered using bolus (push) or other intravenous

Table 10.1	Aseptic Technique

1. Prepare yourself by removing all jewelry and changing into clean clothes with low particulate generation. Wear a cap and mask.
2. Thoroughly scrub, up to the elbows.
3. Clean the hood.
4. Place only essential materials under the airflow hood—no paper, pens, labels, etc. Remove the syringe from its container and discard the waste.
5. Scrub again and glove.
6. Swab or spray needle-penetration closures on vials, injection ports, and other materials.
7. Prepare the sterile product by withdrawing medication from vials or ampules and introducing it into the IV container.
8. Complete a quality check of the product for container integrity and leaks, solution cloudiness, particulates, color of solution, and proper preparation of product.
9. Present the product, containers and devices used, and the label to a pharmacist for verification of the product preparation.

methods. Aseptic technique is treated in this chapter because of the frequency with which parenterals are prepared in hospital and other institutional settings. Table 10.1 summarizes the steps for preparing parenterals using aseptic technique, and the sections that follow explain the procedure in more detail.

When preparing a product in a sterile environment, it is necessary to use an instrument known as a laminar airflow hood. Such an instrument produces parallel layers of highly filtered air that flow across a work area enclosed on all but one side. It is important to note that the clean area created within the hood will provide a very clean environment, but it will not prevent all means of contamination, especially those caused by human error and human touch. There are two types of airflow hoods, horizontal and vertical.

In a horizontal airflow hood (see Figure 10.2), air from the room is pulled into the back of the hood where it is prefiltered with an air conditioner-like filter to remove large particles. The air then passes through a high efficiency particulate air (HEPA) filter, where 99.97% of all particles 0.3 μ or larger are removed. The air flows

Figure 10.2

Horizontal Airflow Hood

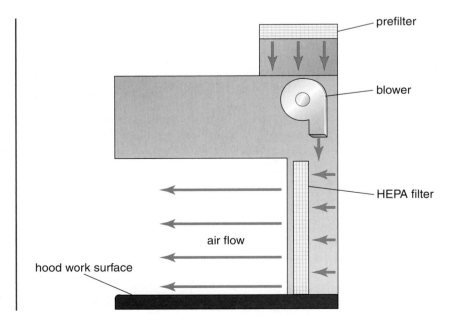

from the back of the hood, across the work surface, and out into the room. It is necessary to work at least six inches into the hood to avoid the mix of filtered and room air at the front of the hood.

In a vertical airflow hood (see Figure 10.3), the air flows from the top of the hood down, through a prefilter and a HEPA filter, and onto the work area. The air is then recirculated through another HEPA filter and out into the room. The front of the hood is partially blocked by a glass shield. This type of hood, because of the extra protection that it provides, is used to prepare hazardous substances, such as parenteral chemotherapy solutions used for treating cancers.

At the start of each shift, the laminar airflow hood should be given a good cleaning with an agent that acts both as a detergent (for cleaning) and as a germicide, fungicide, and virucide. A commonly used agent for cleaning the hood is 70 percent isopropylalcohol. The hood should be cleaned several times during a shift, or as needed (e.g., after a spill), with 70 percent alcohol. The clear Plexiglas sides should be cleaned with warm, soapy water instead of alcohol. The hood should be cleaned in such a way as to work contamination from the back out toward the room. The cleaning motion should be a back-and-forth motion, with each stroke further out than the previous stroke. The parts of the hood should be cleaned in this order: top, back, sides (top to bottom), and work area or bench (back to front using side-to-side strokes).

PREPARING PARENTERALS

Pharmacy personnel, pharmacists and technicians, prepare drugs and IV solutions in a form ready to be administered to patients. Solutions and drug products are delivered to the patient where other health professionals, generally a nurse or physician, administer the therapy.

The intravenous route of administration is used to reach appropriate serum levels, to guarantee compliance, for drugs with unreliable GI absorption, for the patient

Figure 10.3

Vertical Airflow Hood

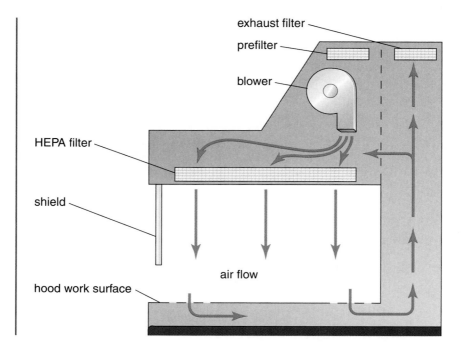

who can have nothing by mouth, for the unconscious or uncooperative patients, and for rapid correction of fluid or electrolytes.

Parenterals, including intravenous push (bolus) and intravenous infusion (IV) dosage forms should be prepared in laminar airflow hoods using aseptic techniques. Products used during the preparation must always be sterile and handled in such a manner as to prevent contamination. The ASHP (American Society of Health System Pharmacists) provides training material and instructional videos that new pharmacy employees study prior to working in the sterile area. Preparation should always be done under the supervision of a licensed pharmacist.

Web Link

Visit the ASHP Web site at www.ashp.org

Equipment Used in Parenteral Preparation

A wide variety of equipment is used in the preparation and administration of parenteral medications. Pharmacies utilize plastic disposable products in order to save time and money and to provide the patient with an inexpensive sterile product. Often the entire system sent out to the patient floors is composed of plastic. Thin, flexible plastic catheters are replacing metal shafts that deliver the medication into the vein. In many cases the only durable, nondisposable product used to deliver parenteral medication is the IV pump or controller.

SYRINGES Syringes, used for intravenous push and in the preparation of infusions, are made of glass or plastic. Glass syringes are more expensive and are used with medications that are absorbed by plastic. Plastic syringes, besides being less expensive, also have the advantages of being disposable and come from the manufacturer sterile and in a sterile package. Figure 10.4 shows the parts of a syringe.

A needle consists of two parts, the cannula, or shaft, and the hub, the part that attaches to the syringe (see Figure 10.5). Needles are made of stainless steel or aluminum. Needle lengths range from ⅜ of an inch to 6 inches and come in gauges ranging from 30 (highest) to 13 (lowest). The higher the gauge, the smaller the lumen, or bore, of the needle. Commonly used gauges in pharmacy range from 18 to 22.

FILTERS Filters are devices used to remove contaminants such as glass, paint, fibers, and rubber cores. Filters will not remove virus particles or toxins. Filter sizes are as follows:

◇ 5.0 micrometers (microns): Random Path Membrane (RPM) filter, removes large particulate matter
◇ 0.45 micrometers: in-line filter for IV suspension drug
◇ 0.22 micrometers: filter that removes bacteria and produces a sterile solution

IV SETS IV sets are devices used to deliver fluids, intravenously, to patients. Nurses generally have the responsibility for attaching IV tubing to the fluid container, establishing and maintaining flow rate, and overall regulation of the system.

Figure 10.4

Components of a Syringe

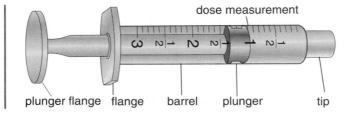

dose measurement

plunger flange   flange   barrel   plunger   tip

Figure 10.5

Components of a Needle

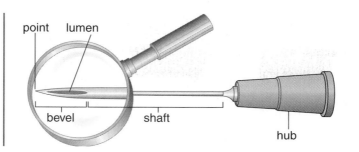

Pharmacy personnel should also have a knowledge of intravenous sets. Changes in regulations have forced pharmacy workers to assess aspects of IV systems, including infusion sets. Pharmacists need a complete understanding of IV sets and their operation for the following reasons:

⬦ Pharmacists may be required to select sets optimal for prevention of incompatibilities in certain drug-drug or drug-fluid combinations.
⬦ Pharmacists and other pharmacy personnel serving on CPR teams may need to calculate doses and drip rates for medications and to prepare IV infusions, attach sets, and prime tubing.
⬦ Pharmacy personnel may become involved in administration of IV meds to patients, including checking and changing lines according to established guidelines.
⬦ Pharmacy personnel may have to provide in-service training for nurses to familiarize them with the proper use of IV sets.
⬦ Pharmacy personnel use IV sets when transferring fluids from container to container under a laminar airflow hood.

IV sets are individually wrapped and then sterilized using either radiation or ethylene oxide. These practices guarantee that the fluid pathway is sterile and nonpyrogenic. However, in an operating room, it is desirable that the entire IV unit be sterile. Such a unit is supplied in packaging that ensures the maintenance of sterility, generally in packages with peel-off top cardboard and sealed plastic wrap. Some packaging has a clear wrap for viewing the contents, while other packaging has instead an opaque package with a diagram of the enclosed set printed on the outside.

A damaged package cannot ensure sterility, although all protectors are in place. It is best to discard sets that are found to be not original, opened, or in damaged packages. Sets do not carry expiration dates. Sets do carry the legend for medical devices: "Federal law restricts this device to sale by or on the order of a physician."

Flanges (Y-sites) and other rigid parts of an IV set are molded from tough plastic. Most of the length of the tubing is molded from a pliable polyvinyl chloride (PVC). PVC sets should not be used for nitroglycerin, which is absorbed by the tubing, nor for IV fat emulsions, which may leach out of the tubing. Therefore, other types of plastic sets are used for such infusions.

The length of sets varies from six-inch extensions up to 110–120-inch sets used in surgery. The priming of tubing depends on its length, from 3 mL for the short extension up to 15 mL for longer sets. The tubing's interior lumen generally contains particles that flush out when fluid is run through the set. Use of final filtration, a filter in the set, has reduced the need for flushing the line with the IV fluid before attaching the set to the patient.

Standard sets have a lumen diameter of 0.28 cm. Varying the size of the lumen diameter achieves different flow rates. Regulation of flow rates is especially critical in neonates and infants but may also be useful in limiting fluid flow to any patient.

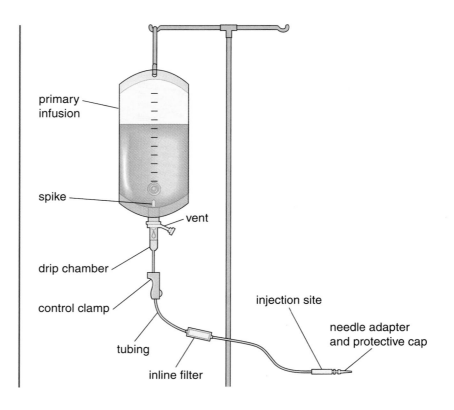

Figure 10.6

Basic Components of an IV Set

primary infusion

spike

vent

drip chamber

control clamp

tubing

inline filter

injection site

needle adapter and protective cap

Regardless of manufacturer, sets have certain basic components (see Figure 10.6), which include a spike to pierce the rubber stopper or port on the IV container, a drip chamber for trapping air and adjusting flow rate, a control clamp for adjusting flow rate or shutting down the flow, flexible tubing to convey the fluid, and a needle adapter for attaching a needle or a catheter. A catheter, or tube, may be implanted into the patient and fixed with tape to avoid having to repuncture the patient each time an infusion is given. In addition to these parts, most IV sets contain a Y-site, or injection port, a rigid piece of plastic with one arm terminating in a resealable port that is used for adding medication to the IV. Some IV sets also contain resealable in-line filters that offer protection for the patient against particulates, including bacteria and emboli. Intravenous infusion may employ any of a variety of pumps to regulate amount, rate, and timing of flow.

The spike is a rigid, sharpened plastic piece used proximal to the IV fluid container. The spike is covered with a protective unit to maintain sterility and is removed only when ready for insertion into the IV container. The spike generally has a rigid area to grip while it is inserted into the IV container.

If an air vent is present on a set, it is located below the spike. The air vent points downward and has a bacterial filter covering. The vent allows air to enter the bottle as fluid flows out. Some glass bottles do not have an air tube. For these, a vented set is necessary.

A transparent, hollow chamber, the drip chamber, is located below the set's spike. Drops of fluid fall into the chamber from an opening at the uppermost end, closest to the spike. An opening that provides 10, 15, or 20 gtt/mL is commonly used for adults. An opening that provides 60 gtt/mL is used for pediatric patients. The drip chamber serves to prevent air bubbles from entering the tubing. Air bubbles generally rise to the top of the fluid if they do form and will not enter the patient. The chamber allows the attending nurse or pharmacy worker to set the flow rate by counting the drops.

Figure 10.7

Attaching the IV Set to the IV Container

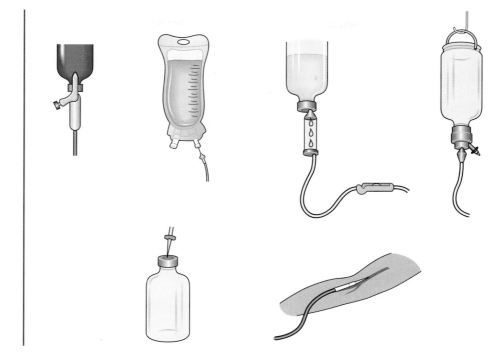

The person administering the fluid starts the flow by filling the chamber with fluid from an attached inverted IV container (see Figure 10.7). The chamber sides are squeezed and released. Then fluid flows into the chamber. The procedure is repeated until an indicated level is reached or approximately half the chamber is filled. The entering drops are then counted for 15 seconds. Adjustments are made until the approximate number of drops desired is obtained. The rate should be checked five times, at 30-second intervals, and again for a last count of one full minute.

Clamps allow for adjusting the rate of the flow and for shutting down the flow. Clamps may be located at any position along the flexible tubing. Usually a clamp moves freely, allowing its location to be changed to one that is convenient for the administrator.

Clamp accuracy is affected by creep, which is a tendency of some clamps to return, slowly, to a more open position with increased fluid flow. Accuracy is also affected by the phenomenon known as cold flow—the tendency of PVC tubing to return to its previous position. Tubing clamps are open during packaging and shipping. As a result, the tube tends to expand when the clamp constricts it. If, on the other hand, the tubing clamp has previously constricted the tubing, then as it is adjusted open, it tends to constrict with the reduced fluid flow, moving in the direction of its original position.

A slide clamp has an increasingly narrow channel that constricts IV tubing as it is pressed further into the narrowed area. Slide clamps do not allow for accurate adjustment of flow rate but may be used to shut off flow while a more accurate clamp is regulated.

A screw clamp consists of a thumbscrew that is tightened or loosened to speed or slow the flow.

A roller clamp is a small roller that is pushed along an incline. The roller, when moved down the incline, constricts the tubing and reduces the fluid flow. Moving the roller up the incline, in contrast, increases the flow.

A needle adapter is usually located at the distal end of the IV set, close to the patient. A needle or catheter may be attached to the adapter. The adapter has a standard taper to fit all needles or catheters and is covered by a sterile cover prior to removal for connection.

A set may have a built-in, in-line filter, which provides a final filtration of the fluid before it enters the patient. Final filtration should protect the patient against particulate, bacteria, air emboli, and phlebitis. A 0.22 micrometer filter is optimal. A 5 micrometer filter removes particles that block pulmonary microcirculation but will not ensure sterility.

A Y-site is an injection port found on most sets. The "Y" is a rigid plastic piece with one arm terminating in a resealable port. The port, once disinfected with alcohol, is ready for the insertion of a needle and the injection of medication.

CATHETERS Intravenous administration can be accomplished through needlelike devices called catheters and is a standard way to gain IV access for fluid and drug therapy. Catheters are devices that are inserted into veins for direct access to the blood vascular system and are used in two primary ways: close to the surface, peripheral venous catheters, and deeper in the body, central venous catheters.

Peripheral venous catheters are inserted into veins close to the surface and used for up to 72 hours. The unit is inserted into a vein, the needle portion is withdrawn, and a flexible Teflon catheter is left in place. Peripheral catheters are easy to insert and most nurses can do this at a patient's bedside. Although various brand names of catheters are available, the Jelco is commonly used and is accepted terminology. (This is similar to the term *tissue;* there are many brands of tissues but the term *Kleenex* is often requested when asking for a tissue.) Peripheral venous catheters are usually inserted in sites on the arms, hands, feet and scalp veins.

Peripheral venous catheters will likely cause problems for 20–50% of patients such as pain and irritation. Some drugs cause vein irritation due to the drug pH or osmolarity and because the blood flow in peripheral veins is slow, allowing drug and fluid to stay in contact with the vessel wall longer. Another problem is infiltration. Infiltration is a breakdown of a vein that allows drug to leak into tissues surrounding the catheter site, causing edema and/or tissue damage.

Central venous catheters are placed deeper in the body, are more complicated to place, and should be placed by a physician. Central catheters are used for therapy of one to two weeks. Common sites of insertion are the subclavian vein, lying below the clavicle, and the jugular vein, in the neck. The femoral vein, in the groin area, is also used but is the least desirable site due to risk of infection. Subclavian catheters are placed deep in the vein so that the end enters the superior vena cava close to the heart where the blood flow is the greatest. A larger blood flow will dilute a more concentrated solution such as total parenteral nutrition (TPN), chemotherapy, or phenytoin. Problems with subclavian catheters are the possibility of subclavian vein laceration (i.e., missing the vein and puncturing a lung), and a greater risk of infection as the procedure is more invasive.

There are instances when several incompatible drugs must be given. Multiple-lumen catheters can be utilized to administer these drugs together. Each lumen exits the catheter at a different location so there is no opportunity for the drugs to mix before being diluted in the blood stream.

Central venous catheters come with one, two, three, or four lumens. The triple and quad catheters will be used with sicker patients.

Some patients may be on TPN therapy for months or even years. Infusion devices are surgically implanted to provide long-term therapy and also reduce the risk of infection. Implantable infusion devices include the external catheters, Hickman or Broviac, which are also called

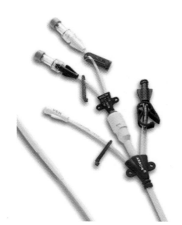

An example of a multiple lumen central venous catheter.

tunnel catheters. The surgeon inserts the catheter below the breast and tunnels it under the skin into the subclavian vein. The catheter has a cuff to which the body's connective tissue heals, thus sealing off bacterial entry into the surgical area. The lower point of body insertion makes the catheter easier for the patient to see and clean. Another form of implantable device is the internal port, such as the Port-A-Cath, Life Port. When implanted the only evidence is a bump in the skin. Drugs are administered by a small needle through the skin in an injection port in the device.

Midline catheters are longer peripheral catheters that go from insertion site into a deep vein. These catheters are designed to stay in place a week or longer. The peripherially inserted central line (PIC) is a very fine line that is threaded through the peripheral vein into the subclavian vein. This catheter has the same characteristics as a central line, however a skilled nurse can insert it at the bedside.

PUMPS AND CONTROLLERS Fluids and drugs are often delivered to catheters by some form of device, including electronic devices, to control infusion rate. These devices are the pumps and controllers.

The first system to deliver a drug IV was the syringe system. The patient must have an IV line or direct entry into a vein, the drug is injected in a port, and it goes directly into the vein. One of the problems with this system is safety. Care must be taken when administering drugs that have to be diluted or given very slowly. The syringe system is very nurse labor-intensive because a nurse has to stand by the bedside and push the drug in. This system is also pharmacy labor-intensive because the pharmacy has to fill the syringe with drugs.

The Buretrol or the Soluset has a built in graduated cylinder. Fluid is run into the cylinder, and the nurse can add a drug in the top of the cylinder injection port for dilution and mixing of the drug before it is infused. The Buretrol or Soluset was in use before infusion pumps and replaced the syringe system. This is a better system than the syringe system because the drug is being diluted in the cylinder and it can be infused over a long period of time. A problem with the use of this system is that all drugs have to be drawn up in syringes and it is very labor intensive. Another problem in using this system is drug compatibility. The drug can not be identified once it is injected into the cylinder.

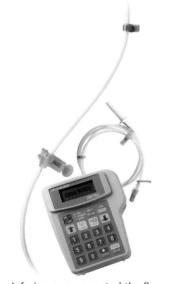

Infusion pumps control the flow of IV medications.

Controllers are low-pressure devices of two to three pounds per square inch. The pressure of the controller is generated by gravity. Flow rate is controlled by the rate of fluid drops falling through a counting chamber. Maximum flow rate is 400 mL/hr. The low pressure of controllers is less likely to cause vein breakdown or infiltration. A problem with controllers is alarms. An alarm will sound with a kink in a line or even the interruption of blood flow when the patient bends an elbow. These devices are used little today.

More popular devices are the infusion pumps used in institutional and home therapy. These devices produce a positive pressure of ten to twenty-five pounds per square inch, are more accurate than controllers, and have fewer flow interruptions, which causes both nurses and physicians to prefer them. Maximum flow is 999 mL/hr, therefore providing a higher rate of infusion; higher pressure, however, presents the problem of infiltration.

Another type of medication delivery that utilizes a parenteral route is the patient controlled analgesia (PCA) device. The PCA device allows the patient to administer analgesics by pressing a button. The device controls the medication so that the patient can not overdose or give the medication too soon after the previous dose. Often, after surgery or severe injuries, a physician will order a PCA for the patient for

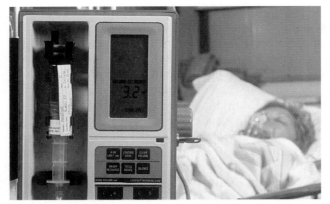

A patient-controlled analgesia pump can allow the patient to regulate the amount of pain medication she receives. This results in better pain control with less drug used.

24–72 hours, after which time the patient may be treated adequately with alternative analgesics.

IV Solutions

The two main types of IV solutions are small-volume parenterals (SVPs) of 100 mL or less and large-volume parenterals (LVPs) of more than 100 mL. Small-volume parenterals are typically used for delivering medications at a controlled infusion rate. Large-volume parenterals are used to replenish fluids, to provide electrolytes (essential minerals), and to provide nutrients such as vitamins and glucose. In some cases, a patient can not or will not eat and so must be fed intravenously. The provision of the entire nutritional needs of a patient by such means is known as total parenteral nutrition (TPN). In some cases, an infusion is prepared specifically to deliver a medication. In other cases, a medication is piggybacked on a running IV. A piggyback involves the preparation of a small amount of solution, usually 50 to 100 mL, in a minibag or bottle. Some IV piggybacks are prepared in 250 mL solution because they contain an additive that is irritating and thus requires a larger volume of solution. The piggybacked solution is infused into the tubing of the running IV, usually over a short time, from half an hour to one hour. In some cases, syringes are used instead of piggyback containers to deliver medication into a running IV.

Table 10.2 provides some typical abbreviations common in parenteral therapy. Table 10.3 shows some commonly used IV fluids and electrolytes. Figure 10.8 shows some typical physician's orders for intravenous infusions. Figure 10.9 shows a typical order form for adult parenteral nutrition.

Table 10.2	Abbreviations Related to Parenteral Therapy
Abbreviation	**Meaning**
$D_{2.5}W$	dextrose 2.5% in water
D_5W	dextrose 5% in water
HEPA	high efficiency particulate air (filter)
IM	intramuscular
IV	intravenous
LR	lactated Ringer's solution
LVP	large-volume parenteral
NS	normal saline (0.9%)
½NS	half-strength normal saline (0.45%)
PCA	patient controlled analgesia
RL	Ringer's lactate
SVP	small-volume parenterals
SW	sterile water
SWI	sterile water for injection
TPN	total parenteral nutrition

Table 10.3	Commonly Used IV Fluids, Electrolytes, and Additives	

IV Components	Abbreviation
Fluids	
5% dextrose in water	D_5W
5% dextrose and normal saline	D_5NS
5% dextrose and 0.45% normal saline	$D_50.45NS$ (½ normal saline)
normal saline	NS
0.45% normal saline	0.45NS
5% dextrose and lactated Ringer's	D_5RL
lactated Ringer's	RL
10% dextrose in water	$D_{10}W$
sterile water for injection	SW for Injection
sterile water for irrigation	SW for Irrigation
normal saline for irrigation	NS for Irrigation
2.5% dextrose in water	$D_{2.5}W$
2.5% dextrose and 0.45% normal saline	$D_{2.5}0.45NS$
Electrolytes	
potassium chloride	KCl
potassium phosphate	K phos
magnesium sulfate	$MgSO_4$
potassium acetate	K acet
sodium phosphate	Na phos
sodium chloride	NaCl
Additives	
multivitamin for injection	MVI
trace elements (combinations of essential trace elements such as chromium, manganese, copper, etc.)	TE
zinc (a trace element)	Zn
selenium (a trace element)	Se

Parenteral Preparation Guidelines

Begin any parenteral preparation by washing your hands thoroughly using a germicidal agent such as chlorhexidine gluconate or povidone-iodine. Wear gloves during the procedure. Make sure the laminar airflow hood has been running for at least 30 minutes before beginning the preparation. Laminar airflow hoods are normally kept running. Should the hood be turned off for installation, repair, maintenance, or relocation, it should be operated at least 30 minutes before being used to prepare sterile products. It is the responsibility of the institution to ensure proper positioning of the hood away from high traffic areas, doorways, air vents, or other locations that could produce air currents contaminating the hood working area. Eating, drinking, talking, or coughing are prohibited in the laminar airflow hood. Follow these guidelines to ensure proper parenteral preparation:

1. Before making the product, thoroughly clean all interior working surfaces. Also make sure that the inside of the airflow hood has been thoroughly cleaned with disinfectant. All jewelry should be removed from the hands and wrists before scrubbing and while making a sterile product. To ensure topical antimicrobial

Figure 10.8

Physician's Orders for IV Infusions
(1 of 2)

✓	START HERE →	DATE 12/10	TIME	A.M. P.M.	PROFILED BY:	FILLED BY:	CHECKED BY:	PATIENT NAME AND I.D.
	Mefoxin	*1 g*	*IV*	*q6h*				
			Davis, MD					

✓	START HERE →	DATE 12/10	TIME 1:00	A.M. P.M.	PROFILED BY:	FILLED BY:	CHECKED BY:	PATIENT NAME AND I.D.
	nafcillin	*1 g*	*IV*	*q4h*				
			Jones, MD					

✓	START HERE →	DATE	TIME	A.M. P.M.	PROFILED BY:	FILLED BY:	CHECKED BY:	PATIENT NAME AND I.D.
	PCN	*2 million units*		*q4h*				
			Harris, MD					

action of chlorhexidine, iodine, or other acceptable scrubs, use 3 to 5 mL and scrub vigorously the hands, nails, wrists, and forearms for at least 30 seconds.

2. Gather all the necessary materials for the operation and check these to make sure they are not expired and are free from particulate. Only essential objects/materials necessary for product preparation should be placed in the airflow hood. If you are using plastic solution containers, check for leaks by squeezing them. Work in the center of the work area within the laminar airflow hood, at least six inches inside the edge of the hood and making sure that nothing obstructs the flow of air from the HEPA filter over the preparation area. Nothing should pass behind a sterile object and the HEPA filter in a horizontal airflow hood or above a sterile object in a vertical airflow hood.

Figure 10.8

Physician's Orders for IV Infusions —continued
(2 of 2)

(✓)	START HERE →	DATE	TIME	A.M. P.M.	PROFILED BY:	FILLED BY:	CHECKED BY:	PATIENT NAME AND I.D.

*add 100 units Humulin Regular Insulin
to D₅W 500 mL @20 mL/hr
(label concentration 0.2 units/mL)*

Jennings, MD

(✓)	START HERE →	DATE	TIME	A.M. P.M.	PROFILED BY:	FILLED BY:	CHECKED BY:	PATIENT NAME AND I.D.

*begin magnesium sulfate 5 g in
500 mL NS to run over 5 hours
x 1 dose only*

Dr. T. Jones

(✓)	START HERE →	DATE	TIME	A.M. P.M.	PROFILED BY:	FILLED BY:	CHECKED BY:	PATIENT NAME AND I.D.

*Δ fluids to 0.45 NS with 20 mEq KCl
@125 ml/hr*

Byrd, MD

3. Follow proper procedure for handling sterile devices and medication containers to ensure an accurate microbial-free product. Remember that the plunger and tip of the syringe are sterile and must not be touched. For greatest accuracy, use the smallest syringe that can hold the desired amount of solution. In any case, the syringe should not be larger than twice the volume to be measured. A syringe is considered accurate to one-half the smallest measurement mark on its barrel. To get an accurate dose, observe closely the calibrations on the syringe barrel. Count the number of marks between labeled measurement units. If there are ten marks, each mark measures off one-tenth of the unit. If there are five marks, each mark measures two-tenths of the unit. The volume of solution drawn into a syringe is measured at the point of contact between the rubber piston and the side of the syringe barrel. The measurement is not read at the tip of the piston.

Figure 10.9

**Order for Adult
Parenteral
Nutrition**
(Front)

Adult Parenteral Nutrition Order Form
Mt. Hope Hospital
My Town, SC

Patient: _____
Room: _____

Date: _____ Time: _____ PM _____ AM

☐ Consult Nutritional Support Service (Beeper 0349)

☐ Conduct Indirect Calorimetry Test

Central Formula (per liter)		Peripheral Formula (per liter)	
Amino Acids	40 g	Amino Acids	25 g
Dextrose	17.5% (600 Kcals)	Dextrose	6% (200 Kcals)
Fat 20%	125 mL (250 Kcals)	Fat 20%	200 mL (400 Kcals)
Standard Electrolytes*		Standard Electrolytes*	
Trace Elements-4: 1 mL/day		Trace Elements-4: 1 mL/day	
Multivitamins-12: 10 mL/day		Multivitamins-12: 10 mL/day	
		Osmolarity: 740 mOsm/L	
Total Volume _____ mL/day		Total Volume _____ mL/day	

*Standard Electrolytes (per liter) Na: 50 mEq, Ca: 7.5 mEq, Cl: 45 mEq, Acetate: 45 mEq, Phos: 9 mM

Special Formulation (Indicate Total Daily Requirements)	Guidelines	General Rule
1. Amino Acids _____ g/day	0.5–2.5 g/kg/day	1 g/kg/day
Type _____		
2. Total Nonprotein		
Calories _____ Kcals/day*	10–40 Kcals/kg/day	25 Kcals/kg/day
Dextrose _____%	0–100%	65%
Fat _____%	0–65%	35%
100%		100%
3. Total Volume _____ mL/day	Minimum Volume: 1 Kcal/1.0 mL	

*Substrate must equal 100%.

Special Formulation—Electrolytes (check one)

☐ Standard Electrolytes/Liter   ☐ Standard Electrolytes plus
                                                    Additional Electrolytes

☐ Standard Electrolytes/Liter—No Potassium   ☐ Custom Electrolytes

Sodium Acetate	_____ mEq/day	Potassium Acetate	_____ mEq/day
Sodium Chloride	_____ mEq/day	Potassium Chloride	_____ mEq/day
Sodium Phosphate	_____ mEq/day	Potassium Phosphate	_____ mEq/day
Magnesium Sulfate	_____ mEq/day	Calcium Gluconate	_____ mEq/day

Multivitamins-12: (10 mL) per _____   Other _____
Trace Elements-4: (1 mL) per _____   Other _____

HUMAN REGULAR INSULIN _____ units/day

Phytonadione (Vit. K) 10 mg IM per _____

OTHER _____

Special Instructions _____
_____

M.D.   **Pharmacy Must Receive TPN Orders by 12 Noon**
76016153

VIALS Vials are closed systems; therefore, the amount of air introduced should be equal to the volume of fluid removed. An exception to this guideline is the withdrawal of cytotoxic drugs from vials where a volume of air less than the solution volume is introduced, producing a vacuum and preventing an aspirate when the needle is withdrawn from the rubber closure. Reconstituting a powder by introducing a diluent produces a positive pressure inside the vial.

Table 10.4 details the procedures generally followed for using a syringe to draw liquid from a vial. You begin by first swabbing the rubber stopper with an alcohol

Figure 10.9

Order for Adult Parenteral Nutrition —continued
(Back)

M.V.I.-12 10 mL* contains: (indicates adult RDA)

1. Ascorbic Acid	100.0 mg	(45 mg)
2. Vitamin A	3,300.0 units	(4,000–5,000 units)
3. Vitamin D	200.0 units	(4,000–5,000 units)
4. Thiamine	3.0 mg	(1.0–1.5 mg)
5. Riboflavin	3.6 mg	(1.1–1.8 mg)
6. Pyridoxine	4.0 mg	(1.6–2.0 mg)
7. Niacin	40.0 mg	(12–20 mg)
8. Pantothenic Acid	15.0 mg	(5–10 mg)
9. Vitamin E	10.0 units	(12–15 units)
10. Biotin	60.0 mg	(150–300 mcg)
11. Folic Acid	400.0 mcg	(400 mcg)
12. Vitamin B_{12}	5.0 mcg	(3 mcg)

*Provides 100% of AMA guidelines for parenteral vitamin supplementation.

Trace Elements 1 mL contains: (AMA daily recommendations)

1. Zinc 5.0 mg (2.5–4 mg)   3. Manganese 0.5 mg (0.15–0.8 mg)
2. Copper 1.0 mg (0.5–1.5 mg)   4. Chromium 10.0 mcg (10–15 mcg)

INSTRUCTIONS FOR USING ORDER FORM

1. Check N.S.S. CONSULT or INDIRECT CALORIMETRY (Metabolic Cart) if desired.

2. Order STANDARD CENTRAL or STANDARD PERIPHERAL FORMULAS by total mLs per day. Nutritional components listed on form as per liter. Standard formulas include MVI, TE, and standard electrolytes.

3. Use SPECIAL FORMULATION section for any orders other than standard formulas including addition of electrolytes and other than standard lytes.

4. AMINO ACIDS ordered in mLs per day. If a change in rate is desired, place a new order for acid products (i.e., renal, hepatic, or HBC).

5. TOTAL NONPROTEIN CALORIES ordered as kcals per day. Specify percentage of total calories to be supplied by dextrose and percentage to come from lipids.

6. TOTAL VOLUME ordered in mLs per day. If a change in rate is desired, a new order form needs to be filled out to ensure the change is acknowledged by the IV pharmacy.

7. If either STANDARD LYTES or STANDARD LYTES—NO POTASSIUM are desired, check the appropriate box.

8. If CUSTOM ELECTROLYTES are desired, check the box and order total mEq per day. If STANDARD ELECTROLYTES PLUS ADDITIONAL ELECTROLYTES are desired, check the appropriate box and specify additional electrolytes in mEq/day.

   Use standard electrolytes (per liter) listed under standard formulas as a guide. Note: 4.0 mEq of Na phosphate or 4.4 mEq K phosphate provides 3 mM phosphate.

9. MULTIVITAMINS and TRACE ELEMENTS should be ordered per day.

10. Specify INSULIN (in units/day) and VITAMIN K if desired; then outline any SPECIAL INSTRUCTIONS if applicable.

ALL TPN ORDERS RECEIVED IN THE PHARMACY BY 12:00 NOON WILL BE HUNG BETWEEN 6:00 P.M. AND 10:00 P.M. THE SAME DAY.

Pharmacy Use

swab using firm strokes, of the same direction, or by spraying with 70% alcohol. The needle bevel tip should penetrate the rubber closure at an angle, which is then straightened to 90° so that as additional pressure is applied to the syringe, the bevel heel enters the closure at the same point as the tip. This technique prevents coring or introducing a small chunk of the rubber closure into the solution.

AMPULES The glass ampule offers another challenge because one must first break the top off the ampule to access the medication. The contents in the top of the ampule must be moved into the body by swirling the ampule in an upright position, inverting

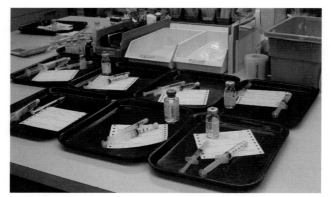

Medication that is prepared by the technician must be reviewed and approved by the pharmacist.

it quickly, and then turning it back upright, or by tapping the top with a finger. Clean the neck with an alcohol swab; then grasp the ampule between the thumb and index finger at the neck with the swab still in place. The glass around the top is scored to make such breaking easy and clean. Use a quick motion to snap off the top (see Figure 10.11). The ampule will generally snap at the neck. Do not break in the direction of the HEPA filer. Tilt the ampule, place the needle bevel of a filter needle or tip of a filter straw in the corner near the opening, and withdraw the medication. Use a needle equipped with a filter for filtering out any tiny glass particles, fibers, or paintchips that may have fallen into the ampule. Before injecting the contents of a syringe into an IV, the needle must be changed to avoid introducing glass or particles into the admixture. A standard needle could be used to withdraw the drug from the ampule; it is then replaced with a filter device before the drug is pushed out of the syringe.

Preparing a Label for an IV Admixture

When making an IV admixture, a label must also be prepared. The label should contain the following information:

- ◇ patient's name and identification/account number
- ◇ room number
- ◇ fluid and amount
- ◇ drug name and strength (if appropriate)
- ◇ infusion period
- ◇ flow rate (e.g., 100 mL/hr or infuse over 30 min)
- ◇ expiration date and time
- ◇ additional information as required by the institution or by state or federal guidelines, including auxiliary labeling, storage requirements, and device-specific information

Figure 10.12 shows examples of labels prepared for a minibag and for a large-volume parenteral.

Table 10.4	Using a Syringe to Draw Liquid from a Vial

1. Choose the smallest gauge needle appropriate for the task and avoid coring the rubber top of the vial and thus introducing particulate into the liquid within.
2. Attach the needle to the syringe.
3. Draw into the syringe an amount of air equal to the amount of drug to be drawn from the vial.
4. Swab or spray the top of the vial with alcohol; allow the alcohol to dry. Puncture the rubber top of the vial with the needle bevel up. Then bring the syringe and needle straight up, penetrate the stopper, and depress the plunger of the syringe, emptying the air into the vial. See Figure 10.10(a).
5. Invert the vial with the attached syringe.
6. Draw up from the vial the amount of liquid required. See Figure 10.10(b).
7. Withdraw the needle from the vial. In the case of a multidose vial, the rubber cap will close, sealing the contents of the vial.
8. Remove and dispose of the needle and cap the syringe. A new needle will be attached at the time of injection.

Figure 10.10

Withdrawing Medication from a Vial
(a) Inject air into the vial, equal to the volume of liquid needed.
(b) Withdraw the desired amount of medication into the syringe from the inverted vial.

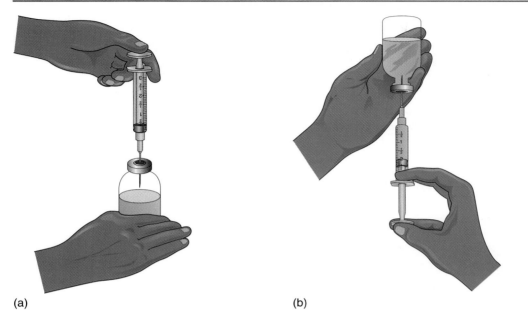

(a)

(b)

Figure 10.11

Opening an Ampule
(a) Gently tap the top of the ampule to bring the medication to the lower portion of the ampule. (b) Wrap gauze around the neck and top of the ampule. (c) Forcefully snap the neck away from you.

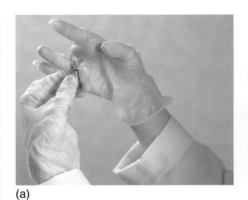

(a)

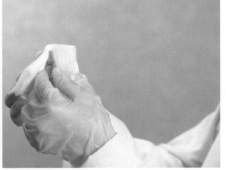

(b)

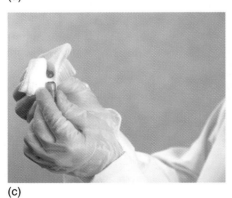

(c)

Figure 10.12

Minibag Label and Large-Volume Parenteral Label

PATIENT NAME	ROOM NUMBER
IDENTIFICATION NUMBER	DATE
FLUID VOLUME	
DRUG DOSE	
DRUG DOSE	
INFUSION RATE (for minibags)	
SCHEDULE (times due)	RATE (for LVPs)
EXPIRATION DATE & TIME	

John Brown	815-2
04596875	10/10/XX
D$_5$0.4NS 1000 mL	
potassium chloride 20 mEq	
MVI-12 10 mL	
q13h 6P 7A/11	75 mL/hr
EXP: 10/11/XX 5P	

MEDICATION ORDERS AND UNIT DOSE DISTRIBUTION

In a hospital or other institution, the pharmacy receives prescriptions in the form of medication orders. Figure 10.13 shows some examples of such medication orders.

Hospitals and other institutions typically make use of a unit dose system for dispensing medications. A unit dose is an amount of a drug prepackaged for a single administration. In other words, it is an amount of medication in a dosage form ready for administration to a particular patient at a particular time. Unit dose preparation increases efficiency by making the drug form as ready to administer as possible, rather than requiring nurses to prepare dosages from multiple dose containers.

Tablets and capsules are labeled, liquids are premeasured, injections are diluted as ordered and accurately measured into syringes, parenteral admixtures are compounded, and oral powders and other dosage forms are prepared appropriately.

A unit dose system saves time and money. It provides increased security for medications, reducing medication errors; reducing nursing time; and making administration, charging, and crediting easier. It also ensures that proper institutional and departmental policies will be followed.

Because manufacturers do not, in all instances, prepare drugs in single-dose form, and because individual medication orders may call for nonstandard dosages, preparing unit doses often involves repackaging. Repackaging may involve the use of a variety of equipment, such as counting trays, automated packaging machines, and liquid filling apparatuses. Typical unit dose packaging includes heat-sealed zip-lock bags, adhesive sealed bottles, blister packs, and heat-

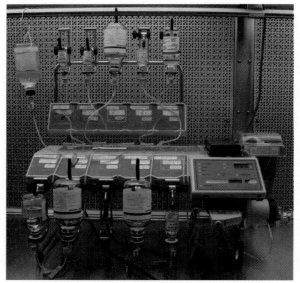

This micro-mix admixture machine adds micronutrients to IV solutions. This procedure is done within a laminar airflow hood.

sealed strip packages for oral solids, and plastic or glass cups, heat-sealable aluminum cups, and plastic syringes labeled "For Oral Use Only" for liquid orals. Oral medication specials (preparations made for a particular patient), IV specials, intramuscular injections, and suppositories are examples of drug forms typically provided in unit dose form. Ointments, creams, ear drops, and eye drops are not unit dose. These are bulk items that are not resupplied daily. They are provided only on request. When repackaging, a record is kept of what is done in order to track each dose for purposes of recall and quality assurance. Such a record is known as a repackaging control log and contains the following information:

- ◇ internal control or lot number
- ◇ drug, strength, dosage form
- ◇ manufacturer's name
- ◇ manufacturer's lot number and expiration date
- ◇ assigned expiration date
- ◇ resulting concentration
- ◇ quantity of units
- ◇ the initials of the repackager
- ◇ the initials of the pharmacist who has checked the repackaging

Additional information may be required, depending on institutional policy and state guidelines. An example of such a log appears in Figure 10.14.

Figure 10.13

Medication Orders
(1 of 4)

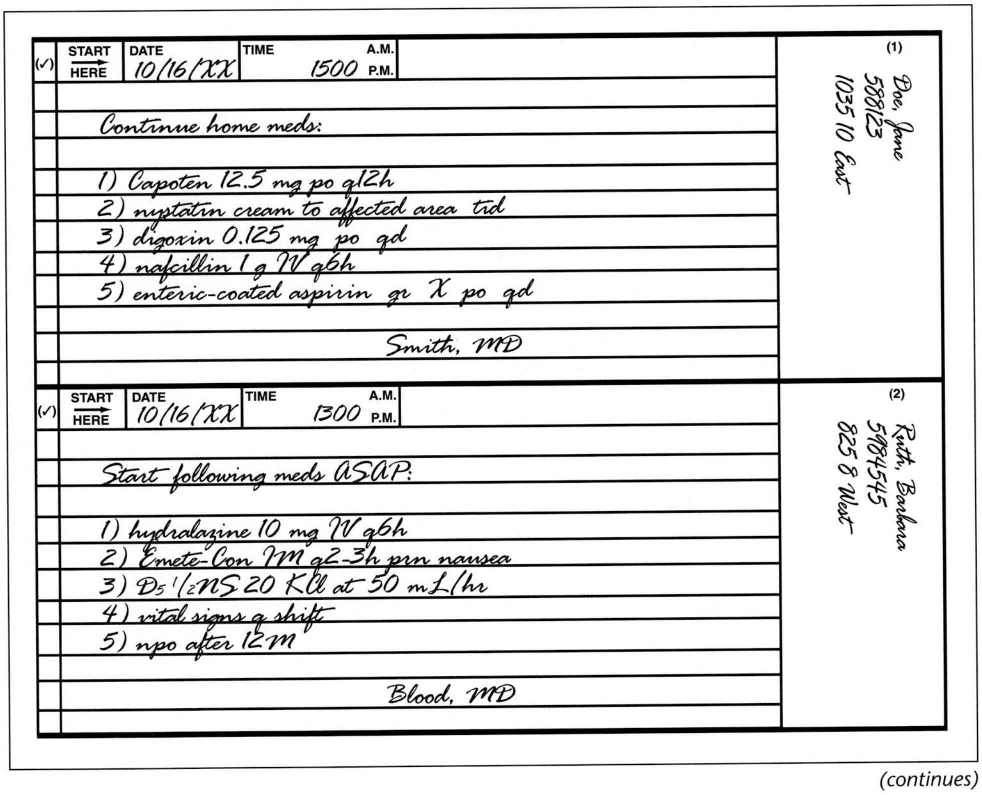

☑	START HERE →	DATE 10/16/XX	TIME 1500	A.M. P.M.		(1) *Doe, Jane* 508123 1035 10 East

Continue home meds:

1) Capoten 12.5 mg po q12h
2) nystatin cream to affected area tid
3) digoxin 0.125 mg po qd
4) nafcillin 1 g IV q6h
5) enteric-coated aspirin gr X po qd

Smith, MD

☑	START HERE →	DATE 10/16/XX	TIME 1300	A.M. P.M.		(2) *Ruth, Barbara* 5784545 825 8 West

Start following meds ASAP:

1) hydralazine 10 mg IV q6h
2) Emete-Con IM q2-3h prn nausea
3) D5 ½NS 20 KCl at 50 mL/hr
4) vital signs q shift
5) npo after 12M

Blood, MD

(continues)

Figure 10.13

**Medication
Orders—continued**
(2 of 4)

NAME	ROOM #	ADMIT TIME
John H. Jones Nalfon 300 mg po q8h Benadryl elixir 5 mL po hs Mucomyst 10% 10 mL on call	235	
Billy Martin MOM 30 mL po prn hs lithium carbonate 300 mg po tid ASA gr X po q4h	821	
Hilda Hornblower Vistaril 25 mg po q4h Tagamet 300 mg po tid acetaminophen 650 mg po q6h	822	
Vera Long Elixophyllin 250 mg po bid give 1 now ascorbic acid po daily Lufyllin 400 mg po q6h	121	
John Henry Garamycin 20 mg IM tid baby powder ASA gr V po q6h	432	
Casey Jones Mellaril 100 mg po bid 1 now Nitrostat SL prn Vasodilan 10 mg po tid	333	
Dolly Madison Principen 500 mg po bid 1 now Oretic 50 mg po bid Senokot po hs and bid	242	
Neil Buckner Colace 150 mg po q AM Decadron 0.75 mg po Motrin 600 mg po q6h	383	
Darla Molari Endep 100 mg po bid Folvite po qd Feosol po qd	422	
Larry Brindle Dilantin 30 mg po qid 1 now Dimetapp po bid Oretic 25 mg po	246	

Figure 10.13

Medication
Orders—continued
(3 of 4)

NAME	ROOM #	ADMIT TIME
Oscar Wilder	503	
Nitrostat SL prn		
Apresoline 50 mg po tid now		
Susan Anthony	610	
Catapres 0.3 mg po tid		
Coumadin 5 mg po qd		
MOM 20 mL po prn hs		
Raul Garcia	111	
Oretic 50 mg po tid I now		
K-Lor po qd		
Medrol 16 mg po		
Tom Smith	230	
ascorbic acid po qd		
Basaljel po prn ac and hs		
Toradol 10 mg po q4-6h		
Tim Turner	407	
10,000 units heparin IV now		
gentamicin 60 mg IVPB tid		
Donnatal po prn pc		
Rick Bono	606	
Compazine 25 mg rectal prn		
Benylin Cough Syrup 2 tsp po q4h		
V-Cillin K 500 mg po q6h		
Marc Janzen	414	
Elixophyllin 125 mg po qd I now		
EES granules 280 mg po q6h		
triamterene 100 mg po AM		
Julia Shriver	409	
Orinase 250 mg po bid		
prednisone 15 mg po qd 8 AM		
Antivert 12.5 mg po tid		
Marian Carter	520	
PPD test with syringe		
Robaxin po tid		
Naprosyn 500 mg po q12h		
Natalie Wang	311	
Diamox 125 mg po q6h		
Dimetapp po q4h		
MOM 30 mL po prn		

(continues)

Figure 10.13

Medication
Orders—continued
(4 of 4)

NAME	ROOM #	ADMIT TIME
Ray Stevens Nitrostat SL prn Aldactone 100 mg po tid Lasix 40 mg po bid	230	
Deborath Gunther acetaminophen elixir 160 mg po q6h Mylicon 80 mg po q pc	143	
George Milar Oretic 25 mg po bid 1 now Klotrix 10 mEq po qd Sudafed 60 mg q12h	502	
Kathy Sooner dexamethasone 100 mg po q AM Dulcolax 5 mg po qd Robaxin po q8h	402	
Gloria Kramer Pen. Vee K 375 mg po q6h Parafon Forte po q6h MOM 30 mL po hs	433	
Wesley Adams Inderal 60 mg po bid 1 now MOM 10 mL po q pc Colace 150 mg po hs	321	
Jennie Conners nitro patch 10 cm² qd send now Fleet prep kit ASA 600 mg po q4h	401	
Jeffrey Hart Ceclor 250 mg po q6h baby oil Esidrix 75 mg po bid	213	
Jennifer Hightower Darvon 100 mg po q6h Mylanta 60 mL po ac & hs Motrin 800 mg po q6h if react to Darvon	334	
Serena Sarles Larodopa 500 mg po qd AM captopril 12.5 mg po tid Tylenol 650 mg po q4h	416	

Each day, a medication fill list is generated by computer. This is a complete list of all the patients' current medications. From this list, a unit dose profile is prepared. The unit dose profile provides the information necessary to prepare the unit doses and includes patient name and location, medication and strength, frequency or schedule of administration, and quantity, as follows:

Figure 10.14

**Repackaging
Control Log**

REPACKAGING CONTROL LOG

DEPARTMENT OF PHARMACEUTICAL SERVICES

PHARMACY LOT NUMBER	DRUG-STRENGTH DOSAGE FORM	MANUFACTURER AND LOT NUMBER	EXP. DATE MANUF. MTC	RESULTING CONC.	QUANTITY	PREP. BY / CK'D

John Doe	Room 535
ampicillin 250 mg	
q6h	5P 11P 5A 11A
Joanne Riggs	Room 532
Nalfon 300 mg	
q8h	8A 4P 12A

Doses are prepared, labeled, and placed in patient drawers on carts that are taken to the wards. Labels include the following information:

- ◇ nonproprietary (generic) name or proprietary (trade) name of the drug
- ◇ dosage form (if special or other than oral)
- ◇ strength of the dose and the total contents delivered (e.g., the number of tablets and their total dose)

◇ any special notes (e.g., "Refrigerate")
◇ internal expiration date
◇ internal control number

A fill list is needed in order to stock patient drawers in a medication cart. This list is used to check medications left in the drawers and to provide needed medications. A 12-hour or 24-hour supply is stocked. If some meds are left in the drawer, these are subtracted from the 12-hour or 24-hour supply, and the difference is placed in the drawer. So, for example, if the fill list called for

medication	sch	Daily Quantity	Post/Add
Tagamet 300 mg	q 8h	3	2

and the drawer had one 300 mg Tagamet tablet from the previous day, two tablets would be added to the drawer.

AUTOMATION IN THE PHARMACY

In many institutional pharmacies, automated pharmacy services are replacing some of the tedious filling procedures. The basic automated service available in almost every institutional pharmacy includes computerized generation of prescription orders that have been entered into the computer, and repackaging of bulk items into unit dose blister packs or heat-sealed foil and plastic packaging. Larger pharmacies have installed robotic equipment to perform the routine filling process. Both pharmacists and technicians are responsible for operating the equipment and maintaining supplies used in the automation process.

Prescription orders that have been keyed into the computer are often filled on a regular twenty-four-hour basis until the patient is released or an order of a change in medication is received. A pharmacist or technician will pull orders from the computer database once daily and begin the fill process for the upcoming day. As new orders arrive in the pharmacy they are keyed into the computer system and the first day's medication are prepared. Orders for "stat" medications are filled immediately according to protocol. Maintenance medications are then included into the following days' automated report.

Pharmacies may utilize a variety of different time- and cost-saving devices to assist in the preparation of medications. As mentioned earlier, most medications in the pharmacy are purchased in unit dose packaging. However some medications are not available or are cost prohibitive in this packaging. Pharmacies may purchase the product in bulk and use a machine in the pharmacy to place the individual doses into a single dose, heat-sealed package. This process is very labor intensive, and is often the responsibility of a pharmacy technician. Repackaging and labeling of medications must be performed according to set guidelines regarding the record keeping and new labeling that must be printed on the unit dose.

Larger automated robots are being utilized to perform some of the filling procedures with

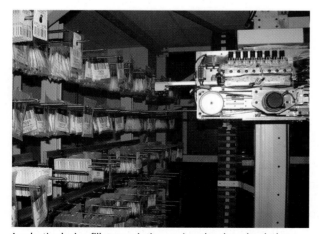

A robotic device fills prescriptions using the downloaded prescription orders and bar coded unit dose packaged medications.

100% accuracy. Patients are assigned a bar code with their patient ID, and the computer matches the needed prescription medications with the patient. All of the unit dose medications are packaged with an identifying bar code and placed on pegs. Both solid and liquid oral medications as well as prefilled syringes and vials are packaged in the bar coded plastic devices. The arm of the robotic device uses suction devices and pneumatic air to pull the medication from a peg on the wall and transfer it to a collection area.

Patients' individualized prescription orders may be collected by the robot and placed in an envelope or plastic tray for delivery. By using technology such as this, the pharmacist is able to spend more time reviewing the patient's medical records and make hospital rounds. The technician's responsibilities are also changed in that much time will be spent keeping the robotic area well stocked with medications. Using technology such as this has allowed the pharmacy to operate more efficiently and significantly reduces the amount of inventory.

FLOOR STOCK

The floor stock system provides medications for each nursing unit. Floor stock distribution deals with those medications that are dispensed frequently on a prn (*pro re nata,* or as needed) basis. It would be impractical, of course, to dispense such drugs on a unit dose basis. Typical floor stock consists of emergency medications and bulk items such as antacids, cough syrup, Tylenol elixir or drops, ointments, creams, inhalers, and narcotics. Advantages of the floor stock system are a quick turnaround time from the writing of the order to the administration of the medication and the convenience of immediate availability of medications to the nursing staff. Disadvantages include increased diversion, increased medication errors, and expense due to lost charges and revenue.

The pharmacy assumes responsibility for maintaining inventory through a floor stock replacement system. Pharmacy personnel maintain the inventory according to predetermined levels. Floor stock must be inspected regularly for proper storage, expired drugs, narcotic control, and removal of discontinued drugs and/or recalled drugs. Medications administered to patients by nursing units are charged to the appropriate records by manual and/or electronic data processing systems.

As with any distribution system, checks are necessary to determine usage and levels of remaining supply. When checking floor stock, it is important to check for expired drugs, to remove excess meds, to ensure items requiring refrigeration are refrigerated, to ensure that the refrigerator temperature is correct, to see that all medications are stored properly, and to confirm that all controlled substances are accounted for.

In many institutions, floor stock items are kept in automated dispensing machines rather than in a stock room or on shelf space on the patient care unit. Automated dispensing machines keep an electronic record of bulk, floor stock, and items utilized by each patient.

HANDLING AND DISPOSAL OF HAZARDOUS AGENTS

In all pharmacy settings, but particularly in hospital and other institutional settings, workers bear the risk of coming into contact with hazardous medications and other chemicals. Many kinds of dangerous drugs and chemicals are encountered in pharmacy, including corrosive materials (materials that can dissolve or eat away at bodily tissues) and cytotoxic materials (materials that are poisonous to cells), as is the case with antineoplastic drugs (used in the treatment of cancer). These materials require special handling and preparation. Table 10.5 lists some commonly used cytotoxic and hazardous drugs.

Four routes of exposure to hazardous substances include trauma, inhalation, direct skin contact, and ingestion, illustrated by the following examples:

◇ *Trauma, or injury.* A technician using a syringe to add a drug to an IV bag might accidentally prick himself or herself with the needle or receive a cut from a broken container of the substance.

◇ *Inhalation, or breathing in, of the hazardous substance.* A technician might drop and break a bottle containing a volatile substance, or poor manipulation technique may release a fine mist or aspirate of the medication from the container.

◇ *Direct skin contact.* A technician might accidentally spill a medication when pouring it from a large container into a smaller container or flask. Direct contact with some cancer drugs can cause immediate reactions.
  • Asparaginase may cause skin irritation.
  • Doxorubicin can cause tissue death and sloughing if introduced into a skin abrasion. Nitrogen mustards can cause irritation of the eyes, mucous membranes, and skin.
  • Streptozocin is a potential carcinogen when it is exposed to skin. Accidental exposures in the pharmacy may result in trauma, direct skin contact, and inhalation.

◇ *Ingestion.* A technician might ingest dust when crushing an oral tablet or cleaning a counting tray.

In any of these acute exposure examples, the exposure incident may produce symptoms or signs of sensitivity, eye irritation, vesicles on the skin, coughing, headache, and dizziness.

All personnel in an institution should have proper training in procedures involving identification, containment, collection, segregation, and disposal of cytotoxic and other hazardous drugs. Any organization involved with cytotoxic or other hazardous drugs should have written procedures for proper handling and disposal of such drugs and should provide access to medical care and methods for documentation in the case of incidents of exposure. All personnel involved should have specialized training on policies and procedures, individual instruction, use of equipment, and check-off on competencies of technique. Any pharmacy worker who is pregnant, breast-feeding, or trying to conceive should notify her supervisor so that extra precautions can be taken to minimize contact with hazardous substances.

Table 10.5	Commonly Used Cytotoxic and Hazardous Drugs		
asparaginase	dacarbazine	hydroxyurea	mitotane
bleomycin	dactinomycin	idarubicin	mitoxantrone
busulfan	daunorubicin	ifosfamide	plicamycin
carboplatin	doxorubicin	lomustine	procarbazine
carmustine	estramustine	mechlorethamine	streptozocin
chlorambucil	etoposide	melphalan	thioguanine
cisplatin	floxuridine	mercaptopurine	thiotepa
cyclophosphamide	fluorouracil	methotrexate	vinblastine
cytarabine	ganciclovir	mitomycin	vincristine

Receipt and Storage of Hazardous Agents

Hazardous drugs should be delivered directly to the storage area, checked, and, if necessary, refrigerated. The inventory should be separated to reduce the potential error of pulling a look-alike container from an adjacent shelf or bin. Equipment for storage and transport should minimize container breakage. For example, storage shelves should have a barrier at the front, carts should have rims, and hazardous drugs should be stored at eye level or lower. Hazardous drugs requiring refrigeration should be stored separately from other drugs in bins that prevent breakage and to contain leakage, should it occur. The person checking a shipment should wear gloves.

A list of cytotoxic and otherwise hazardous drugs should be compiled and posted in appropriate locations in the workplace. Storage areas, such as drug cartons, shelves, bins, counters, and trays should carry appropriate warning labels and should be designed in such a way as to minimize the possibility of falling and breakage. Access to storage areas and work areas for hazardous materials should be limited to specified trained personnel.

Protective Clothing

Damaged packages should be inspected in an insulated area, such as a vertical airflow hood. Broken vials of unreconstituted drugs should be treated as drug spills. Protective clothing like eye protection, respirator, utility and latex gloves, disposable gown or coveralls, and shoe covers should be worn when disposing of damaged packages.

A disposable, lint-free, nonabsorbent, closed-front gown with cuffed sleeves should be worn. Hair covers and shoe covers should be worn to reduce the potential for particulate contamination.

Double gloves should be put on following a thorough washing of the hands. Factors that influence glove permeability are thickness of the glove and time of exposure. All glove sizes should be available so each worker has a good fit. The first pair of gloves should be tucked under the sleeve cuff while the second pair should be placed over the top of the cuff. Gloved hands should then be washed to remove any powder that may be present, so as to prevent unnecessary particles in the hood. Gloves should be changed every 20 to 30 minutes with continuous use or immediately when there is contamination or puncture. Gloves should be turned inside out as they are taken off.

After exposure to cytotoxic or hazardous drugs, no protective clothing should be taken outside the area where exposure occurred. Caution should be taken, including warning others, so as not to contaminate other persons or objects. In case of an accidental exposure or skin contact, the area should be thoroughly washed with soap and large amounts of water. Report any incident to a supervisor and complete an incident report (Figure 10.15).

Technique for Handling Hazardous Agents

Rapid movements should be avoided to minimize air flow disturbances. Cytotoxic drugs should be prepared in a vertical laminar airflow hood (biological safety cabinet). The construction and operation of a vertical laminar airflow hood was introduced earlier in this chapter. This instrument should be cleaned and disinfected on a regular basis, at least every eight hours or immediately when there is a visible spill.

During cleaning, the blower should be left on. The area underneath the tray and the spillage trough should also be thoroughly cleaned. The technician should wear eye protection, a respirator, and proper apparel—gown, gloves, and hair cover when cleaning the vertical laminar airflow hood. Avoid excessive use of alcohol to

Figure 10.15

Cytotoxic and
Hazardous
Materials Incident
Report Form

MT. HOPE HOSPITAL
CYTOTOXIC AND HAZARDOUS MATERIALS INCIDENT REPORT

Date:	Time		Dept.

Person/persons Involved Name:		Sex	Date of birth

Home Address		Phone	

Name:		Sex	Date of birth

Home Address		Phone	

Witness:

Description of Incident:

Agent and Amount of Spill:

Actions Taken:

Was Medical Treatment Necessary?
If Yes, Physician Name and Address.

Diagnosis:

Follow-up:

Suggestions for Prevention of Future Incidences:

Signature: _____

Title: Date:

disinfect the work surface to avoid build-up of alcohol vapors in the cabinet. Allow the disinfectant to dry before medication preparation. Often, a lint-free plastic-lined pad will be used to absorb small particles or spills in the hood.

When preparing cytotoxic agents, proper aseptic technique should be followed. All syringes and IV containers should be labeled according to institutional guidelines. Syringes should be large enough so that they will not be full when the full dose is drawn into them. Therefore when syringes are filled with the full dose, the plunger will not separate from the barrel. Because drugs in vials may build up pressure causing the drug to spray out around the needle, a slight negative pressure should be maintained. To prevent excessive negative pressure, inject into the vial enough air to equal about 75 percent of the volume of drug to be withdrawn. Do not inject a volume of air that is equal to or greater than the amount of drug to be withdrawn.

Excessive negative pressure may cause leakage from the needle when it is withdrawn. The use of a chemo venting pin also will equalize air pressure in the vial.

When adding diluent to a vial, one should do so slowly, allowing pressure in the vial and syringe to equalize. The needle should be kept in the vial while gently swirling the vial until the contents are dissolved. The vial is inverted and the drug solution is gradually withdrawn while equal amounts of air are exchanged for solution. The vial is then inverted into an upright position, and a small amount of air is drawn from the needle and syringe hub before the needle is drawn out of the vial. Vials should not be vented unless one is using a filter device.

When opening an ampule, one should tap the drug from the top of the ampule, wrap a pad around the ampule, and hold the ampule away from the face before breaking off the top. A 5 micron filter needle should be placed on the syringe to withdraw the solution from the ampule. The fluid should be drawn through the syringe hub. A regular needle is placed on the syringe. Excess drug and any air is ejected into the sterile vial until the correct volume is left.

If the medication is to be dispensed from the syringe, the solution should be cleared from the needle and hub and the needle replaced with a locking cap. The syringe should be wiped with a moistened wipe and then labeled. If the medication is to be added to an IV bag, care should be used to prevent a puncture of the bag. The injection port and the bag should be wiped with a moistened wipe. The bag should be placed in a sealable container, a bag, to contain leakage.

Priming of IV administration sets should be done in the vertical laminar airflow hood where the cytotoxic agent can be captured in an appropriate container. If the set is not primed in the cabinet, then other priming techniques should be followed.

1. Retrograde priming, with the fluid from the primary IV solution (without the cytotoxic drug) is used to fill the tubing of the set.
2. The set is attached to the drug container.
3. The priming fluid is run through the set into the port of the drug container.
4. A gauze is placed in a sealable container and fluid is run through the set onto the gauze to prevent splashing.

Hazardous Agent Spills

The goal for the containment of a cytotoxic or hazardous material spill is to ensure that the healthcare setting, staff, patients, visitors, and the environment (both inside and outside of the medical facility) are not contaminated.

All spills should be dealt with immediately. Cleanup and decontamination should be done with a spill kit. Spill kits will contain materials to control and clean up spills of up to 1,000 mL. A commercially available spill kit may be used or one may be assembled with the following contents:

- ◇ nonabsorbent, lint-free gown
- ◇ gloves, two pair
- ◇ respirator mask
- ◇ goggles, one pair
- ◇ absorbent towels
- ◇ chemo hazard labels
- ◇ incident report form (Figure 10.15)
- ◇ spill control pillows, or towels folded to work as pillows
- ◇ scoop and brush (for collecting glass fragments)
- ◇ plastic disposal bags labeled "Chemo Waste"
- ◇ "CAUTION: Chemo Spill" sign

A spill outside the airflow hood should be posted with a warning sign. Proper attire should be worn, including gown, double gloves, goggles, and a mask or respirator. Broken glass should be placed in the appropriate container, but never with the hands. When cleaning up the spill, one should start from the edge of the spill and work inward, using absorbent sheets, spill pads, or pillows for the liquids or damp cloths or towels for solids. Use spill pads and water to rinse the area. Detergent should be used to remove residue.

Spills in the airflow hood require additional steps. The spill is removed as previously described. The drain trough should be thoroughly cleaned and the cabinet decontaminated. All contaminated materials from a spill should be sealed in hazardous waste containers and placed in leak-resistant containers. The spill and cleanup must be documented.

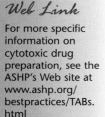

Web Link

For more specific information on the handling of cytotoxic and hazardous agents, ASHP's Web site at www.ashp.org/bestpractices/TABs.html

Procedures in Case of Exposure

Any body area exposed should be flooded with water and thoroughly cleansed with soap and water. Normal saline for irrigation should be used to cleanse the eyes. The exposed person should be sent or escorted to the employee health or emergency room. If the substance comes in contact with the skin, wash the skin thoroughly with soap and water and seek appropriate medical attention. If the substance comes in contact with the eyes, flush the affected eye with large amounts of water, or use an eye flush kit and seek appropriate medical attention. Remove contaminated garments and/or gloves, and wash hands after removing the gloves. Dispose of contaminated garments appropriately in biohazard materials containers.

Nonparenteral Hazardous Dosage Forms

Web Link

For more specific information on cytotoxic drug preparation, see the ASHP's Web site at www.ashp.org/bestpractices/TABs.html

Tablets and capsule forms of hazardous nonparenterals should not be placed in any automated counting or packaging machine. During routine handling of these drugs, workers should wear one pair of gloves of good quality and thickness. The counting and pouring of these drugs should be done carefully, and contaminated equipment should be cleaned with detergent and rinsed. Compounding with any of these drugs should be done in a protected area away from drafts and traffic. The worker should wear a gown and respirator in addition to gloves. When one is crushing a hazardous drug in a unit-of-use package, the package should be placed in a small, sealable plastic bag and crushed with a spoon or pestle, using caution not to break the plastic bag.

Chapter Summary

Hospital and other institutional pharmacies carry out many functions of community pharmacies but also undertake a number of activities unique to or especially common in the institutional setting. These activities include, but certainly are not limited to, the preparation of a formulary, or list of drugs approved for use; maintenance of a drug information center; training of staff in universal precautions; preparation, using sterile techniques, of parenteral admixtures; filling of medication orders using unit dose systems; stocking of nursing stations; and proper handling and disposal of hazardous agents.

Chapter Review

Knowledge Inventory

Choose the best answer from those provided.

1. A formulary is a
   a. list of approved drugs.
   b. description of contents and pharmacological characteristics of manufactured drugs.
   c. set of formulae for extemporaneous compounding.
   d. set of formulae for preparation of common parenteral admixtures.

2. Universal precautions deal with infections by disease-causing microorganisms found in
   a. tap water and other liquid sources.
   b. blood and other bodily fluids.
   c. emergency rooms.
   d. pharmacies.

3. A unit dose is
   a. a supply prepared for a hospital ward, or unit.
   b. an amount and dosage form appropriate for a single administration to a single patient.
   c. the average recommended dosage for an adult male.
   d. the dosage recommended by the United States Pharmacopeia.

4. The term used to describe a person confined to a hospital bed is
   a. outpatient.
   b. ambulatory patient.
   c. peripatetic patient.
   d. inpatient.

5. A pathogen causes
   a. a desired therapeutic outcome.
   b. an embolism.
   c. a thrombosis.
   d. a disease.

6. The germ theory of disease is credited to
   a. Robert Hooke.
   b. Edward Jenner.
   c. Anton Van Leeuwenhoek.
   d. Louis Pasteur.

7. People used to believe that life forms, such as microorganisms and maggots, could arise miraculously out of decayed or other matter in a process known as
   a. spontaneous combustion.
   b. spontaneous generation.
   c. zoomorphogenesis.
   d. parthenogenesis.

8. Small microorganisms that consist of little more than some genetic material surrounded by a protein case are known as
   a. bacteria.
   b. protozoa.
   c. viruses.
   d. fungi.

9. The absence of disease-causing microorganisms is known as
   a. sterilization.
   b. asepsis.
   c. aseptic technique.
   d. mechanical sterilization.

10. The provision of the entire nutritional needs of a patient by means of intravenous infusion is known as
    a. LVP.
    b. PRN.
    c. SVP.
    d. TPN.

Pharmacy in Practice

1. Write out a complete description, not using abbreviations, of the medication orders given in Figure 10.13. Refer to Chapter 3, Pharmaceutical Terminology and Abbreviations, as necessary.

Using the orders below and the reconstitution chart in the workbook, answer the medication questions.

2.

(✓)	START → HERE	DATE	TIME	A.M. P.M.	PROFILED BY:	FILLED BY:	CHECKED BY:	PATIENT NAME AND I.D.
	acyclovir 1 g q12h							
			Welby, MD					

   a. What fluid is the drug mixed in?
   b. What is the expiration time at room temperature?
   c. Can it be refrigerated?

3.

(✓)	START HERE	DATE	TIME	A.M. P.M.	PROFILED BY:	FILLED BY:	CHECKED BY:	PATIENT NAME AND I.D.
	vancomycin 1.5 g q8h							
	Johnson, MD							

a. What size of bag is used?
b. What is the infusion time?
c. What is the room temperature expiration?

4.

(✓)	START HERE	DATE	TIME	A.M. P.M.	PROFILED BY:	FILLED BY:	CHECKED BY:	PATIENT NAME AND I.D.
	Primaxin 500 mg q6h x 3 days							
	Marsh, MD							

a. What fluid is the drug mixed in?
b. What size of bag is needed?
c. How many bags will be needed?

5.

(✓)	START HERE	DATE	TIME	A.M. P.M.	PROFILED BY:	FILLED BY:	CHECKED BY:	PATIENT NAME AND I.D.
	oxacillin 1 g x 5 days							
	Docigrio, MD							

a. What size of bag is needed?
b. What fluid?
c. If all bags are prepared today, will the last one expire before the end of
    therapy?
d. What is the infusion rate?

Improving Communication Skills

1. Communicating in the hospital or institutional setting often means working with a wide variety of other healthcare providers. Understanding what role they play in the patients' healthcare is essential in effective communication. What duties do each of the following have?
   a. primary care physician
   b. anesthesiologist
   c. registered nurse
   d. practical nurse
   e. nurse's aide
   f. housekeeping aide
   g. social services aide or worker
   h. respiratory therapist
   i. phlebotomist
   j. medical lab technician
   k. pharmacist
   l. pharmacy technician

Internet Research

1. Visit the ASHP Web site.
   a. What types of training do they offer?
   b. What are the benefits of technician membership?
   c. How do you become a member?

2. Visit the ASHP Web site again, and find the link to your state affiliate organization.
   a. Where are they located?
   b. What is the phone number to contact the state organization?
   c. What services are offered to members?

Your Future in Pharmacy Practice

Chapter

11

Learning Objectives

◇ Explain some ways in which the job of the pharmacy technician is changing.

◇ Describe the format and content of the Pharmacy Technician Certification Examination.

◇ Explain the criteria for recertification for pharmacy technicians.

◇ Enumerate a wide variety of strategies for successful adaptation to the work environment.

◇ Make a plan for a successful job search.

◇ Write a résumé.

◇ Write a cover letter.

◇ Prepare for and successfully complete an interview.

◇ Enumerate some trends for the future of the pharmacy profession.

The past century has seen dramatic changes in the pharmacy profession, but nothing compared with the changes in the coming years. Exciting changes are afoot, including a movement toward national certification of pharmacy technicians and the placement of technicians in new roles and responsibilities. This chapter provides useful information and skills to prepare you for becoming a pharmacy technician.

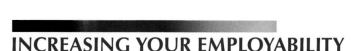

INCREASING YOUR EMPLOYABILITY

As learned in Chapter 1, the pharmacy technician career field is presently undergoing dramatic changes. Throughout the country, pharmacy technicians are gaining recognition for the vital role they play in providing a wide range of pharmaceutical services in a wide range of employment settings. The occupational outlook for the pharmacy paraprofessional is quite bright. Some estimates put the number of new pharmacy technicians to be employed over the coming years in the tens of thousands. In many parts of the country, technicians are now receiving official recognition from state boards of pharmacy and are being required to register with the state. At least one state is experimenting with having technicians check the work of other technicians in institutional settings. Chain drugstores and other employers are increasingly calling for technicians to become certified by taking the national Pharmacy Technician Certification Examination. Some people and organizations within the profession, including the Pharmacy Technicians Educators Council, are calling for the development of a two-year associate degree standard for technician training. All of these developments point to an increase in the presence, responsibilities, and status of the technician within the pharmacy community.

The elevation of the career of pharmacy technician to paraprofessional status brings with it increasing demands upon the technician. Today's employers expect more (and deliver more) to their technician employees. This section provides some useful information to help you to meet these increased demands and to place your best foot forward as you enter the field.

Certification and the National Certification Examination

In January of 1995, the Pharmacy Technician Certification Board (PTCB) was created by the American Pharmaceutical Association (APhA), the American Society of Health-System Pharmacists (ASHP), the Illinois Council of Health-System Pharmacists (ICHP), and the Michigan Pharmacists Association (MPA). The mission of the PTCB is to establish and maintain criteria for certification and recertification of pharmacy technicians on a national basis. A nonprofit testing company, the Professional Examination Service (PES), administers the Pharmacy Technician Certification Examination (PTCE), which candidates must pass in order to become certified and receive the title of CPhT, or certified pharmacy technician. While institutional and retail pharmacies do not uniformly require their pharmacy technicians to be certified, employers are increasingly encouraging certification. Often an employer is willing to pay for training pharmacy technicians must take in preparation for the certification exam and may even pay the exam fee. Of course, technicians often receive higher pay once they are certified.

The PTCE is a multiple-choice examination containing a total of 125 questions organized into three sections, each of which is weighted differently. Candidates for certification are given three hours to complete the exam. Points are not deducted for incorrect answers on the exam, so it pays to answer every question. Candidates must receive a score of 650 or higher to pass and receive certification. A technician may retake the exam as many times as is necessary to achieve a passing score.

Candidates should bring with them to the examination photo identification; a silent, hand-held, nonprogramable, battery-operated calculator; and a supply of No. 2 pencils. No reference materials, books, papers, or other materials may be taken into the examination room. The PTCB recommends that persons taking the exam be familiar with the material in "any of the basic pharmacy technician training manuals."

The goal of the PTC exam is to verify the candidate's knowledge and skill base for activities performed by pharmacy technicians under the supervising pharmacist. Table 11.1 details the content of the examination as specified by the PTCB. (Functions and responsibilities of pharmacy technicians may also be specifically defined by state laws and regulations and job-center policies and procedures.) These activities are characterized under three broad function areas:

⬥ Assisting the Pharmacist in Serving Patients—64% of Examination
⬥ Maintaining Medication Distribution and Inventory Control Systems—25% of Examination
⬥ Participating in the Administration and Management of Pharmacy Practice—11% of Examination

Web Link

Sample questions from the certification examination are available on the PTCB Web site at www.ptcb.org

Recertification

Recertification is required by the PTCB every two years. To be recertified, one must earn a total of 20 hours credit in pharmacy-related continuing education, with at least one of these hours being in pharmacy law. Certified technicians receive notification of the need for recertification approximately 60 days before their certification lapses.

Table 11.1	The Contents of the Pharmacy Technician Certification Examination

I. Assisting the Pharmacist in Serving Patients

1. Receive prescription or medication order(s) from patient/patient's representative, prescriber, or other healthcare professional:
   - Accept new prescription or medication order from patient/patient's representative, prescriber, or other healthcare professional.
   - Accept new prescription or medication order electronically (e.g., by telephone, fax, or computer).
   - Accept refill request from patient/patient's representative, prescriber, or other healthcare professional.
   - Accept refill request electronically (e.g., by telephone, fax, or computer).
   - Contact prescriber/originator for clarification of prescription or medication order refill.
2. At the direction of the pharmacist, assist in obtaining from the patient/patient's representative such information as diagnosis or desired therapeutic outcome, medication use, allergies, adverse reactions, medical history and other relevant patient information, physical disability, and reimbursement mechanisms.
3. At the direction of the pharmacist, assist in obtaining from prescriber, other healthcare professionals, and/or the medical record such information as diagnosis or desired therapeutic outcome, medication use, allergies, adverse reactions, medical history and other relevant patient information, physical disability, and reimbursement mechanisms.
4. At the direction of the pharmacist, collect data (e.g., blood pressure and glucose) to assist the pharmacist in monitoring patient outcomes.
5. Assess prescription or medication order for completeness (e.g., patient's name and address), accuracy (e.g., consistency with products available), authenticity, legality, and reimbursement eligibility.
6. Update the medical record/patient profile with such information as medication history, allergies, medication duplication, and/or drug-disease, drug-drug, drug-laboratory, and drug-food interactions.
7. Process a prescription or medication order:
   - Enter prescription or medication order information onto patient profile.
   - Select the product(s) for a generically written prescription or medication order.
   - Select the product(s) for a brand-name prescription or medication order (consulting established formulary as appropriate).
   - Obtain medications or devices from inventory.
   - Measure, count, or calculate finished dosage forms for dispensing.
   - Record preparation of prescription or medication, including any special requirements, for controlled substances.
   - Package finished dosage forms (e.g., blister pack, vial).
   - Affix label(s) and auxiliary label(s) to container(s).
   - Assemble patient information materials.
   - Check for accuracy during processing of the prescription or medication order (e.g., matching NDC number).
   - Verify the measurements, preparation, and/or packaging of medications produced by other technicians.
   - Prepare prescription or medication order for final check by pharmacist.
8. Compound a prescription or medication order:
   - Assemble equipment and/or supplies necessary for compounding the prescription or medication order.
   - Calibrate equipment (e.g., scale or balance, TPN compounder) needed to compound the prescription or medication order.
   - Perform calculations required for usual dosage determinations and preparation of compounded IV admixtures.
   - Compound medications (e.g., ointments, reconstituted antibiotic suspensions) for dispensing according to prescription formula or instructions.
   - Compound medications in anticipation of prescription or medication orders (e.g., bulk compounding for a specific patient).
   - Prepare sterile products (e.g., TPNs, piggybacks).
   - Prepare chemotherapy.
   - Record preparation and/or ingredients of medications (e.g., lot number, control number, expiration date).
9. Provision of medication to patient/patient's representative:
   - Store medication prior to distribution.
   - Provide medication to patient/patient's representative.
   - Place medication in dispensing system (e.g., unit-dose cart, robotics).
   - Deliver medication to patient-care unit.

(continues)

◇ Record distribution of prescription medication.
◇ Record distribution of controlled substances.
◇ Record distribution of investigational drugs.
10. Determine charges and obtain reimbursement for services.
11. Communicate with third-party payers to determine or verify coverage and obtain prior authorizations.
12. Provide supplemental information (e.g., patient package leaflets, computer generated information, videos) as requested/required.
13. Ask patient if counseling by pharmacist is desired.
14. Perform drug administration functions under appropriate supervision (e.g., perform drug/IV rounds, anticipate refill of drugs/IVs).
15. Assist the pharmacist in monitoring patient laboratory values (e.g., blood pressure, cholesterol values).

II. Maintaining Medication and Inventory Control Systems

1. Identify pharmaceuticals, durable medical equipment, devices, and supplies to be ordered (e.g., want book).
2. Place orders for pharmaceuticals, durable medical equipment, devices, and supplies (including investigational and hazardous products and devices), and expedite emergency orders in compliance with legal, regulatory, professional, and manufacturers' requirements.
3. Receive goods and verify against specifications on original purchase orders.
4. Place pharmaceuticals, durable medical equipment, devices, and supplies (including hazardous materials and investigational products) in inventory under proper storage conditions.
5. Perform non-patient-specific distribution of pharmaceuticals, durable medical equipment, devices, and supplies (e.g., crash carts, nursing station stock, automated dispensing systems).
6. Remove from inventory expired/discontinued/slow-moving pharmaceuticals, durable medical equipment, devices, and supplies.
7. Remove from inventory recalled pharmaceuticals, durable medical equipment, devices, and supplies.
8. Communicate changes in product availability (e.g., formulary changes, recalls) to pharmacy staff, patient/patient's representative, physicians, and other healthcare professionals.
9. Implement and monitor policies and procedures to deter theft and/or drug diversion.
10. Maintain a record of controlled substances received, stored, and removed from inventory.
11. Perform required inventories and maintain associated records.
12. Maintain record-keeping systems for repackaging, bulk compounding, recalls, and returns of pharmaceuticals, durable medical equipment, devices, and supplies.
13. Compound medications in anticipation of prescription/medication orders (e.g., bulk compounding).
14. Perform quality assurance tests on compounded medications (e.g., for bacterial growth; for sodium, potassium, dextrose levels; for radioactivity).
15. Repackage finished dosage forms for dispensing.
16. Participate in quality assurance programs related to products and/or supplies (e.g., orange book equivalence, formulary revision, nursing unit audits, performance evaluations of wholesalers).
17. Communicate with representatives of pharmaceutical and equipment suppliers.

III. Participating in the Administration and Management of Pharmacy Practice

1. Coordinate written, electronic, and oral communications throughout the practice setting (e.g., route phone calls, faxes, verbal and written refill authorizations; disseminate policy changes).
2. Update and maintain information (e.g., insurance information, patient demographics, provider information, reference material).
3. Collect productivity information (e.g., the number of prescriptions filled, fill times, money collected, rejected claim status).
4. Participate in quality improvement activities (e.g., medication error reports, customer satisfaction surveys, delivery audits, internal audits of processes).
5. Generate quality assurance reports.
6. Implement and monitor the practice setting for compliance with federal, state, and local laws, regulations, and professional standards (e.g., Materials Safety Data Sheet [MSDS], eyewash centers, JCAHO standards).
7. Implement and monitor policies and procedures for sanitation management, handling of hazardous waste (e.g., needles), and infection control (e.g., protective clothing, laminar flow hood, other equipment cleaning).
8. Perform and record routine sanitation, maintenance, and calibration of equipment (e.g., automated dispensing equipment, balances, robotics, refrigerator temperatures).

Table 11.1	The Contents of the Pharmacy Technician Certification Examination—continued

9. Maintain and use manual or computer-based information systems to perform job-related activities (e.g., update prices, generate reports and labels, perform utilization tracking/inventory).
10. Maintain software for automated dispensing technology, including point-of-care drug dispensing cabinets.
11. Perform billing and accounting functions (e.g., personal charge accounts, third-party rejections, third-party reconciliation, census maintenance, prior authorization).
12. Communicate with third-party payers to determine or verify coverage.
13. Conduct staff training.
14. Aid in establishing, implementing, and monitoring policies and procedures.

Source: Pharmacy Technician Certification Board, <http://www.ptcb.org/exam/content.asp> (18 March 2002). Used with permission.

ADJUSTING TO THE WORK ENVIRONMENT

If you have not worked before, or if your work experience has been sporadic, then getting used to your job as a technician might seem like getting used to life in a foreign country. You will have to adjust to a new "work culture," to different behaviors, to unfamiliar customs, and even to a new "language," the technical jargon of the profession. The following list provides some advice for making your adjustment to the job a comfortable one.

- ◇ **Attitude** Do not give in to the temptation to behave in ways that are elitist or superior. Remember you are part of a healthcare team, and cooperation is extremely important.
- ◇ **Reliability** Healthcare, like teaching, is one of those industries in which standards for reliability are very high. One simply cannot show up late for work, take days off arbitrarily, without good reason, and so on. Unreliable employees in the healthcare industry do not keep their jobs for long. Therefore, make sure that your employer can always depend on you to arrive at work on time. Staying late does not make up for a tardy arrival. Remember that tardiness can play havoc with other people's work schedules and work loads. Finish your grooming and eating before you enter your work area.
- ◇ **Accuracy and Responsibility** In a pharmacy, one rarely has the leeway to be partially correct. An error, even a small one, can have dire consequences for a patient or customer and/or the pharmacy itself. Develop work habits to ensure accuracy, and expect to be held responsible for what you do on the job. Work steadily and methodically. Keep your attention on the task at hand, and always double-check everything you do.
- ◇ **Relating to Your Supervisor** Always show your supervisor a reasonable degree of deference and respect. Ask your supervisor how he or she prefers to be addressed. Be respectful of your supervisor's experience and knowledge. If tensions arise between you and your supervisor, take positive steps to lessen them. Remember that your supervisor has power over your raises, promotions, benefits, and references for future employment.
- ◇ **Personality** It may come as some surprise to you, but personality is one of the greatest predictors of job success. Be positive, cooperative, self-confident, and enthusiastic.
- ◇ **Performance** Demonstrate that you can get things done and that you put the job first.

- **Questioning** Sometimes people are afraid to ask questions because doing so might make them appear less intelligent or knowledgeable. Nothing could be further from the truth. When you do not know how something should be done, always ask.
- **Dress** Follow the dress code of the company or institution for which you work.
- **Receptivity** Listen to the advice of others who have been on the job longer. Accept criticism gracefully. If you make a mistake, own up to it. If you are criticized unfairly, adopt a nondefensive tone of voice and explain your view of the matter calmly and rationally.
- **Etiquette** Every workplace has its unique culture. Especially at first, pay close attention to the details of that culture. Pick up on the habits of interaction and communication practiced by other employees and model the best of these.
- **Alliances** In all organizations, two kinds of power systems exist—formal, or organizational ones, and informal ones, based upon alliances. Cultivate alliances on the job, but make sure that you are not seen as part of a clique. Even as a new employee, you will begin to build power through making alliances. If a problem or an opportunity arises, you will probably hear about it first through your allies on the job. If a change in the workplace affects you, advance notice may give you the time to plan a strategic response.
- **Reputation** Many people assume that if they work hard and are loyal, they will be rewarded. This is often but not necessarily always true. Management personnel may be so involved with their own concerns that you remain little more than a face in the crowd. Being pleasant to others will help you to be noticed, as will making helpful or useful suggestions. Do not keep your professional qualifications a secret. Join professional organizations. Serve on committees within the institution. When you have won an award or achieved some other success, see that your name is publicized in, for example, institutional newsletters, community newspapers, or the newsletters of professional organizations. Give presentations at professional meetings, civic groups, churches, or synagogues. Write articles for publication in professional publications. In short, avoid hiding your light under a bushel.
- **Luck** Most of the big lucky breaks in life come through knowing the right people at the right time. So, by cultivating alliances, you can, more than you might expect, control your luck.

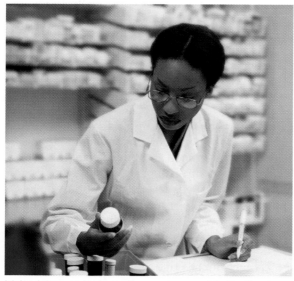

Maintaining medical supplies requires careful attention to detail and accurate documentation.

- **Crisis** When a crisis occurs, do not overreact. Take time, if you can, to think and then act, and do not keep the crisis a secret from your supervisor.
- **Learning** Pharmacy is a rapidly changing field. Accept the idea of continuing education as a way of life. You need not take formal course work every year (unless you are doing so to maintain your certification), but do make a point to read and to attend professional meetings to learn about the latest trends. Think of the job-related learning that you do as a regular "information workout," as necessary to your employment fitness as aerobic workouts are to your physical fitness.
- **Expertise** How can you become a person who makes things happen? Become highly knowledgeable about a specialty within your field. Become the most expert technician that you can become in that area. Then move on and

master another area. Soon, others will be asking your advice, and your reputation will build.

◇ **Reflectiveness about Your Career** There will never be a time in your career to coast and relax. Good career chances can come your way at any time in life, so make a regular habit of taking the time to think about your career and where you are headed. Planning lends structure and substance to your career management.

THE JOB SEARCH

Before you can implement the excellent strategies introduced in the preceding section, you must, of course, find the right job. Many people find the prospect of job hunting overwhelming. Avoid such negative thinking. Instead, think of the job hunt as an adventure, a period of exploration that can lead to exciting new possibilities. Taking the following steps can make the job search successful.

Clarify Your Career Goals

It will be very difficult to find a job if you are not sure what you are looking for. Do you want to work in a community pharmacy? in a hospital? in a long-term care facility? in a home infusion pharmacy? If you have uncertainties about the setting in which you wish to work, arrange to interview some people who work in these settings. Also do some thinking about what you want out of the job. Are you interested in jobs with opportunities for advancement in retail management? Are you more interested in the R component of the job? Do you want to master the preparation of parenterals? compounding? ordering and inventory? billing? maintenance of a drug information library? Think about what you want to do. Then look for jobs that suit your ambitions. Many schools have career counselors who can help you to answer such questions. Make an appointment to visit and talk to one of these people.

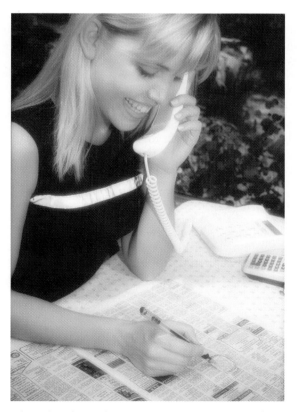

Taking the job search process one step at a time can help you successfully find a position as a pharmacy technician.

Write a Good Résumé

Make use of some of the excellent résumé-writing software now available, or contact a résumé-writing service. A résumé is a brief written summary of what you have to offer an employer. It is a sales tool, and the product you are selling is yourself. A résumé is an opportunity to present your work experience, your skills, and your education to an employer. Table 11.2 outlines the general topics to be included in a chronological résumé:

Make sure that your résumé follows a consistent, standard format, like that shown in Figure 11.1. Limit it to a single page. Type it, or print it on a high-quality printer, using high-quality 8½ × 11-inch paper. Many special résumé papers are available from stationary and office supply shops. However, ordinary opaque white paper is acceptable. Be sure

Table 11.2	The Parts of a Résumé
Heading	Give your full name, address, and telephone number. Remember to include your zip code and area code.
Employment Objective	This is the first thing an employer wants to know. The objective should briefly describe the position you are seeking and some of the abilities you would bring to the job. Identify the requirements of the position. Then tailor the employment objective to match those requirements.
Education	Give your college, city, state, degree, major, date of graduation, and additional course work related to the job, to the profession, or to business in general. State your cumulative grade point average if it is 3.0 or higher.
Experience	In reverse chronological order, list your work experience, including on-campus and off-campus work. Do not include jobs that would be unimpressive to your employer. Be sure to include cooperative education experience. For each job, indicate your position, employer's name, the location of the employment, the dates employed, and a brief description of your duties. Always list any advancements, promotions, or supervisory responsibilities.
Skills	If you do not have a lot of relevant work experience, include a skills section that details the skills that you can use on the job. Doing so is a way of saying, "I'm really capable. I just haven't had much opportunity to show it yet."
Related Activities	Include any activities that show leadership, teamwork, or good communication skills. Include any club or organizational memberships, as well as professional or community activities.
References	State that these are "Available on request."

to check your résumé very carefully for errors in spelling, grammar, usage, punctuation, capitalization, and form. No one wants to hire a sloppy technician. Once your resume is complete, you should always have another person read through it and check for errors in spelling, grammar, and vocabulary, as it is easy to overlook such things.

Establish a Network

Tell everyone you know that you are looking for a job. Identify faculty, acquaintances, friends, and relatives who can assist you in your job search. Identify persons within employers' organizations who can give you insight into their needs. Join professional associations. Attend meetings, and network with colleagues and potential employers.

Identify and Research Potential Employers

Your school may have a career placement office. Use the services of that office. Check the classified ads in newspapers. Go to a career library and look up employers in directories. Look up potential employers in telephone directories. Make use of career opportunities posted on Web sites and job-search Web sites. Many local hospitals also have a Web site that is used to post job vacancies as well.

Web Link

Rx Trek: rxtrek.net
Pharmacy Technician Certification Board: www.ptcb.org
America's Job Bank: www.ajb.dni.us
Health Care Jobs Online: www.hcjobsonline.com

Write a Strong Cover Letter

The cover letter, or letter of application, is the first letter that you send to an employer. It is generally sent in response to a job ad or posting or prior to a cold call to a potential employer. The résumé should accompany the cover letter. Both the cover letter and the résumé should be typed or printed on the same stock, or kind, of paper, and both should be placed in a matching business envelope addressed by means of typing or printing on an inkjet or laser printer. The letter should be single-

Figure 11.1

Sample Résumé

Ronald Cashman
1700 Beltline Blvd.
My Town, SC 29169
(345) 555-3245

Objective: Position as pharmacy technician that makes use of my training in dispensing and compounding medications, ordering and inventory, patient profiling, third-party billing, and other essential functions

Education	My Town Technical College My Town, South Carolina Diploma in Health Science—Pharmacy Program Accredited by the American Society of Health-System Pharmacists Dean's List

Skills	Converting units of measure
	Setting up ratios and proportions for proper
	  performance of pharmacy calculations
	Aseptic preparation of intravenous solutions
	Proper interpretation of prescriptions and
	  physician's orders
	Proper interpretation and updating of
	  prescription records
	Attention to clerical detail
	Operation of pharmacy computer systems

Employment 2002–03	Clerk Arborland Pharmacy Erewhon, SC

References available on request.

spaced, using a block or modified block style. In the block style, all items in the letter begin at the left margin. In the modified block style, the sender's address, the complimentary close, and the signature are left-aligned from the center of the paper, and all other parts of the letter begin at the left margin.

The cover letter should highlight your qualifications and call attention to your résumé. Remember that a sloppy cover letter will detract from even the most professional résumé. As with your résumé, proofread the cover letter carefully for errors in spelling, grammar, usage, punctuation, capitalization, and form. Address the letter, when possible, to a particular person, by name and by title, and make sure to identify the position for which you are applying. If necessary, call the employer to get the correct spelling of the recipient's name. Use the format shown in Table 11.3 for your letter. Figure 11.2 shows a sample cover letter.

Prepare for the Interview

Review your research on the employer and role-play an interview situation. Get plenty of sleep and eat well on the day before the interview. Find out everything that you can about the company or institution before you go for an interview. Better yet,

Table 11.3	Suggested Format for Cover Letters
First Paragraph	In your initial paragraph, state why you are writing, what specific position or type of work you are seeking, and how you learned of the opening (e.g., from the placement office, the news media, or a friend).
Second Paragraph	Explain why you are interested in the position, the organization, or the organization's products and services. State how your academic background makes you a qualified candidate for the position. If you have had some practical experience, point out your specific achievements.
Third Paragraph	Refer the reader to the enclosed résumé, a summary of your qualifications, training, and experience.
Fourth Paragraph	Indicate your desire for a personal interview and your flexibility as to the time and place. Repeat your telephone number in the letter. Close your letter with a statement or question to encourage a response, or take the initiative by indicating a day and date on which you will contact the employer to set up a convenient time for a personal meeting.

Figure 11.2

Sample Cover Letter

February 1, 20XX

James Green, Pharm.D.
Main Street Community Pharmacy
1500 Main Street
My Town, SC 29201

Dear Dr. Green:

I learned of Main Street Community Pharmacy's need for a pharmacy technician through the Placement Office at My Town Technical College. I was pleased to learn of an opening for a technician at the very pharmacy that my family has frequented for years.

I believe that my education and experience would be an asset to Main Street Community Pharmacy. This May, I will be graduating from My Town Technical College's superb pharmacy technician training program. I would welcome the opportunity to apply what I have learned to a career with your pharmacy. I bring to the job a number of assets, including a 3.4 grade point average, commitment to continuing development of my skills as a technician, a willingness to work hard, and a desire to be of service.

I am a responsible person, concerned with accuracy and accountability, someone whom you can depend upon to carry out the technician's duties reliably. I have enclosed my résumé for your consideration.

I would appreciate an opportunity to discuss the position with you. I will call next week to inquire about a meeting. Thank you for considering my application.

Sincerely,

Ronald Cashman
1700 Beltline Blvd.
My Town, SC 29169

Enc.: résumé

do this work before you write the cover letter that you send with your résumé. Knowing details about a potential employer can help you to assess whether the employer is right for you and can win points in your cover letter or interview.

During the interview, follow the guidelines provided in Table 11.4 and be prepared to answer the questions listed in Table 11.5. Rehearse answers to these questions before the interview. When coming up with answers to such questions, bear in mind the employer's point of view. Try to imagine what you would want if you were the employer, and take the initiative, during the interview, to explain to the employer how you can meet those needs.

After the interview, follow up with a thank-you note and, within an appropriate time, a telephone call. Be persistent but not pushy.

TRENDS IN PHARMACY PRACTICE

One of the wonderful things about a career in pharmacy is that the profession changes continually. Consider how different the average community pharmacy of today is from the druggist's shop at the turn of the century, in which premanufactured medicines were novelties and rows of bottled tonics and elixirs vied for customers' attention with open barrels of hard candies. Doubtless the profession will change as much or more in the next 30 years as it did in the past one hundred, and that is a lot of change. The following are but a few of the exciting developments that lie in store.

Table 11.4	Guidelines for Job Interviews

1. Find out the exact place and time of the interview.
2. Know the full name of the company, the address, the interviewer's full name, and the correct pronunciation of the interviewer's name. Call the employer, if necessary, to get this information.
3. Know something about the company's operations.
4. Be courteous to the receptionist, if there is one, and to other employees. Any person with whom you meet or speak may be in a position to influence your employment.
5. Bring to the interview your résumé and the names, addresses, and telephone numbers of people who can provide references.
6. Arrive ten to fifteen minutes before the scheduled time for the interview.
7. Wear clothing and shoes appropriate to the job.
8. Greet the interviewer and call him or her by name. Introduce yourself at once. Shake hands only if the interviewer offers to do so. Remain standing until invited to sit down.
9. Be confident, polite, poised, and enthusiastic.
10. Look the interviewer in the eye.
11. Speak clearly, loudly enough to be understood. Be positive and concise in your comments. Do not exaggerate, but remember that an interview is not an occasion for modesty.
12. Focus on your strengths. Be prepared to enumerate these, using specific examples as evidence to support the claims you make about yourself.
13. Do not hesitate to ask about the specific duties associated with the job. Show keen interest as the interviewer tells you about these.
14. Avoid bringing up salary requirements until the employer broaches the subject.
15. Do not chew gum or smoke.
16. Do not criticize former employers, co-workers, working conditions.
17. At the close of the interview, thank the interviewer for his or her time and for the opportunity to learn about the company.

Table 11.5	Interview Questions

1. Why did you apply for a job with this company?
2. What part of the job interests you most and why?
3. What do you know about this company?
4. What are your qualifications?
5. What did you like the most and the least about your work experience? (Note: Explaining what you liked least should be done in as positive a manner as possible. For example, you might say that you wish that the job had provided more opportunity for learning about this or that and then explain, further, that you made up the deficiency by study on your own. Such an answer indicates your desire to learn and grow and does not cast your former employer in an unduly negative light.)
6. Why did you leave your previous job? (Again, avoid negative responses. Find a positive reason for leaving, such as returning to school or pursuing an opportunity.)
7. What would you like to be doing in five years? How much money would you like to be making? (Keep your answer reasonable, and show that you have ambitions consistent with the employer's needs.)
8. What are your weak points? (Again, say something positive, such as "I am an extremely conscientious person. Sometimes I worry too much about whether I have done something absolutely correctly, but that can also be a positive trait.")
9. Why do you think you are qualified for this position?
10. Would you mind working on the weekends? overtime? traveling?
11. Do you prefer working with others or by yourself? in a quiet or a noisy environment?
12. If you could have any job you wanted, what would you choose and why?
13. Tell me a little about yourself.
14. What are your hobbies and interests?
15. Why did you attend [the college that you attended]?
16. Why did you choose this major?
17. What courses did you like best? least? (Again, couch your responses to both questions in positive ways.)
18. What have you learned from your mistakes?
19. What motivates you to put forth your greatest efforts?
20. Do you plan to continue your education?

New Medicines and New Drug Development Technologies

Every day, new medicines come to market, many involving new drug development technologies such as genetic engineering. To work in pharmacy is to be at the front lines when new medications are introduced to combat AIDS, cancer, heart disease, cystic fibrosis, Parkinson's disease, and other scourges.

New Dosage Forms and Drug Delivery Mechanisms

New dosage forms and drug delivery mechanisms are not introduced as often as new drugs, but here, as well, the pace of innovation is increasing rapidly. The past few years have seen the introduction of such innovations as transdermal patches, conjunctival discs, and wearable intravenous infusion pumps. What the future holds is anyone's guess, but the one certainty is that new dosage forms and delivery mechanisms will emerge.

Robotics

Robotic machinery is already used in many institutional settings for unit dose repackaging procedures. It is likely that in the future robotics will play a larger role in pharmacy, providing, for example, automated compounding, filling, labeling, and record keeping in a single device.

Higher Professional Standards

In the near future, the entry level degree for the pharmacist will be the Pharm.D., and the national certification movement for pharmacy technicians is growing rapidly.

Continued Growth in Clinical Applications

The clinical pharmacy movement also continues to grow. In the future, more and more of the pharmacy professional's time and energies will be given to educational and counseling functions.

Increased Emphasis on Home Healthcare

The home healthcare industry is one of the most rapidly growing of all industries in the developed world. The reasons behind this growth include reduced cost, improvements in technology that make home care more practical, and the preference of individuals for remaining at home rather than in institutions. The growth of the home-care industry shows no signs of abating, and so, in the future, more pharmacists and technicians will find themselves servicing that industry.

Increased Technician Responsibility and Specialization

Some states are already experimenting with allowing trained technicians to check the work of other technicians. Expect, in the future, for technicians to be given ever more responsibility and for more and more technicians to become specialized in particular areas of service, such as radiopharmaceuticals or pediatric or geriatric pharmacy.

Web Pharmacies

A very recent development with much promise is the emergence of the online pharmacy, allowing patients and healthcare professionals to access records, communicate or refill prescriptions, monitor drug regimens, order nonprescription drugs and medical supplies, and conduct many other functions via the World Wide Web.

Online Reference Works

Already, many standard reference works in pharmacy are available in CD-ROM format. In the future, expect to see the most important reference works all become available in easily accessible and searchable online form via the World Wide Web.

Increase in Geriatric Applications

As the population of the United States ages, the importance of geriatric pharmacy will increase. The aging of the population will place great financial burdens on the healthcare system as a whole and on pharmacy in particular, leading inevitably to political decisions that will affect the functions of the pharmacist and the technician.

Chapter Summary

The occupational outlook for the pharmacy technician is promising. Increasingly, states are requiring certification or registration with the state board of pharmacy. Certification is offered through the Pharmacy Technician Certification Board (PTCB), an organization created by the American Pharmaceutical Association and other pharmacy groups in 1995. Persons who pass the certification examination receive the title of CPhT, or certified pharmacy technician.

Preparing to work in an institutional or community-based pharmacy requires serious thought about one's attitude, reliability, accuracy, sense of responsibility, personal appearance, organizational skills, and the ability to relate to others, particularly the supervisor. Cultivating alliances and making acquaintances across the profession plays a role, too, as does the desire to learn throughout life. After carefully planning a job search, you are ready to write a comprehensive, attractive résumé and cover letter that will result in interviews and, eventually, one or more job offers.

New medicines and drugs are continually being developed. Other trends to watch for include the use of robotics in drug manufacturing and compounding, higher professional standards, an increased emphasis on home healthcare, increased technician responsibility, and healthcare changes brought about by the expansion of the senior population.

Chapter Review

Knowledge Inventory

Choose the best answer from those provided.

1. The organization that certifies pharmacy technicians is the
   a. Pharmacy Technician Certification Board.
   b. Committee for the Certification of Pharmacy Technicians.
   c. Pharmacy Technician Review Council.
   d. American Society of Pharmacy Technicians.

2. The Pharmacy Technician Certification Examination is
   a. an essay examination.
   b. a multiple-choice examination.
   c. a true/false examination.
   d. All of the above

3. When taking the Pharmacy Technician Certification Examination, the candidate is allowed to bring into the room
   a. two reference works of his or her choosing.
   b. scrap paper on which to do calculations.
   c. a calculator.
   d. one pharmacy technician training manual.

4. The person legally responsible by virtue of state licensure for the care and safety of patients served by a pharmacy is the
   a. pharmacy technician.
   b. pharmacist.
   c. supervising pharmacist.
   d. pharmacologist.

5. The Pharmacy Technician Certification Examination tests candidates on
   a. assisting the pharmacist in serving patients.
   b. medication distribution and inventory control systems.
   c. operations.
   d. All of the above

6. A standard résumé does not list
   a. the job objective.
   b. employment history.
   c. name, address, and telephone number of the applicant.
   d. names, addresses, and telephone numbers of references.

7. A candidate without a great deal of work experience can compensate for this deficiency by emphasizing the
   a. employment history section of the résumé.
   b. references section of the résumé.
   c. job objective section of the résumé.
   d. skills section of the résumé.

8. The cover letter sent with a résumé should highlight one's
   a. qualifications.
   b. personality.
   c. network of connections.
   d. need for the job.

9. The transdermal patch is an example of a recently developed
   a. dosage form.
   b. drug.
   c. drug delivery mechanism.
   d. drug development technology.

10. In the future, it is likely that most pharmacy reference works will become available via
    a. microfiche.
    b. microfilm.
    c. CDi or CD interactive.
    d. the World Wide Web.

Pharmacy in Practice

1. Using reference texts and the Internet, compile a list of three potential employers of pharmacy technicians in each of the following areas: community pharmacy, hospital pharmacy, long-term care, and home infusion. Each list should include the name of the employer, the address, the telephone number, and a contact person. Collect the lists prepared by students in the class to make a master list.
2. Choose one potential employer of pharmacy technicians and research to find more information about the employer. Write a brief report providing information that might be of interest to a potential employee of this pharmacy or institution.
3. Write a résumé and cover letter that you might use to apply for a job as a pharmacy technician.

Improving Communication Skills

1. Practice role-playing an interview situation with other students in your class. Use the interview questions supplied in this chapter.
2. Share your résumé with another student. Ask that student to identify your strengths from your résumé.

Internet Research

1. Visit the Web site of the Pharmacy Technician Certification Board at http://www.ptcb.org and study the sample test questions available on that site. Print the sample questions and work with other students in small groups to answer them. To answer some of these questions, you may have to refer to reference works or to more advanced texts in pharmacology or pharmacy calculations.

2. Write an e-mail to the Pharmacy Technician Certification Board and order information on the PTCE.
3. Search the Web for the Association of Pharmacy Technicians (APT). Some areas have a local chapter with a Web site. Locate the contact person's name and the next meeting dates, and times.

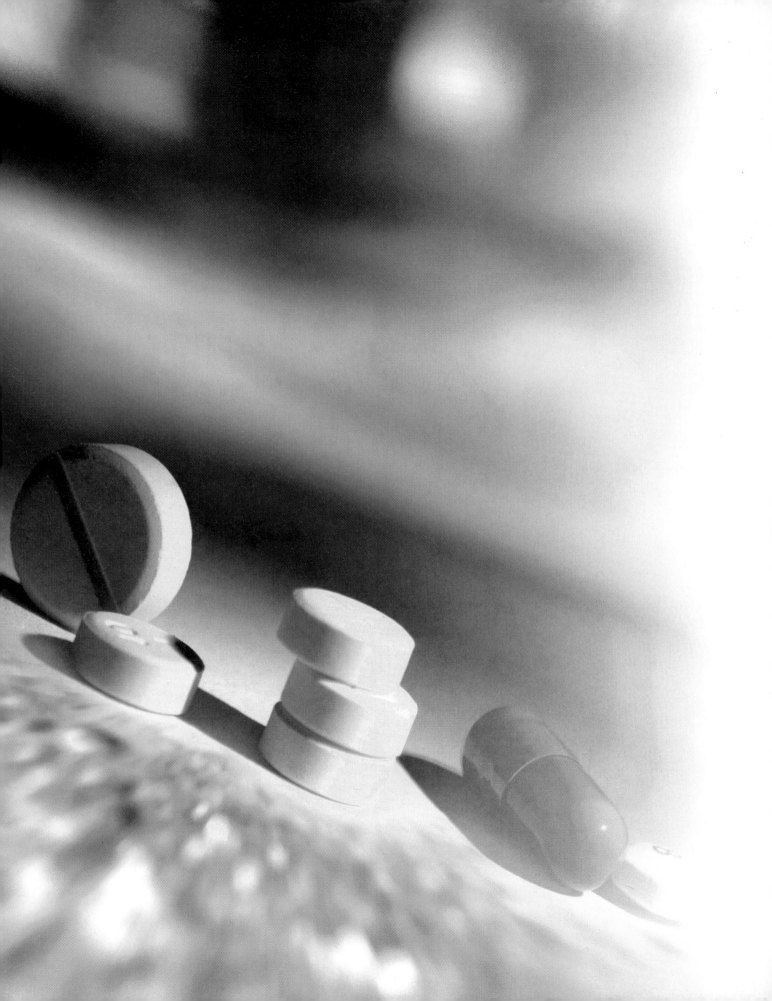

Common Prescription Abbreviations

This table is a quick reference of some of the common prescription abbreviations. Some prescribers may write abbreviations using capital letters or periods.

Abbreviation	Meaning	Abbreviation	Meaning
ac	before meals	os	left eye
ad	right ear	ou	both eyes
am	morning, before noon	per	by or through
amp	ampule	pc	after meals
aq	water	pm	evening, after noon
as	left ear	po	by mouth
au	both ears	prn	as needed
bid	twice daily	q	each, every
BSA	body surface area	qd	every day
$\bar{c}$	with	qh	every hour
cap	capsule	qid	four times a day
cc	cubic centimeter, milliliter	qod	every other day
D/C	discontinue	qs	a sufficient quantity
dil	dilute	R	by rectum, rectal
DW	distilled water	RL	Ringer's lactate
D_5W	5% dextrose in water	$\bar{s}$	without
elix	elixir	sig	write on label
fl	fluid	sol	solution
g	gram	$\bar{ss}$	one-half
gr	grain	stat	immediately
gtt	drop(s)	SC	subcutaneous
h, hr	hour	supp	suppository
hs	bedtime	susp	suspension
IM	intramuscular	syr	syrup
IV	intravenous	tab	tablet
IVP	intravenous push	tbsp	tablespoonful
IVPB	intravenous piggyback	tsp	teaspoonful
mcg	microgram	tid	three times a day
mEq	milliequivalent	ud	as directed
mg	milligram	ung	ointment
mL	milliliter		
N&V, N/V	nausea and vomiting	*Symbols*	
noct	at night	Δ	change by, change to
NS	normal saline, 0.9%	ʒ	dram
½NS	half normal saline, 0.45	fʒ	fluid dram
od	right eye	ʒ	ounce

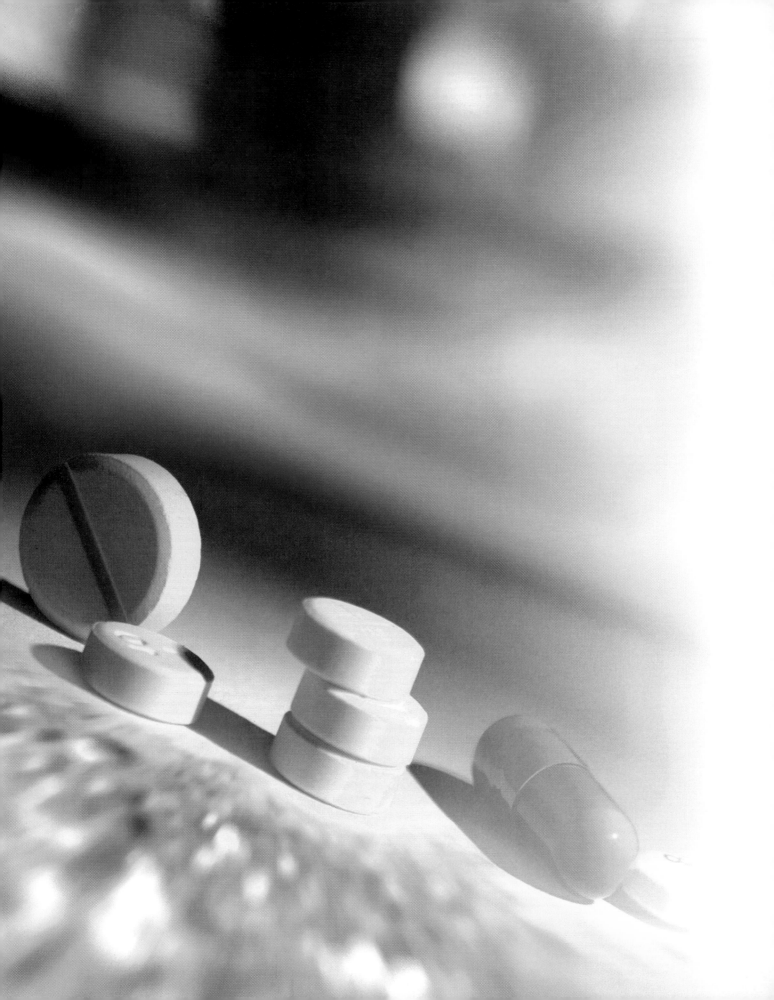

Common Prescription Abbreviations

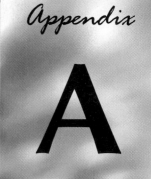

Appendix

A

This table is a quick reference of some of the common prescription abbreviations. Some prescribers may write abbreviations using capital letters or periods.

Abbreviation	Meaning	Abbreviation	Meaning
ac	before meals	os	left eye
ad	right ear	ou	both eyes
am	morning, before noon	per	by or through
amp	ampule	pc	after meals
aq	water	pm	evening, after noon
as	left ear	po	by mouth
au	both ears	prn	as needed
bid	twice daily	q	each, every
BSA	body surface area	qd	every day
$\bar{c}$	with	qh	every hour
cap	capsule	qid	four times a day
cc	cubic centimeter, milliliter	qod	every other day
D/C	discontinue	qs	a sufficient quantity
dil	dilute	R	by rectum, rectal
DW	distilled water	RL	Ringer's lactate
D_5W	5% dextrose in water	$\bar{s}$	without
elix	elixir	sig	write on label
fl	fluid	sol	solution
g	gram	$\bar{ss}$	one-half
gr	grain	stat	immediately
gtt	drop(s)	SC	subcutaneous
h, hr	hour	supp	suppository
hs	bedtime	susp	suspension
IM	intramuscular	syr	syrup
IV	intravenous	tab	tablet
IVP	intravenous push	tbsp	tablespoonful
IVPB	intravenous piggyback	tsp	teaspoonful
mcg	microgram	tid	three times a day
mEq	milliequivalent	ud	as directed
mg	milligram	ung	ointment
mL	milliliter		
N&V, N/V	nausea and vomiting	*Symbols*	
noct	at night	Δ	change by, change to
NS	normal saline, 0.9%	ʒ	dram
½NS	half normal saline, 0.45	fʒ	fluid dram
od	right eye	℥	ounce

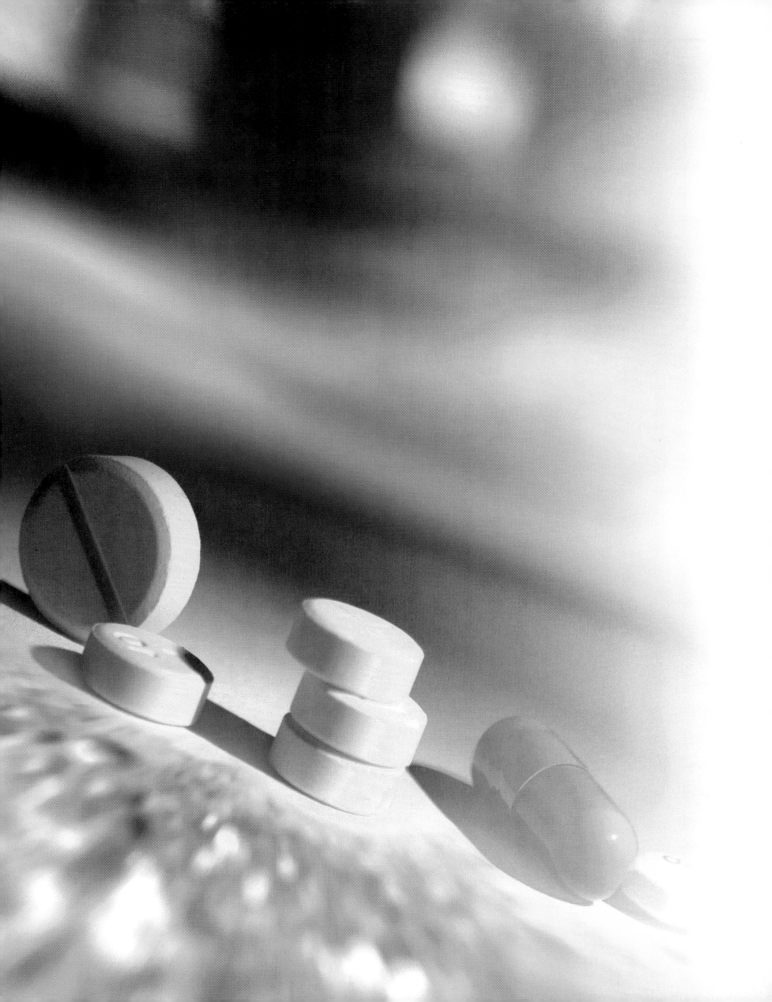

Common Categories of Drugs

Drug Category	Action or Indication	Example
absorbent	absorbs, or takes up, other chemicals of a toxic nature; often added to tablets and capsules	polycarbophil, a gastrointestinal absorbent
adrenergic	activates organs affected by the sympathetic nervous system	epinephrine (Adrenalin)
adsorbent	binds other chemicals to its surface; reduces amount of toxic chemical in the body	kaolin and pectin (Kaopectate)
alcohol abuse inhibitor	raises internal pH, making the blood and tissues more alkaline	disulfiram (Antabuse)
alkalinizer	disassociates to provide bicarbonate ion which causes systemic and urinary alkalinization	sodium bicarbonate
anabolic steroid	for treatment of catabolic disorders, in which living tissue is turned into energy and waste products	oxymetholone (Anadrol-50)
analeptic	stimulates central nervous system	doxapram hydrochloride (Dopram Injection)
analgesic	suppresses pain without rendering the patient unconscious	morphine sulfate, aspirin
androgen	hormone that affects male reproductive functions and sexual characteristics	testosterone (Depo-testosterone)
anesthetic	reduces or eliminates pain; general anesthetic renders the patient unconscious; local anesthetic affects pain in a particular location; topical anesthetic is a local anesthetic that affects the mucous membranes	enflurane, procaine, tetracaine
anorexic	elevates mood to suppress appetite	phendimetrazine
antacid	neutralizes excess gastric acid	aluminum hydroxide (Amphojel)
anthelmintic	eradicates intestinal worms	thiabendazole (Mintezol)
anti-infective	kills microorganisms and sterilizes wounds	hexachlorophene liquid soap
anti-inflammatory	reduces inflammation	ibuprofen (Advil)
antiacne	controls acne vulgaris	isotretinoin (Accutane)
antiamoebic	eradicates or inhibits amoebic parasites	metronidazole (Flagyl)
antiandrogen	reduces conversion of testosterone to dihydrotestosterone	finasteride (Proscar)
antianginal	dilates blood vessels; used to treat angina pectoris, pain in chest	nitroglycerin (Nitrostat Sublingual)
antiarrhythmic	depresses the action of the heart to combat irregularities in its rhythm	procainamide (Pronestyl)
antiarthritic	reduces inflammation of joints	diclofenac (Voltaren)
antibacterial	kills bacteria (topical)	bacitracin

Drug Category	Action or Indication	Example
antibiotic	kills bacteria or otherwise fights or prevents infection	penicillin g benzathine (Bicillin L-A)
anticholesterol	lowers cholesterol levels	colestipol hydrochloride (Colestid)
anticoagulant	slows the clotting of blood; for treatment of thrombosis and embolism or for storage of collected blood	heparin (for internal use); anticoagulant citrate dextrose solution (for collected blood)
anticonvulsant	prevents or arrests seizures	phenytoin (Dilantin)
antidepressant	elevates mood	amitriptyline hydrochloride (Elavil)
antidiabetic	for treatment of diabetes	insulin (Humulin L)
antidiarrheal	for treatment of diarrhea	diphenoxylate (Lomotil)
antidiuretic	reduces volume of urine produced	desmopressin acetate (Stimate Nasal)
antidote	reverses effects of poisoning	activated charcoal (general antidote); dimercaprol (antidote for arsenic and mercury poisoning)
antiemetic	suppresses vomiting	prochlorperazine (Compazine)
antiepileptic	prevents epileptic seizures	ethosuximide (Zarontin)
antiflatulent	reduces gastrointestinal gas	simethicone (Maalox Anti-Gas)
antifungal	eradicates or suppresses fungi	griseofulvin (systemic); tolnaftate (local)
antiglaucoma	for treatment of glaucoma	methazolamide (Neptazane)
antihemophilic	for treatment of hemophilia; allows blood to clot	antihemophilic factor (Bioclate)
antiherpes	for treatment of herpes	acyclovir (Zovirax)
antihistaminic	for treatment of allergies	chlorpheniramine maleate (Chlor-Trimeton)
antihypertensive	lowers blood pressure	guanethidine monosulfate (Ismelin)
antihypoglycemic	for treatment of hypoglycemia	glucagon
antimalarial	for treatment of malaria	chloroquine phosphate (Aralen Phosphate)
antimanic	for treatment of manic psychosis	lithium (Lithane)
antimigraine	for treatment of migraine headaches	sumatriptan (Imitrex)
anti-motion sickness	for treatment of motion sickness	dimenhydrinate (Dramamine Oral)
antinarcotic	reverses effects of a narcotic	naloxone (Narcan)
antineoplastic	attacks and destroys malignant cells	chlorambucil (Leukeran)
antipruritic	suppresses itching	hydrocortisone (Procort), diphenhydramine hydrochloride (Benadryl Oral)
antipsychotic	reduces effects of psychotic disorders	promazine (Sparine)
antipyretic	reduces fever	acetaminophen (Tylenol)
antispasmodic	reduces spasms	glycopyrrolate (Robinul)
antithyroid	reduces amount of thyroid hormone produced	methimazole (Tapazole)
antitubercular	fights tuberculosis	isoniazid (Laniazid)

Drug Category	Action or Indication	Example
antitussive	suppresses coughing	dextromethorphan (Vicks Formula 44)
antiviral	kills or suppresses viruses, or prevents viral infection	amantadine (Symmetrel)
anxiolytic	reduces anxiety	diazepam (Valium)
astringent	causes contraction locally after topical application	aluminum acetate (Otic Domeboro)
barbiturate	type of sedative	pentobarbital (Nembutal)
beta blocker	decreases heart rate, myocardial contractility, blood pressure, and myocardial oxygen demand	propranolol (Inderal)
bronchodilator	expands the bronchial passages; for treatment of asthma	salmeterol (Serevent)
bulk-forming	promotes evacuation from bowel	methylcellulose (Citrucel)
calcium channel blocker	blocks flow of calcium ions in the heart for treatment of angina pectoris, arrhythmia, and hypertension	verapamil (Isoptin)
cardiotonic	strengthens heartbeat; for treatment of congestive heart failure	digoxin (Lanoxin)
cathartic	*see purgative*	
chelating agent	for treatment of poisoning	edetate calcium disodium (for lead poisoning) (Calcium Disodium Versenate)
choleretic	increases secretion of bile by liver	dehydrocholic acid (Cholan-HMB)
contraceptive	prevents conception	norethindrone (Micronor)
corticosteroid	relieves inflammation and manages autoimmune diseases	dexamethasone (Decadron)
diagnostic	given to determine functioning of body or to discover presence of a disease	Tuberculin Partial Protein Derivative (PPD)
digestive	aids digestion	pancreatin (Creon)
diuretic	increases production of urine	furosemide (Lasix)
emetic	causes vomiting	ipecac syrup
estrogen	hormone that affects female reproductive functions and sexual characteristics	ethinyl estradiol (Estinyl)
expectorant	increases secretions of the respiratory tract and lowers their viscosity	potassium iodide (Pima)
fertility	promotes ovulation or creation of sperm	clomiphene citrate (Clomid)
gonadotropin	a type of fertility drug	luteinizing hormone
growth hormone	stimulates growth	somatrem (Genotropin Injection)
hemostatic	stops bleeding	aminocaproic acid (systemic)
hypnotic	causes sleep	flurazepam (Dalmane)
immunization	*see vaccine*	
keratolytic	applied topically to soften and remove superficial skin layer	salicylic acid (Compound W)
miotic	constricts the pupils of the eyes	pilocarpine (Adsorbocarpine Ophthalmic)
muscle relaxant	inhibits muscle contraction	dantrolene (Dantrium)
mydriatic	dilates the pupils of the eyes	atropine sulfate (Alcon)

Drug Category	Action or Indication	Example
narcotic	often addictive; relieves pain and induces sleep; includes opium and its derivatives	codeine
nasal decongestant	constricts vessels in nasal passages	naphazoline (Privine)
opiate	narcotic derived or related to opium	morphine sulfate (Astramorph PF Injection)
oxytocic	begins production of milk after childbirth	oxytocin (Pitocin)
parasiticide	destroys parasites on the skin *See scabicide and pediculicide*	
pediculicide	kills lice	lindane (G-well)
psychotherapeutic	for treatment of psychological disorders	chlorpromazine hydrochloride (Thorazine)
radiopharmaceutical	contains a radioactive isotope; for diagnosis or for therapy	ioxilan (Oxilant); technetium TC-99M (Lympho Scan)
scabicide	destroys skin mites and their eggs	lindane (G-well)
sedative	depresses the central nervous system, causing relaxation	phenobarbital (Luminal)
tranquilizer	reduces anxiety or disturbance	trifluoperazine hydrochloride (Stelazine)
urinary acidifier	lowers internal pH (level of acidity or alkalinity), making the blood and tissues more acidic	ammonium chloride
vaccine	introduces an antigen into the body to stimulate the production of antibodies for protection against a disease-causing microorganism	tetanus immune globulin
vasoconstrictor	narrows vessels and increases blood pressure	norepinephrine bitartrate (Levophed Injection)
vasodilator	expands vessels and lowers blood pressure	nitroglycerin (Nitroglyn Oral)
vitamin	chemical or mineral necessary in small amounts for proper metabolism	vitamin C, present in citric acid

Reference Lab Values

These are just a few of the reference lab values for adults that the technician may have to look up for the pharmacist. These normal ranges are for reference only. The laboratory doing the tests will provide normal ranges for the results provided.

Serum Plasma
    Albumin 3.2–5 g/dL
    Calcium 8.6–10.3 mg/dL
    Chloride 98–108 mg/L
    Creatinine 0.5–1.4 mg/dL
    Glucose 60–140 mg/dL
    Hemoglobin, glycosylated 4–8%
    Magnesium 1.6–2.5 mg/dL
    Potassium 3.5–5.2 mEq/L
    Sodium 134–149 mEq/L
    Urea Nitrogen (BUN) 7–20 mg/dL

Cholesterol
    Total <220 mg/dL
    LDL 65–170 mg/dL
    HDL 40–60 mg/dL
    Triglycerides 45–150 mg/dL

Liver Enzymes
    GGT
        Male 11–63 IU/L
        Female 8–35 IU/L
    SGOT (AST) <35 IU/L (20–48)
    SGPT (ALT) (10–35) <35 IU/L

CBC
    Hgb (hemoglobin)
        Male 13.5–16.5
        Female 12.0–15.0
    Hct (hematocrit or "crit")
        Male 41–50
        Female 36–44
    WBC with differential 4.5–11.0 (×10 to the third power over mm cubed)

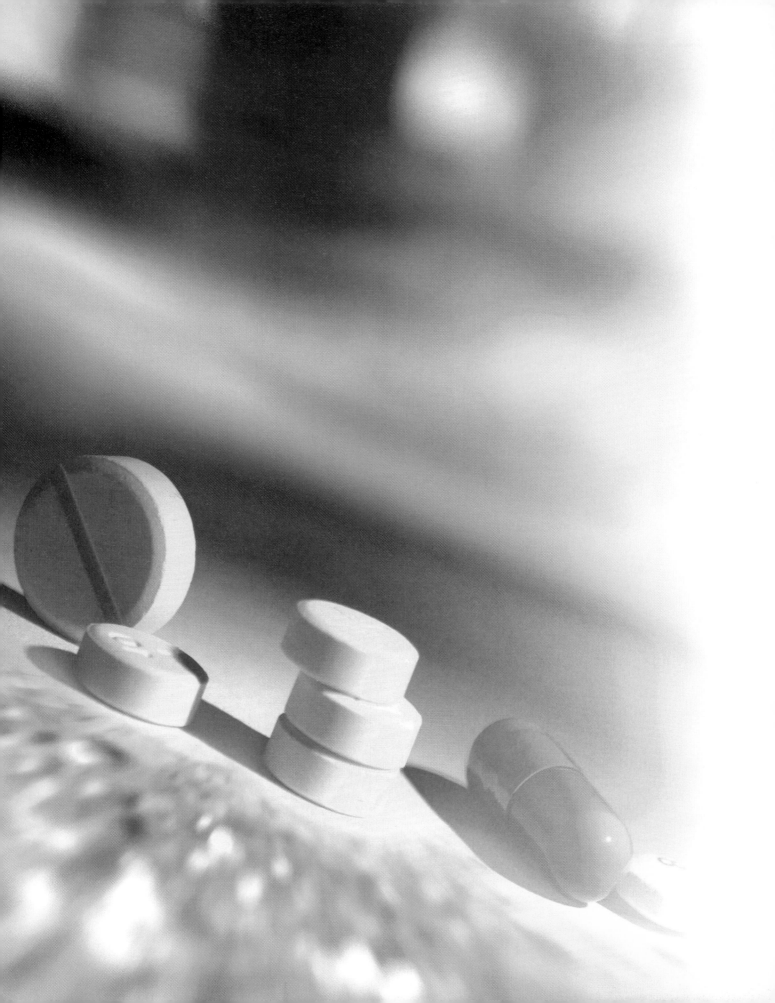

Resources

Appendix

D

PHARMACY ORGANIZATIONS AND THEIR JOURNALS

Since the days of the medieval guilds, when craftspeople and artisans such as silver-smiths and carpenters joined together to oversee apprenticeships, training, and business affairs, professional people have created organizations or associations to advance the purposes of their professions. Contemporary pharmacy is no exception. Listed below are some of the most important organizations in the pharmacy profession.

American Association of Colleges of Pharmacy (AACP) The AACP, founded in 1900, represents all 79 pharmacy colleges and schools in the United States and is the national organization representing the interests of pharmaceutical education and educators. The AACP publishes the journals *American Journal of Pharmaceutical Education, Roster of Faculty and Professional Staff, Profile of Pharmacy Faculty, Profile of Pharmacy Students,* and a monthly newsletter, the AACP News. The address of the *AACP* on the World Wide Web is http://www.aacp.org.

American Association of Pharmaceutical Scientists (AAPS) The AAPS, formerly an academy of the APhA, represents pharmaceutical scientists employed in academia, industry, government, and other research institutions. It has sections related to such fields as pharmaceutical quality, biotechnology, medicinal and natural products chemistry, pharmaceutics and drug delivery, pharmacokinetics, pharmacodynamics, and regulatory affairs. Its publications include the journals *Pharmaceutical Research, Pharmaceutical Development and Technology, Journal of Pharmaceutical and Biomedical Analysis, Journal of Pharmaceutical Marketing and Management,* and the *AAPS Newsletter.* The address of the AAPS on the World Wide Web is http://www.aaps.org.

American Association of Pharmacy Technicians (AAPT) Formerly called the APT, the AAPT, founded in 1979, is a national organization, with chapters in many states, representing pharmacy technicians and promoting certification of technicians. The association has established a Code of Ethics for Pharmacy Technicians. The address of the national headquarters is P.O. Box 1447, Greensboro, NC 27402. Its telephone numbers are: toll free phone (877) 368-4771; fax (336) 275-7222. The addess of the AAPT on the World Wide Web is http://www. pharmacytechnician.com.

American College of Apothecaries (ACA) The ACA, a professional association representing community-based pharmacists, publishes the quarterly *Voice of the*

Pharmacist and the ACA Newsletter. The address of the ACA on the World Wide Web is http://www.acainfo.org.

American College of Clinical Pharmacy (ACCP) The ACCP is a professional and scientific society that provides leadership, education, advocacy, and resources for clinical pharmacists. The ACCP publishes the journal *Pharmacotherapy.* The address of the ACCP on the World Wide Web is http://www.accp.com.

American Council on Pharmaceutical Education (ACPE) Founded in 1932, the ACPE is the national accrediting agency for pharmacy education programs recognized by the Secretary of Education. The ACPE is located in East Brunswick, New Jersey, and can be reached at (732) 238-1600. The address of the ACPE on the World Wide Web is http://www.cfpa.com/accreds/acpe.html.

American Pharmaceutical Association (APhA) The largest of the national pharmacy organizations, the APhA consists of three academies: the Academy of Pharmacy Practice and Management (APhA-APPM), the Academy of Pharmaceutical Research and Science (APhA-APRS), and the Academy of Students of Pharmacy (APhA-ASP). The APhA publishes the bimonthly *Journal of the American Pharmaceutical Association,* the monthly *Pharmacy Today* newsletter, and the monthly *Journal of Pharmaceutical Sciences.* The APhA also operates a political action committee, or PAC. According to the APhA, its mission is "to advocate the interests of pharmacists; influence the profession, government, and others in addressing vital pharmaceutical care issues; promote the highest professional and ethical standards; and foster science and research in support of the practice of pharmacy." The address of the APhA on the World Wide Web is http://www.aphanet.org.

American Society of Consultant Pharmacists (ASCP) The ASCP is a professional organization representing consultant pharmacists, practitioners who provide, on a contractual basis, medication distribution and pharmacy expertise to nursing homes and other long-term care facilities, including subacute care and assisted living facilities, psychiatric hospitals, facilities for the mentally retarded, correctional facilities, adult day care centers, hospices, alcohol and drug rehabilitation centers, ambulatory and surgical care centers, and home care providers. The ASCP publishes a journal, *The Consultant Pharmacist,* and *Update—The Monthly Newsletter of the American Society of Consultant Pharmacists.* The address of the ASCP on the World Wide Web is http://www.ascp.com.

American Society of Health-System Pharmacists (ASHP) The ASHP is a large organization that represents pharmacists who practice in hospitals, health maintenance organizations (HMOs), long-term care facilities, home care agencies, and other institutions. The ASHP is a national accrediting organization for pharmacy residency and pharmacy technician training programs. The ASHP publishes the *American Journal of Health-System Pharmacy.* The address of the ASHP on the World Wide Web is http://www.ashp.org. The society's Practice Standards are available online at http://www.ashp.org/bestpractices/index.html.

Drug Enforcement Administration (DEA) The DEA enforces federal laws and regulations related to controlled substances. The address of the DEA on the World Wide Web is http://www.usdoj.gov/dea.

Food and Drug Administration (FDA) The FDA is the federal government agency charged with primary responsibility for creating regulations governing the safety of foods, drugs, and cosmetics. The FDA enforces the Food, Drug, and Cosmetic Act of 1938 and its subsequent amendments, oversees new drug development, approves or disapproves applications to market new drugs, monitors reports of adverse reactions, and has the authority to recall drugs deemed dangerous. The address of the FDA on the World Wide Web is http://www.fda.gov.

Healthcare Distribution Management Association (HDMA) The HDMA is an association representing those companies that provide pharmacies with drugs and supplies. The address of the HDMA on the World Wide Web is http://www. healthcaredistribution.org.

Institute for Safe Medication Practices (ISMP) The ISMP is a nonprofit organization that provides education about adverse drug events and their prevention. It independently reviews medication error events that have been voluntarily submitted to the Medication Errors Reporting Program (MERP) operated by the United States Pharmacopeia (USP). ISMP is a partner with the FDA MEDWATCH and communicates with the FDA on a regular basis. The address of the ISMP is 1800 Byberry Road, Suite 810, Huntington Valley, Pennsylvania 19006. The telephone number is (215) 947-7797. The address of the ISMP on the World Wide Web is http:// www.ismp.org.

National Association of Boards of Pharmacy (NABP) The NABP is an association of state boards of pharmacy. State boards of pharmacy are the organizations, in the individual states, with the responsibility of licensing pharmacists, conducting inspections, and ensuring compliance with regulations and ethical standards. The NABP supports the rights of states to determine their own pharmacy regulations and guidelines but has worked toward standardizing licensing, especially through the promotion of a national licensing examination, the North American Pharmacist Licensure Examination, or NABPLEX. The address of the NABP is 700 Busse Highway, Park Ridge, Illinois 60068. The telephone number is (847) 698-6227. The address of the NABP on the World Wide Web is http://www.nabp.net.

National Association of Chain Drug Stores (NACDS) Founded in 1933, the NACDS is an association representing the large number of community pharmacies that are parts of chain retail operations. This well-funded public relations and political action organization includes as members chief executives of retail chains that include pharmacies. The address of the NACDS on the World Wide Web is http://www.nacds.org.

National Community Pharmacists Association (NCPA) Formerly known as the National Association of Retail Druggists, or NARD, the NCPA is an association representing independent community pharmacies. The NCPA publishes *America's Pharmacist, NCPA Newsletter, Inside Pharmacist Care, Alternate Site Pharmacist,* and *Regimen: An Update on Long-Term Care Drug Therapy.* The address of the NCPA on the World Wide Web is http://www.ncpanet.org.

National Home Infusion Association (NHIA) Located in Alexandria, Virginia, this association, created by NARD (now NCPA), provides information and support related to the fast-growing field of home infusion. The address of the NHIA on the World Wide Web is http://www.nhianet.org.

National Pharmaceutical Association (NPA) The NPA is the professional organization representing the community pharmacies of Great Britain. Its address on the World Wide Web is http://www.npa.co.uk.

Pharmaceutical Research and Manufacturers of America (PhRMA) PhRMA is an association of companies involved in pharmaceutical research. The address of PhRMA on the World Wide Web is http://www.phrma.org.

Pharmacy Technician Certification Board (PTCB) The PTCB publishes the Pharmacy Technician Certification Examination, or PTCE, for those wishing to become Certified Pharmacy Technicians (CPhTs). The PTCE has been taken, voluntarily, by thousands of technicians around the country and is required for certification in some states. In addition to publishing the PTCE, the PTCB oversees a recertification program for technicians. The address of the PTCB is 2215 Constitution Avenue, NW, Washington, DC, 20037. The telephone number is (202) 429-7576. The address of the PTCB on the World Wide Web is http://www.ptcb.org.

Pharmacy Technician Educators Council (PTEC) PTEC is an association of educators who prepare people for careers as pharmacy technicians. Its official publication is the *Journal of Pharmacy Technology.* The PTEC address on the World Wide Web is http://www.rxptec.org.

Proprietary Association of Great Britain (PAGB) The PA is a British association representing manufacturers of over-the-counter medications and related products. The address of the PA on the World Wide Web is http://www.pagb.co.uk.

United States Pharmacopeia (USP) The USP is a nonprofit organization that sets standards for the identity, strength, quality, purity, packaging, and labeling of drug products. The USP provides drug information online. The address of the USP on the World Wide Web is http://www.usp.org.

REFERENCE WORKS

A wide variety of reference works on topics related to pharmacy are available. A complete description of these references is beyond the scope of this book. However, some of the most important reference works are described under appropriate topical headings below.

Medicine and Anatomy

A.D.A.M. Interactive Anatomy. CD-ROM. Atlanta, GA. A.D.A.M. Software, 1998. A new, professional version of the acclaimed human anatomy software. Less expensive teaching versions of this software are available. See the company's site on the World Wide Web at http://www.adam.com.

The Charles Press Handbook of Current Medical Abbreviations. Philadelphia: Charles Press, 1997. A standard reference work on symbols and abbreviations used in medicine. The address of the Charles Press on the World Wide Web is http://www.charlespresspub.com.

Davis, Neil M. *Medical Abbreviations: 15,000 Conveniences at the Expense of Communications and Safety.* 10th ed. Huntingdon Valley, PA: N.M. Davis Assoc., 2001. A guide to medical abbreviations.

Dorland's Illustrated Medical Dictionary. 29th ed. Philadelphia: Saunders, 2000. A standard medical dictionary. The address of W. B. Saunders on the World Wide Web is http://www.harcourthealth.com/WBS/index.html.

Gray's Anatomy: The Anatomical Basis of Medicine and Surgery. 38th ed. New York: Churchill Livingstone, 1998. The classic reference work on human anatomy.

Harrison's Principles of Internal Medicine. 15th ed. New York: McGraw-Hill, 2001. A standard, authoritative overview of the field of internal medicine. See McGraw-Hill Professional Publications on the World Wide Web at http://www.pbg. mcgraw-hill.com.

The Merck Manual of Diagnosis and Therapy. 17th ed. Whitehouse Station, NJ: Merck, 1999. This is a comprehensive survey of diseases, diagnosis, prevention, symptoms, and treatments. The manual is available in book form; it is searchable online at http://www.merck.com/pubs/mmanual; it is available on CD-ROM or diskette from Keyboard Publishing; and in a handheld electronic version from Franklin Electronic Publishers at http://www.franklin.com or (800) 266-5626.

The Merck Manual of Medical Information: Home Edition. Whitehouse Station, NJ: Merck, 1997. A simplified and updated version of the Merck Manual for use by lay people. It is available in an online version at the company's World Wide Web site at http://www.merck.com.

Nelson Textbook of Pediatrics. 16th ed. Philadelphia: W.B. Saunders, 2001. A standard textbook on pediatric medicine. The address of W.B. Saunders on the World Wide Web is http://www.harcourthealth.com/WBS/index.html.

Stedman's Medical Dictionary: Illustrated in Color. 27th ed. Baltimore: Williams & Wilkins, 2000. A standard medical dictionary. The address of Lippincott Williams & Wilkins on the World Wide Web is http://www.lww.com.

Drugs, Dosage Forms, Patient Counseling, Pharmacology, and Adverse Reactions

American Drug Index 2002. St. Louis, MO: Facts and Comparisons, 2002. This standard reference work contains more than 20,000 entries on drugs and drug products, including alphabetically listed drug names, cross-indexing, phonetic pronunciations, brand names, manufacturers, generic and/or chemical names, composition and strength, pharmaceutical forms available, package size, use, and common abbreviations. It also contains a listing of orphan drugs. The work is available in hardbound and CD-ROM editions. The address of Facts and Comparisons on the World Wide Web is http://www.factsandcomparisons.com.

American Hospital Formulary Service Drug Information 2002 (AHFS). Bethesda, MD: American Society of Health-System Pharmacists, 2002. The complete text of roughly 1,400 monographs covering about 50,000 commercially available and experimental drugs, including information on uses, interactions, pharmacokinetics, dosage, and administration. The address of the American Society of Health-System Pharmacists on the World Wide Web is http://www.ashp.org.

Ansel, Howard C., et al. *Pharmaceutical Dosage Forms and Drug Delivery Systems.* 7th ed. Baltimore: Williams & Wilkins, 1999. A superb survey of contemporary dosage forms and delivery systems. The address of Lippincott Williams & Wilkins on the World Wide Web is http://www.lww.com.

Drug Facts and Comparisons. St. Louis, MO: Facts and Comparisons, 2002. This comprehensive source of information about 16,000 prescription and 6,000 over-the-counter drugs contains monographs about individual drugs and groups of related drugs; product listings in table format providing information on dosage forms and strength, distributor names, costs, package sizes, product identification codes, flavors, colors, and distribution status; and information on therapeutic uses, interactions, and adverse reactions. The publication includes an index of manufacturers and distributors and controlled substance regulations. This reference work is available in hardbound form, on CD-ROM, or in a loose-leaf form that is updated monthly. The address of Facts and Comparisons on the World Wide Web is http://www.factsandcomparisons.com.

Drug Information Fulltext (DIF). Norwood, MA: Silverplatter. A searchable computer database combining two publications: the *American Hospital Formulary Service Drug Information* and the *Handbook on Injectable Drugs.* This database is available on a hard disk, on CD-ROM, or via the Internet. Silverplatter's address on the World Wide Web is http://www.silverplatter.com.

Drug Interaction Facts. St Louis, MO: Facts and Comparisons, 2002. This reference, available as a hardbound book, CD-ROM, or loose-leaf book that is updated quarterly, provides comprehensive information on potential interactions that can be reviewed by drug class, generic drug name, or trade name. Provides information on drug/drug and drug/food interactions. The address of Facts and Comparisons on the World Wide Web is http://www.factsandcomparisons.com.

Food and Drug Administration. *Approved Drug Products with Therapeutic Equivalence Evaluations.* Washington, DC: U.S. Government Printing Office. Revised annually, with monthly updates, this source lists drug products approved for use in the United States. Also known as the *Orange Book* because of its orange-colored cover, it is available online at http://www.fda.gov/cder/ob/default.htm. The address of the FDA on the World Wide Web is http://www.fda.gov.

Fudyuma, Janice. *What Do I Take? A Consumer's Guide to Nonprescription Drugs.* New York: HarperCollins, 1997. A simple-to-read guide to over-the-counter drugs.

Goodman & Gilman's The Pharmacological Basis of Therapeutics. 10th ed. New York: McGraw-Hill, 2002. An authoritative text on pharmacology and therapeutics containing 67 articles by leading experts in the field. This text provides information for pharmacists to help them answer clinical questions about how drugs work under different conditions in the body. See McGraw-Hill Professional Publications on the World Wide Web at http://www.pbg.mcgraw-hill.com.

Graedon, Joe, and Teresa Graedon. *Deadly Drug Interactions: The People's Pharmacy Guide: How to Protect Yourself from Harmful Drug/Drug, Drug/Food, Drug/Vitamin Combinations.* New York: St. Martin's Press, 1997. An easy-to-read guide to dangerous drug interactions.

Koda-Kimble, Maryanne, and Lloyd Yee Young. *Applied Therapeutics: The Clinical Use of Drugs.* 6th ed. Vancouver, WA: Applied Therapeutics Inc., 1995.

Index Nominum. Geneva: Swiss Pharmaceutical Society, 1995. A compilation of synonyms, formulas, and therapeutic classes of over 7,000 drugs and 28,000 proprietary preparations from 27 countries. Available in text and CD-ROM formats.

The International Pharmacopoeia. 3rd ed. New York: World Health Organization, 1994. Recommended production methods and specifications for drugs, in four volumes. The World Health Organization is on the World Wide Web at http://www.who.ch.

MedCoach CD-ROM (Windows, NT, & Macintosh). Rockville, MD: United States Pharmacopeial Convention, 1997. A database of information for patients on over 6,000 generic and brand-name drug products, over-the-counter drugs, nutritional and home infusion items, test devices, and infant formulas. Provides information for patients on proper drug use and preparation, drug and food interactions, side effects/adverse effects, therapeutic contraindications, and product storage. Information is tailored to particular patients' needs (pediatric, male or female, geriatric, etc.). Subscription includes quarterly updates. The address of the United States Pharmacopeial Convention on the World Wide Web is http://www.usp.org.

Orange Book. See Food and Drug Administration.

Patient Drug Facts, 1996: Professionals Guide to Patient Drug Facts. St. Louis, MO: Facts and Comparisons, 1996. This is a comprehensive guide to patient counseling about drugs, available in loose-leaf format for verbal patient counseling and in PC format (on disk) for creation of patient handouts. The address of Facts and Comparisons on the World Wide Web is http://www.factsandcomparisons.com.

Physician's Desk Reference (PDR). 56th ed. Oradell, NJ: Medical Economics, 2002. Available in hardbound and CD-ROM form, with two supplements published twice a year, this standard reference work contains information from package inserts (see below) for more than 4,000 prescription drugs, as well as information on 250 drug manufacturers. The address of Medical Economics on the World Wide Web is http://www.medec.com.

Smith, C. G. *The Process of New Drug Discovery and Development.* Boca Raton, FL: CRC Press, 1992. Description of the process by which new drugs are developed, tested, and approved for clinical trials and marketing.

Stringer, Janet L. *Basic Concepts in Pharmacology: A Student's Survival Guide.* 2nd ed. New York: McGraw-Hill, 2001. Survey of basic pharmacological concepts for students. See McGraw-Hill Professional Publications on the World Wide Web at http://www.pbg.mcgraw-hill.com.

United States Pharmacopeia, 23rd Rev.—National Formulary. 20th ed. Rockville, MD: United States Pharmacopeial Convention, 2001. Combined compendium of monographs setting official national standards for drug substances and dosage forms *(United States Pharmacopeia)* and standards for pharmaceutical ingredients *(National Formulary).* Available in book or CD-ROM form and in English- and Spanish-language editions. The address of the United States Pharmacopeial Convention on the World Wide Web is http://www.usp.org.

USP Dictionary of USAN and International Drug Names. Rockville, MD: United States Pharmacopeial Convention, 2001. An authoritative guide to drug names, including chemical names, brand names, manufacturers, molecular formulas, therapeutic uses, and chemical structures. The address of the United States Pharmacopeial Convention on the World Wide Web is http://www.usp.org.

USP Drug Information (USP DI). Vol. I. Drug Information for the Health Care Professional. Rockville, MD: United States Pharmacopeial Convention, 2002. A comprehensive source of in-depth drug information, available in book or CD-ROM form and in English- and Spanish-language editions. Describes medically accepted uses of more than 11,000 generic and brand-name products. The address of the United States Pharmacopeial Convention on the World Wide Web is http://www.usp.org.

USP Drug Information (USP DI). Vol. II. Advice for the Patient. Rockville, MD: United States Pharmacopeial Convention, 2002. Contains monographs corresponding to those in the USP DI, Vol. I, but simplified for the purpose of patient education and counseling. Available in English- and Spanish-language editions. The address of the United States Pharmacopeial Convention on the World Wide Web is http://www.usp.org.

USP Drug Information (USP DI). Vol. III. Approved Drug Products and Legal Requirements. Rockville, MD: United States Pharmacopeial Convention, 2002. Therapeutic equivalence information and selected federal requirements that affect the prescribing and dispensing of prescription drugs and controlled substances. Includes the FDA *Orange Book;* USP-NF requirements for labeling, storage, packaging, and quality; federal Food, Drug, and Cosmetic Act provisions relating to drugs for human use; portions of the Controlled Substance Act Regulations; and the FDA's Good Manufacturing Practice regulations for finished pharmaceuticals. The address of the United States Pharmacopeial Convention on the World Wide Web is http://www.usp.org.

Filling Prescriptions, Compounding, Calculations, Preparing Parenteral Admixtures, Drug Interactions, and Toxicology

Benitz, William E., and David S. Tatro. *The Pediatric Drug Handbook.* 3rd ed. St. Louis, MO: Mosby-Year Book, 1995. Information on drugs, dosage forms, and administration for pediatric patients. The address of Mosby on the World Wide Web is http://www.mosby.com.

Davies, D. M. *Textbook of Adverse Drug Reactions.* 5th ed. New York: Oxford University Press, 1999. A standard textbook on the subject. The address of Oxford University Press on the World Wide Web is http://www.oup-usa.org.

Goldfrank's Toxicologic Emergencies. 6th ed. New York: Appleton & Lange, 1998. Information on treating toxicologic emergencies. The medical titles of Appleton & Lange are distributed by McGraw-Hill and may be found at that Web site: http://www.pbg.mcgraw-hill.com.

Handbook of Nonprescription Drugs. 2 vols. 11th ed. Washington, DC: American Pharmaceutical Association, 1996-1997. A reference work on over-the-counter medications. The address of the American Pharmaceutical Association on the World Wide Web is http://www.aphanet.org.

Hunt, Max L., Jr. *Training Manual for Intravenous Admixture Personnel.* 5th ed. Chicago: Bonus Books, 1995. A manual for training people to create parenteral preparations. The address of Bonus Books on the World Wide Web is http://www.bonus-books.com.

The King Guide to Parenteral Admixtures, 2001 Edition. Napa, CA: King Guide Publications, 2001. Available in four loose-leaf volumes, on microfiche, and on CD-ROM, the King Guide provides 350 monographs on compatibility and stability information critical to determining the advisability of preparing admixtures of drugs for parenteral administration. The guide is updated quarterly. The address of King Publications on the World Wide Web is http://www.kingguide.com.

Nahata, Milap C., and Thomas F. Hipple. *Pediatric Drug Formulations.* 3rd ed. Cincinnati, OH: Harvey Whitney, 1997. Information on formulation and compounding of drugs for pediatric patients. You can e-mail Harvey Whitney Books at hwb@eos.net.

Poisindex System. Englewood, CO: Micromedex. A computerized poison information system. The address of Micromedex on the World Wide Web is http://www.mdx.com.

Remington: The Science and Practice of Pharmacology. 20th ed. Lippincott, 2000. The compounding "bible" of the pharmacy profession.

Stoklosa, Mitchell J., and Howard C. Ansel. *Pharmaceutical Calculations.* 11th ed. Baltimore, MD: Williams & Wilkins, 2001. A clear, concise, thorough introduction to pharmaceutical mathematics. The address of Lippincott Williams & Wilkins on the World Wide Web is http://www.lww.com.

Trissel, Lawrence A. *Handbook on Injectable Drugs, with Supplement.* 11th ed. Bethesda, MD: American Society of Health-System Pharmacists, 2000. Provides information on stability and compatibility of injectable drug products, including formulations, concentrations, and pH values. The address of the American Society of Health-System Pharmacists on the World Wide Web is http://www.ashp.org.

Understanding and Preventing Errors in Medication Orders and Prescription Writing. Bethesda, MD: United States Pharmacopeial Convention, 1998. An education resource, consisting of lecture materials, videotapes, and 35 mm slides describing medication errors that arise from poorly written orders and prescriptions, using examples of actual reports received through the USP Medication Errors Reporting

Program. Contains recommendations for preventing errors. The address of the United States Pharmacopeial Convention on the World Wide Web is http://www.usp.org; search within USP Educational Programs.

Pharmaceutical Law, Regulation, Ethics, Communication, and Economics

Abood, Richard R., and David B. Brushwood. *Pharmacy Practice and the Law.* 3rd ed. Gaithersburg, MD: Aspen, 2000. A survey of contemporary pharmacy law, covering the entire range of legal issues in pharmacy, including major acts, regulations, regulatory agencies, torts, malpractice liability, and legal issues related to hospital pharmacies, long-term care, third-party prescription programs, and managed care, with cases. The address of Aspen Publishers on the World Wide Web is http://www.aspenpub.com.

Code of Federal Regulations (CFR), Title 21, Food and Drugs. Washington, DC: U.S. Government Printing Office, Superintendent of Documents. Annually revised compilation of federal Food and Drug Administration regulations. The address of the Government Printing Office on the World Wide Web is http://www.access.gpo.gov.

Cramer, Joyce A., and Bert Spilker. *Quality of Life and Pharmacoeconomics: An Introduction.* Philadelphia: Lippincott Williams & Wilkins, 1997. A general survey of the economics of pharmacy. The address of Lippincott Williams & Wilkins on the World Wide Web is http://www.lww.com.

Federal Register. Washington, DC: U. S. Government Printing Office, Superintendent of Documents. Daily publication listing new federal regulations. The address of the Government Printing Office on the World Wide Web is http://www.access.gpo.gov.

Practice Standards of ASHP, 1997–1998. Bethesda, MD: American Society of Health-System Pharmacists, 1997. Standards for hospital pharmacy practice. The address of the American Society of Health-System Pharmacists on the World Wide Web is http://www.ashp.org.

Smith, Mickey, et al. *Pharmacy Ethics.* Binghamton, NY: Haworth Press, 1991. The address of Haworth Press on the World Wide Web is http://www.haworthpressinc.com.

Tootelian, Dennis H., and Ralph M. Gaedeke. *Essentials of Pharmacy Management.* St. Louis, MO: Mosby-Year Book, 1993. Information on managing a retail pharmacy operation. The address of Mosby on the World Wide Web is http://www.mosby.com.

Training and Certification of Pharmacy Technicians

Ballington, Don A., and Mary M. Laughlin. *Pharmacology for Technicians.* 2nd ed. St. Paul, MN: EMC/Paradigm, 2003. Presents the basic principles of pharmacology and the essential characteristics of commonly prescribed drug classes. The address of EMC/Paradigm on the World Wide Web is http://www.emcp.com.

Ballington, Don A., and Mary M. Laughlin. *Pharmacy Calculation for Technicians.* 2nd ed. St. Paul, MN: EMC/Paradigm, 2003. Offers a review of basic mathematics as applied to common pharmaceutical calculations. The address of EMC/Paradigm on the World Wide Web is http://www.emcp.com.

Idsvoog, Peter B. *Manual for Hospital Pharmacy Technicians: A Programmed Course in Basic Skills.* Bethesda, MD: American Society of Health-System Pharmacists, 1977. The address of the American Society of Health-System Pharmacists on the World Wide Web is http://www.ashp.org.

Manual for Pharmacy Technicians. 2d ed. Bethesda, MD: American Society of Health-System Pharmacists, 1998. The address of the American Society of Helath-System Pharmacists on the World Wide Web is http://www.ashp.org.

Moss, Susan. *Pharmacy Technician Certification Quick Study Guide.* Washington, DC: American Pharmaceutical Association, 1995. A study guide for the Pharmacy Technician Certification Examination. The address of the American Pharmaceutical Association on the World Wide Web is http://www.aphanet.org.

Reifman, Noah. *Certification Review for Pharmacy Technicians.* 5th ed. Harvey Whitney Books, 2000. The address of Harvey Whitney Books on the World Wide Web is http://www.hwbooks.com.

Other References

Gerson, Cyrelle K. *More Than Dispensing: A Handbook on Providing Pharmaceutical Services to Long Term Care Facilities.* Washington, DC: American Pharmaceutical Association, 1980. The address of the American Pharmaceutical Association on the World Wide Web is http://www.aphanet.org.

Journal of Pharmacy Technology is the official publication of the Pharmacy Technician Educators Council. This journal is published by Harvey Whitney Books, which can be contacted by e-mail at hwb@hwbooks.com, by telephone at (513) 793-3555, or by fax at (513) 793-3600. The address of Harvey Whitney Books on the World Wide Web is http://www.hwbooks.com.

Meldrum, Helen. *Interpersonal Communication in Pharmaceutical Care.* Binghamton, NY: Haworth Press, 1994. The address of the Haworth Press on the World Wide Web is http://www.haworthpressinc.com.

RxTrek, a Web site providing information and links for pharmacy technicians, is located at http://www.rxtrek.net.

The World Wide Web Virtual Library maintains a large list of pharmacy links at http://www.pharmacy.org.

Guide to Preventing Prescription Errors

The following simple procedures will help avoid errors in the pharmacy.

- Always keep the prescription and the label together during the fill process.
- Know the common look-alike and sound-alike drugs, and keep them stored in different areas of the pharmacy so they will not be mistaken easily.
- Keep dangerous or high-alert medications in a separate storage area of the pharmacy.
- Always question bad handwriting.
- Make sure prescriptions/orders include the correctly spelled drug name, strength, appropriate dosing, quantity or duration of therapy, dosage form, and route. Missing information should be obtained from the prescriber.
- Use the metric system. A leading zero should always be present in decimal values less than one. Remember that an error of this nature will mean a dosage error of at least tenfold!
- Question the prescription/order that utilizes abbreviations you are not familiar with or that are uncommon. Avoid using abbreviations that have more than one meaning, and verify the meaning of these abbreviations with the prescriber.
- Be aware of insulin mistakes. Insulin brands should be clearly separated from one another. Educate patients to always verify their insulin purchase.
- Clear stock bottles no longer needed away from the work area in a timely fashion. Only keep what is needed for immediate use in the work area.
- The label should always be compared to the original prescription by at least two people. If an error occurs at this stage, the refills may be filled incorrectly as well!

What can the technician do to reduce errors?

- Use the triple check system, discussed in Chapter 7.
- Verify your own data entry before processing.
- Do a mental check on dosage appropriateness.
- Observe and report pertinent OTC purchases.
- Keep your work area free of clutter.

What can the pharmacist do to reduce errors?

- Check prescriptions in a timely manner.
- Initial checked prescriptions.
- Visually check the product in the bottle.
- Encourage OTC and herbal remedy documentation.
- Document all clarifications on orders.

What can the pharmacy do to reduce errors?

- ◇ Automate and bar code all fill procedures.
- ◇ Maintain a safe work area.
- ◇ Provide adequate storage areas.
- ◇ Encourage physicians to use common terminology.
- ◇ Provide adequate computer applications and hardware.

Index

Italicized page locators denote figures or photos; *t* denotes table.

A

AACP. *See* American Association of Colleges of Pharmacy
AAPT. *See* American Association of Pharmacy Technicians
Abbreviations, 39, 40, 59
  for amounts, 54*t*
  for bodily functions or conditions, 55*t*
  dosage forms, solutions, and delivery systems, 55-56*t*
  for drugs and drug references, 56*t*
  for metric units, 104
  for parenteral therapy, 212*t*
  for pharmacy and provider instructions, 57-58*t*
  on prescriptions, 53, 145
  for sites of administration/parts of the body, 57*t*
  for time and time of administration, 56-57*t*
Absorption, distribution, metabolism, and excretion of drugs, 51
Acacia, 177
Accreditation, 16. *See also* Certification
Accuracy, 241
Acetaminophen: in Children's Tylenol Elixir, 77
Acetic acid solution (1%), 77
Acetonide dental paste, 79
Acetylsalicylic acid (aspirin), 71
Acidic solutions, 95
Acute, 59
Addition
  of decimals, 113
  of fractions, 109, 136
Additives: commonly used, 213*t*
Addresses: on prescriptions, 145-146
Adhesive sealed bottles, 220
Adjudication, 151, 159
ADME. *See* Absorption, distribution, metabolism, and excretion of drugs
Admixtures, 155
Adrenaline, 67
Adult day-care services, 9
Adult dosages, 121
Adulterated drugs, 17-18
Adult parenteral nutrition
  order for (back), *217*
  order for (front), *216*
Adverse drug interactions/reactions, 4, 162
  information about, 8
  and parenteral administrations, 94
  warnings about, 153
Adverse reaction reports, 151
Advice for the Patient: Volume 2—*USP Drug Information*, 66
Aerosols, 70, 80
Aging of the population: and geriatric pharmacy, 249

AIDS (acquired immunodeficiency syndrome), 199, 201
Air: contamination through, 203
Airflow hoods
  horizontal, *204*
  spills in, 232
  vertical, *205*
Air vent: in IV set, *208*
Albuterol, 80
Alcohol, 203
Alcoholic liniments, 78
Alcoholic solutions, 76, 177
Alkaline solutions, 95
Allergies
  checking on, for prescriptions, 148, 151
  and patches, 83
  warnings about, 162
Alliances: workplace, 242
Alligation method, 129-131, 136
Aluminum hydroxide gel, 79
Amber liquid containers, 155
Ambulatory injection devices, 82
American Association of Colleges of Pharmacy, 4, 16
American Association of Pharmacy Technicians, 31, 33, 51
American Hospital Association, 7
American Pharmaceutical Association, 6, 16, 31, 33, 50, 238, 250
American Society of Health-System Pharmacists, 6, 16, 238
Amino acids, 68
Amoebae, 202
Amoebic dysentery, 202
Amounts in prescriptions/medication orders, 54*t*
Amoxicillin: in capsule form, 72
Ampules, 82, 95
  opening, *219*, 231
  and parenteral preparations, 217-218
Amyl nitrate, 80
Analgesics, 40
Anesthetics, 70, 92
Antacids, 67, 73, 78
Anthrax infection, 201
Antibiotics, 67, 69, 148
Antibodies, 68
Antidepressants, 69
Antifungal agents, 69, 92
Antifungal jellies, 79
Antigens, 68
Anti-inflammatories, 69, 92
Antineoplastic drugs, 228
Antiseptic jellies, 79
Antiseptics, 70, 92
Antiviral agents, 69
APhA. *See* American Pharmaceutical Association
Apothecaries' weights, 170, *171*
Apothecary, 2, 3. *See also* Pharmacists
Apothecary measurement system, 106,

117, 136
  common symbols from, 58*t*
  converting measurements between metric system and, 117-120
  measurement unit, equivalent within system, metric equivalent, 107*t*
  and metric system equivalents, 118*t*
  and prescriptions/medication orders, 53
Appearance: of pharmacy technicians, 186-187
Applications, 152
Approved Drug Products and Legal Requirements: Volume 3—*USP Drug Information*, 66
Aqueous solutions, 76, 98, 177
Arabic numerals, 53, 106
Aromatic waters, 76, 77, 84
Asepsis: and sterilization, 202
Aseptic technique, 200, 204*t*
  and cytotoxic agent preparation, 230
  and equipment, 203-205
ASHP. *See* American Society of Health-System Pharmacists
Asparaginase, 228
Aspirin, 67, 71
Asthma medications, 80
Astringents: epicutaneous administration of, 92
Athlete's foot, 202
Atomic weights, 123
  and valences of common elements, 122*t*
Attitude, 250
  of pharmacy technicians, 186
  workplace, 241
Autoclave, *202*
Automated compounding, 248
Automated dispensing machines: and floor stock, 227
Automated packaging machines: for repackaging, 220
Automation: in pharmacy, 226-227
Auxiliary labels, 157, 162, 178
Average inventory, 162
Average wholesale price, 131, 133, 136
Avoirdupois measure, 106, 136
Avoirdupois measurement system
  common symbols from, 58*t*
  measurement unit, equivalent within system, metric equivalent, 107*t*
  and prescriptions/medication orders, 53
  weights, 171
AWP. *See* Average wholesale price

B

Bacitracin zinc topical powder, 74
Backing up computer data, 153
Bacteria, 201, 203

E

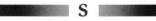

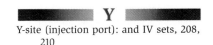

Photo Credits